Physical Health of Adults with Intellectual and Developmental Disabilities

Vee P. Prasher • Matthew P. Janicki
Editors

Physical Health of Adults with Intellectual and Developmental Disabilities

Second Edition

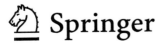 Springer

Editors
Vee P. Prasher
The Greenfields
Birmingham
UK

Matthew P. Janicki
University of Illinois at Chicago
Chicago, IL
USA

ISBN 978-3-030-07930-7   ISBN 978-3-319-90083-4   (eBook)
https://doi.org/10.1007/978-3-319-90083-4

This Springer imprint is published by the registered company Springer Nature Switzerland AG
The registered company address is: Gewerbestrasse 11, 6330 Cham, Switzerland

Foreword to the Second Edition

The health revolution for people with intellectual and developmental disabilities is becoming more impactful and successful. The doors of opportunities have never been more open, which now allow for a much greater ability to show their eagerness, their spirit, their joy, and willingness to be a part of the world community in every village, town, and city. This demonstration of courage and determination has brought great happiness to so many and their families. In the hard work brought forth in creating and living inclusive lives, there has also been shown a continued discrimination and an injustice that has led to great disparities to access healthcare and its various resources. Time and time again we still see many who have poor dentition, continued pain, poor vision and hearing as well as a lack of understanding on where they can best receive their care.

We wish to challenge those providers and our healthcare friends to give the much needed and highly deserved care that those with intellectual differences have been denied and been obstructed in the past from rightly receiving. For the health revolution to continue and grow, education and training must first be available. The materials and content written within this excellent healthcare resource have been complied by an outstanding team of dedicated experts. Each of them has demonstrated their appreciation for the just cause of reducing health disparities. They bring their particular knowledge and experience in the field. It is now up to those who wish to join the movement and to make a difference and not only challenge themselves but others around them including their friends and colleagues as well as their workplace, academic center, clinic, and hospital to take what is presented and help those who are willing, able, and eager to allow them to have a healthy and productive life.

Timothy P. Shriver
Board of the Special Olympics Organization
Washington, DC
USA

Preface to the Second Edition

A number of useful texts have been published focusing on the conditions affecting people with intellectual and developmental disabilities, but most have either focused specifically on psychiatric and psychological problems or addressed the health and functional status of subgroups, such as individuals with Down syndrome, cerebral palsy, or autism. This text *Physical Health of Adults with Intellectual and Developmental Disabilities*, which is the second edition of the book *Physical Health of Adults with Intellectual Disabilities*, focuses on the wide range of physical health conditions, the growing role of genetic influences, on amelioration of health morbidity and on the provision of healthcare systems, which arise in adults with intellectual and developmental disabilities. Developmental, educational, behavioral, psychological, and social issues are not discussed in this text unless they are specifically associated with one or more of the physical disorders covered. The growing role of molecular genetics is touched upon but due to limited space, detailed discussions on recent advances in this field are excluded. Included are the conditions and diseases that may present to a practitioner or diagnostician as part of routine care.

Physical Health of Adults with Intellectual and Developmental Disabilities aims to give professionals and carers working with people with intellectual and developmental disabilities a more detailed and focused text on particular areas of concern that they may experience as part of their day-to-day work. Many internationally recognized experts, from a wide variety of medical specialties and allied health disciplines, have come together to give the latest view on the commonest physical health conditions that occur in this group of individuals. This text promotes early diagnosis and appropriate management of such problems with a view to establishing good health in this population.

The editors are extremely grateful to our colleagues, made up of a group of internationally renowned physicians, researchers, and scientists, who have contributed to this volume with clarity and scholarly knowledge. The contributors to this volume have been actively involved in academic and clinical work in the field of intellectual disabilities and have all published and/or conducted research in their respective areas. They provide their insight and personal experience and understanding of conditions that occur in people with intellectual disabilities that are not readily encountered by generic professionals. We acknowledge the breadth of information, knowledge, and experience of the many countries that are represented in this text.

A comment on terminology adopted for this text. We have adopted the term "intellectual disability" throughout the text; while the adoption of the term has been approved by international authorities (such as the World Health Organization— WHO), it has not yet gained universal acceptance, particularly by some nations. Other terms still in use generally connote what the WHO refers to as an intellectual disability. For example, although the terms "mental retardation," "learning disabilities," "mental handicap," or "intellectual handicap" (or variants) are in use in other nations, it is common belief that these terms are synonymous and generally understood to reflect the same condition. We also recognize that the term "developmental disability" reflects a category of childhood-derived neurodevelopmental, sensory, or physical conditions, only one of which is an intellectual disability. However, where our authors have specifically implied a broader application or usage, we have left this term in place.

Birmingham, UK

Chicago, IL, USA

2019

Vee P. Prasher

Matthew P. Janicki

Contents

Contributors

Tomas J. Ballesteros, DMD Department of Pediatric Dentistry, Special Care Treatment Center, Rutgers School of Dental Medicine, Newark, NJ, USA

Neha Bansal, MRCPsych Greenfields, Birmingham Community NHS Trust, Birmingham, UK

Helen Baxter, PhD Centre for Academic Primary Care, Population Health Sciences, Bristol Medical School, University of Bristol, Bristol, UK

Helen Beange, MD Centre for Developmental Disability Studies, University of Sydney, Sydney, NSW, Australia

Sarah Bent, MPhys (Hons), MSc (Hons), PhD North Wales Audiology Service, Betsi Cadwaladr University Health Board, Wrexham Maelor Hospital, Wrexham, UK

Siobhan Brennan, BEng (Hons), MSc (Hons), PhD Manchester Centre for Audiology and Deafness (ManCAD), University of Manchester, Manchester, UK

Stephen Brown, FRCPsych Professor (Retired) University of Plymouth Medical School, Cornwall, UK

Éilish Burke, PhD School of Nursing and Midwifery and Trinity Centre of Ageing and Intellectual Disability, Trinity College, The University of Dublin, Dublin, Ireland

Carmen E. Capó-Lugo, PT, PhD Department of Physical Therapy, School of Health Professions, University of Alabama at Birmingham, Birmingham, AL, USA

George Capone, MD Pediatrics, Johns Hopkins School of Medicine, Baltimore, MD, USA

Down Syndrome Clinic & Research Center, Kennedy Krieger Institute, Baltimore, MD, USA

Rachael Carroll, PhD School of Nursing and Midwifery, and The Trinity Centre for Ageing and Intellectual Disability, Trinity College, The University of Dublin, Dublin, Ireland

Priya Chandan, MD, MPH Division of Physical Medicine and Rehabilitation, Department of Neurological Surgery, University of Louisville, Louisville, KY, USA

Brian Chicoine, MD Advocate Medical Group, Adult Down Syndrome Center, Park Ridge, IL, USA

Faculty, Family Medicine Residency, Advocate Lutheran General Hospital, Park Ridge, IL, USA

Michelle Cornacchia, MD Department of Internal Medicine, Geisinger Medical Center, Danville, PA, USA

Alexander Curmi, MD Maudsley Hospital, London, UK

Susan C. Danberg, OD, FCOVD Private Practice, Special Olympics Global Health Program, Glastonbury, CT, USA

Lisa A. Ferretti, LMSW The School of Social Work, College of Public Health, Temple University, Philadelphia, PA, USA

Sinéad Foran, PhD Health Sciences Nursing and Health Care, School of Nursing and Health Care, Waterford Institute of Technology, Waterford, Ireland

Robert J. Fortuna, MD, MPH Internal Medicine, Pediatrics, and Community Health, University of Rochester School of Medicine and Dentistry, Rochester, NY, USA

Meindert Haveman, PhD Department of Rehabilitation Sciences, University of Dortmund, Dortmund, Germany

Tamar Heller, PhD Department of Disability and Human Development, University of Illinois at Chicago, Chicago, IL, USA

Patricia C. Heyn, PhD, FGSA, FACRM Department of Physical Medicine and Rehabilitation, School of Medicine, University of Colorado Denver Anschutz Medical Campus, Aurora, CO, USA

Matthew P. Janicki, PhD Department of Disability and Human Development, University of Illinois at Chicago, Chicago, IL, USA

Seth M. Keller, MD Advocare Neurology of South Jersey, Lumberton, NJ, USA

Gerard J. Kerins, MD, MPA, FACP Section of Geriatrics, Department of Internal Medicine, Yale University School of Medicine, Yale New Haven Health System, New Haven, CT, USA

Mike Kerr, FRCPsych Psychiatry at Cardiff University, Wales and an Honorary Professor at the School of Medicine, Swansea University, Swansea, Wales, UK

Caoinhne MacGiolla Phadraig, PhD Special Care Dentistry, School of Dental Science, Trinity College, The University of Dublin, Dublin, Ireland

Beth Marks, PhD, RN, FAAN Department of Disability and Human Development, University of Illinois at Chicago, Chicago, IL, USA

Philip McCallion, PhD School of Social Work, College of Public Health, Temple University, Philadelphia, PA, USA

Mary McCarron, PhD Faculty of Health Sciences and The Trinity Centre for Ageing and Intellectual Disability, Trinity College, The University of Dublin, Dublin, Ireland

Aidan McElduff, PhD, FRACP Discipline of Medicine, University of Sydney, Camperdown, NSW, Australia

Eimear McGlinchey, PhD Global Brain Health Institute and Trinity Centre for Ageing and Intellectual Disability, Trinity College, The University of Dublin, Dublin, Ireland

Andrew McQuillin, MD Molecular Psychiatry Laboratory, Division of Psychiatry, UCL, London, UK

Lynzee McShea, BSc (Hons), MSc (Hons), DProf Audiology Department, City Hospitals Sunderland Foundation Trust, Sunderland Royal Hospital, Sunderland, UK

Dawna Torres Mughal, PhD, RDN, LDN, FADA, FAND Gannon University, Erie, PA, USA

Márie O'Dwyer, PhD School of Pharmacy and Pharmaceutical Science, Trinity College, The University of Dublin, Dublin, Ireland

Vee P. Prasher, MRCPsych, MD, PhD Neuro-Developmental Psychiatry, Birmingham, UK

Mark D. Robinson, DMD Department of Pediatric Dentistry, Special Care Treatment Center, Rutgers School of Dental Medicine, Newark, NJ, USA

Jaclyn K. Schwartz, PhD, OTR/L Occupational Therapy Department, Nicole Wertheim College of Nursing and Health Sciences, Florida International University, Miami, FL, USA

Rohit Shankar, MBE, FRCPsych Cornwall Partnership NHS Foundation Trust, Bodmin, UK

Exeter Medical School, Truro, UK

Jasmina Sisirak, PhD, MPH Department of Disability and Human Development, University of Illinois at Chicago, Chicago, IL, USA

Harriet Slater, MRCPsych Mental Health and Learning Disabilities Delivery Unit, Abertawe Bro Morgannwg University Health Board, Cardiff, UK

Evan Spivack, DDS Department of Pediatric Dentistry, Special Care Treatment Center, Rutgers School of Dental Medicine, Newark, NJ, USA

Ilana Stol, MD Section of Geriatrics, Department of Internal Medicine, Yale University School of Medicine, Yale New Haven Health System, New Haven, CT, USA

Andre Strydom, PhD Department of Forensic and Neurodevelopmental Science, Institute of Psychiatry, Psychology and Neuroscience, King's College London, London, UK

Margaret A. Turk, MD Physical Medicine & Rehabilitation, Pediatrics, and Public Health & Preventive Medicine, SUNY Upstate Medical University, Syracuse, NY, USA

Lance Watkins, MRCPsych Mental Health and Learning Disability Delivery Unit, Neath Port Talbot CLDT, Abertawe Bro Morgannwyg University Health Board, Swansea, Wales, UK

Sunil J. Wimalawansa, PhD, DSc Department of Medicine, Cardio Metabolic Institute (hon.), North Brunswick, NJ, USA

Part I

Introduction

1

Vee P. Prasher and Matthew P. Janicki

The health initiative, Healthy People 2020 [1, 2], defines health disparities as "a particular type of health difference that is closely linked with social, economic, and/ or environmental disadvantage." It goes on to note that "health disparities adversely affect groups of people who have systematically experienced greater obstacles to health based on their racial or ethnic group; religion; socioeconomic status; gender; [sex]; age; mental health; cognitive, sensory, or physical disability; sexual orientation or gender identity; geographic location; or other characteristics historically linked to discrimination or exclusion." The same initiative defines health equity as the "attainment of the highest level of health for all people," positing "achieving health equity requires valuing everyone equally with focused and ongoing societal efforts to address avoidable inequalities, historical and contemporary injustices, and the elimination of health and health care disparities." The World Health Organization [WHO] [3, 4] notes that health disparities reflect that health status between population groups (and apply to both health inequities and health inequalities), and this commentary aptly applies to the disparity issues that confront adults with intellectual and developmental disabilities.

Indeed, the WHO has recognized that adults with disabilities are particularly vulnerable to deficiencies in access to health care services and knowledgeable care. Depending on the group and setting, persons with disabilities may experience greater vulnerability to secondary conditions, co-morbid conditions, age-related conditions, engaging in health risk behaviors and higher rates of premature death [5]. Dr. Margaret Chan, the Director-General of the WHO noted that "More than one billion people in the world live with some form of disability, of whom nearly 200 million experience considerable difficulties in functioning" [3, 4]. In its report

V. P. Prasher (✉)
Neuro-Developmental Psychiatry, Birmingham, UK

M. P. Janicki
Department of Disability and Human Development, University of Illinois at Chicago, Chicago, IL, USA

© Springer Nature Switzerland AG 2019
V. P. Prasher, M. P. Janicki (eds.), *Physical Health of Adults with Intellectual and Developmental Disabilities*, https://doi.org/10.1007/978-3-319-90083-4_1

on people with disabilities, the WHO [3, 4] noted that among this broad group of individuals with disabilities, adults with intellectual and developmental disabilities are included among those considered part of vulnerable sub-populations. Further, adults with intellectual and developmental disabilities experience greater vulnerability to preventable secondary conditions, co-morbidities, and age-related conditions [6]. Adults with intellectual and developmental disabilities are also at substantially higher risk for obesity and other chronic conditions and may be experiencing them at younger ages [7]. As in the general population, the occurrence of multiple chronic conditions compounds the impact on health status. Krahn and Fox [7] further note that with aging there will be a substantial increase in the rates of chronic conditions and their effect on health. Attention has to be given to the prevention and management of conditions such as diabetes, hypertension, and cardiovascular disease so as improve health outcomes in later life.

Others have noted that particular situations of health outcomes and health access disparities affecting adults with intellectual and developmental disabilities. Such situations can include hospital experiences [8], access to critical health services [9], long-term care management [10], and medications [11]. These disparities are also perceived by adults with these disabilities themselves [12]. While the purpose of this text is not to investigate or explore the etiology of health disparities or the overall social and health care environment that contributes to these, it is our intent to drill down into a number of facets of physical health conditions that can affect disparities and use the collective contributions of the authors to help provide the framework and system base of information for practitioners, clinicians, health policy workers and administrators, as well as provider/services management to improve the understanding of conditions contributing to health challenges among adults with intellectual and developmental disabilities. To this end we have assembled a balanced collection of experts in a variety of fields of medical concerns and health care and asked them to delve into various health issues particular to adults with intellectual and developmental disabilities.

In this update of our text, we begin again with the context for health presentations. Philip McCallion and colleagues, in the second chapter on 'Epidemiological Issues in Intellectual Disabilities and Aging Research' help us better understand how health data contribute to the context of health conditions and health provision. Their explanation of the value of data and of challenges that exist in using existing datasets to track adults with intellectual disability help us with putting data in perspective and realistically ascribing value to what is accumulated. Burke et colleagues, in the third chapter on 'Overview of the Important Physical Health Concerns' help put the nature of conditions found among adults with intellectual and developmental disabilities in useful context. The explore how a variety of conditions, such as obesity, poor cardiovascular health, osteoporosis, falls and fractures, gastrointestinal conditions, sensory impairment, oral health compromises, increased dementia prevalence and polypharmacy concerns are further compromising health as adults age. Lastly, completing this introductory section, Kerins and Stol in Chap. 4, cover 'Assessing Physical Health'. They note that identifying and targeting health problems early is key in reducing unnecessary morbidity and mortality in this age group, and make the plea that attention needs to be paid to reviewing symptoms of medical conditions which may disproportionately affect this population, and that the same standard of care for medical work-up and diagnostic testing for age-matched peers in the general population should be applied to adults with intellectual and developmental disabilities.

In the second section, we offer specialty chapters which consider conditions or issues that are explored in-depth and offer clinical and treatment information. In Chap. 5, Strydom and colleagues speak to 'Physical Health and Clinical Phenotypes'. They cover major specific disorders in terms of their genetic cause, approximate incidence, level of intellectual disability, and major phenotypic characteristics. They also outline prevention and management strategies with respect to these disorders. In Chap. 6, Turk and Fortuna, cover the 'Health Status of Adults with Cerebral Palsy' and note that the physical health issues facing adults with cerebral palsy remain complex and assessing health is usually confounded by the overlying motor impairments and associated health conditions. They cover the common health conditions seen in adults with cerebral palsy and offer a review of their risk factors and prevention and health promotion strategies. Chicoine and Capone, in Chap. 7, cover an emerging topic, 'Regression in Adolescents and Adults with Down Syndrome'. This condition affects adults with Down syndrome in their early adult years and is associated with cognitive-executive impairment, social withdrawal, loss of functional language and previously acquired adaptive skills. This 'regression' in function vexes caregivers and practitioners and the authors explanation of this phenomenon is a welcome addition. In Chaps. 8 and 9, Danberg, and Bent and colleagues, respectively, cover vision issues and hearing issues. Sensory impairments and their physical bases often are masked by behavior and providing information to better understand these phenomena can aid in decreasing false assumptions about behavioral etiologies. Shankar and colleagues, in Chap. 10, cover 'Intellectual Disability and Epilepsy'. They address the issue of seizures and the problems of treatment resistance and increased preponderance to side effects and challenging behavior which makes epilepsy management in people with intellectual disability challenging. In Chap. 11, McElduff and Bansal, delve into 'Endocrinological Issues,' and review the endocrine and related disorders which are commonly seen in adults with intellectual disability and can affect behavior and function.

In the third section, our authors explore a range of ancillary issues that have an impact on health. In Chap. 12, Spivak and colleagues, take us into the area of oral health and note that as the presence of dental disease has been shown to have a direct impact on the person's overall systemic health; attending to dental care is a critical component of overall health care. Mughal in Chap. 13 and Wilmalawansa in Chap. 14, explore issues related to 'Nutrition' and 'Malnutrition', delving into select nutrients, their key functions, recommended intakes, effects of deficiencies and excesses, and major food sources, while highlighting select principles of dietary management relevant to persons with intellectual and developmental disabilities. Haveman, in Chap. 14, examines a number of factors related to 'Aging and Physical Health'. With aging, he notes that health inequalities and health disparities become more prevalent as adults grow into older age and are found in health issues and in access to health services. Part of this is caused by genetic predispositions to certain health conditions, less favorable social circumstances, and reluctance or inability to utilize generic health services—another key cause is that many jurisdictions are unprepared for geriatric medicine to also accommodate patients aging with lifelong disabilities. Cornacchia and Chandan, cover a range of concerns in their chapter on 'Psychotropic Polypharmacy'. Given that polypharmacy is a major issue in this population, often due to the multiplicity of co-incident conditions. How to reduce this factor is a question common in general practice, and as such the authors offer strategies for reducing it when prescribing for adults with lifelong disabilities. In Chaps. 17 and 18, Schwartz and colleagues, and Marks and Sisirak, respectively, offer us critical information on 'Health Self-Management' and 'Health Promotion'. Enabling adults to serve as their own health advocates or to help promote greater awareness among health care providers is an important process in reducing health inequities. The concluding Chap. 19, covers 'Barriers to Health Care Services and the Role of the Physician'. The authors, Slater and colleagues, note that the barriers to the delivery of health care to people with intellectual disabilities include challenges with accessibility, mobility, sensory impairment, behavioral problems, communication, knowledge, attitudes and accessing specialist services, and time and resources. Their commentary on overcoming these barriers is welcome.

The last chapter in the text, examines the key findings of our contributors and takes forth into increasing efforts to reduce health disparities and enlist various agents in promoting health equity for adults with intellectual and developmental disabilities. While we can't speak quantitatively to how much health disparities and inequalities will be reduced in time, we are hopeful that the increased awareness of this situation, as noted by the WHO and many national governments, as well as international and national disability advocacy organizations, will lead to minimizing disparities as a health challenge. More knowledge and a better understanding of select disability or impairment conditions and how various physical health systems work and what detracts or contributes to wellness can certainly begin to decrease the dissonance between our current and future understanding of maintaining sound physical health among adults with lifelong disabilities. This text can contribute to a greater mastery of health matters and to raising the level of understanding of how health disparities can be approached and reduced.

Research findings specific to the adults with intellectual and developmental disabilities are allowing more targeted health care systems to be employed rather than, as often was the case in the past, their needs 'added-on' to generic health care provision. Recent developments in molecular genetics with identification of numerous genes for many health conditions mean that during the next decade a greater link between the underlying genetic cause of intellectual and developmental disabilities and health morbidity will be a fascinating area of development. It is not unreasonable in the future to contemplate the prevention of the onset of life limiting disorders in persons with intellectual and developmental disabilities. Prevention of Alzheimer's disease dementia, by gene manipulation in adults with Down syndrome is an excellent example. Finally the role of individual choice and self-determination of one's own health will remain a challenge for persons with intellectual and developmental disabilities.

V. P. Prasher and M. P. Janicki
2019

References

1. Healthy People. Disparities. HealthPeople.gov. 2018. Accessed from: https://www.healthypeople.gov/2020/about/foundation-health-measures/Disparities.
2. U.S. Department of Health and Human Services. The Secretary's Advisory Committee on National Health Promotion and Disease Prevention Objectives for 2020. Phase I report: recommendations for the framework and format of Healthy People 2020 [Internet]. Section IV: Advisory Committee findings and recommendations [cited 2010 January 6]. 2010. Accessed from: http://www.healthypeople.gov/sites/default/files/PhaseI_0.pdf.
3. World Health Organization. Closing the gap: policy into practice on social determinants of health. Geneva: WHO; 2011a. Accessed from: http://www.who.int/sdhconference/Discussion-Paper-EN.pdf?ua=1.
4. World Health Organization. World report on disability. 2011b. Accessed from: http://apps.who.int/iris/bitstream/handle/10665/70670/WHO_NMH_VIP_11.01_eng.pdf;jsessionid=AD31358D0A3A5BAA4324A5658871300D?sequence=1-30-.
5. World Health Organization. Disability and health. 2018. Accessed from: http://www.who.int/news-room/fact-sheets/detail/disability-and-health.
6. Emerson E, Hatton C. Health inequalities and people with intellectual disabilities. Cambridge: Cambridge University Press; 2013. https://doi.org/10.1017/CBO9781139192484.
7. Krahn GL, Fox MH. Health disparities of adults with intellectual disabilities: what do we know? What do we do. J Appl Res Intellect Disabil. 2014;27:431–46. https://doi.org/10.1111/jar/12067.
8. Iacono T, Bigby C, Unsworth C, Douglas J, Fitzpatrick P. A system review of hospital experience of people with intellectual disability. BMC Health Serv Res. 2014;14:505. Accessed from: http://www.biomedcentral.com/1472-6963/14/505.
9. Williamson J, Contreras GM, Rodriguez ES, Smith JM, Perkins EA. Health care access for adults with intellectual and developmental disabilities: a scoping review. Occup Participat Health. 2017;37(4):227–36. https://doi.org/10.1177/1539449217714148.
10. Hanlon P, MacDonald S, Wood K, Allan L, Cooper S-A. Long-term condition management in adults with intellectual disability in primary care: a systematic review. BJGP Open. 2018;2:bjgpopen18X101445. https://doi.org/10.3399/bigpopen18X101445.
11. Salomon C, Britt H, Pollack A, Trollor J. Primary care for people with an intellectual disability — what is prescribed? An analysis of medication recommendations from the BEACH dataset. BJGP Open. 2018; https://doi.org/10.3399/bjgpopen18X101541.
12. Bollard M, Mcleod E, Dolan A. Exploring the impact of health inequalities on the health of adults with intellectual disability from their perspective. Disabil Soc. 2018;33:831. https://doi.org/10.1080/09687599.2018.1459476.

Epidemiological Issues in Intellectual Disability and Aging Research

2

Philip McCallion, Lisa A. Ferretti, Helen Beange, and Mary McCarron

2.1 Introduction

Epidemiology is the study of prevalence, incidence and contributors to chronic conditions and other disorders in a population completed for its own sake, and also because it may inform the knowledge of distributions of conditions, understanding of causes, and indicators of how best to work to manage population level and sub-population level concerns. Such knowledge in turn may (a) inform the setting of priorities for public health initiatives and healthcare planning, targeting and implementation and (b) longitudinally be the basis for measuring changes in the conditions and overall success of initiatives and interventions to improve health or reduce the impact of targeted health concerns.

Epidemiological studies use a variety of designs and may be longitudinal (multiple data points), cross-sectional (one-time data collection on selected health variables), case-control (allowing the measurement of differences between groups), and experimental (large scale randomized trials of interventions targeting health concerns) [1].

Ideally, data is drawn from large scale national and even international data sets with variables that address the demographics of the population, diagnoses of

P. McCallion (✉)
The School of Social Work, College of Public Health, Temple University, Philadelphia, PA, USA
e-mail: philip.mccallion@temple.edu

L. A. Ferretti
School of Social Work, College of Public Health, Temple University, Philadelphia, PA, USA

H. Beange
Centre for Developmental Disability Studies, University of Sydney, Sydney, NSW, Australia

M. McCarron
Faculty of Health Sciences and The Trinity Centre for Ageing and Intellectual Disability, Trinity College, The University of Dublin, Dublin, Ireland

© Springer Nature Switzerland AG 2019
V. P. Prasher, M. P. Janicki (eds.), *Physical Health of Adults with Intellectual and Developmental Disabilities*, https://doi.org/10.1007/978-3-319-90083-4_2

physical and mental health conditions (current and historical), living situations, work circumstances, family and social support structures and experiences, and healthcare utilization including preventive health intervention participation, and medication use (current and historic, prescription and non-prescription). Availability of such variables offers the best opportunity to understand the precursors of current health and well-being, estimate future experiences and compare groups within a population [2]. Examples of such surveys are national census data, household surveys, birth and death records, surveillance surveys, administrative datasets with health encounter, service utilization, and demographic data, registries, electronic health records, and population surveys targeting persons with specific health conditions [3, 4]. There are also, at times, opportunities to combine some of these data sources to produce a more comprehensive picture. However, there are also challenges including differences in definition of key variables, different time frames and challenges presented by missing data, and varying coding systems which make data harmonization difficult [5].

The tracking of health and health related outcomes for people with intellectual disability utilizing population-based surveys such as the U.S. National Health Interview Survey (NHIS) existing population surveys (e.g., the census or administrative datasets such as on medical encounters) offer a number of advantages:

- The only additional costs are for analyses of participants with intellectual disability
- There is often high quality in the sampling, fieldwork and data management
- There may be a built-in opportunity to compare the lives of people with intellectual disability to other groups (e.g., people with other kinds of disabilities) or other health disparity groups, or to the population without identified life-long disabilities.
- Measures are already tested and validated [6]

However, there are many challenges in such use, not least that many such surveys are household based and the person with an intellectual disability may not be the responding adult, and that those living in group homes and other out-of-home situations or accommodations are excluded from the sample; many surveys use phone, email, and in-person measurement approaches that may also exclude persons with intellectual disability; survey implementation may be periodic and may not follow the same individuals; persons with intellectual disability may be excluded because of concerns about ability to give consent, and persons with intellectual disability may interact less with those collecting data for administrative datasets [3, 6]. A large challenge is inconsistency in defining and measuring intellectual disability.

2.2   Defining and Measuring Intellectual Disability

The World Health Organization [7] defines intellectual disability as "a significantly reduced ability to understand new or complex information and to learn and apply new skills (impaired intelligence)" which results in a reduced ability to cope independently (impaired social functioning), and begins before adulthood, with a lasting effect on development. Further, the WHO notes that the disability depends not only on a person's health conditions or impairments, but also and crucially on the extent to which environmental factors support the person's full participation and inclusion in society. The WHO definition includes persons with autism who have intellectual impairments and it also encompasses persons who have been placed in institutions because of perceived disabilities or family rejection and who consequently acquire developmental delays and psychological problems.

Although the term "intellectual disability" has widely replaced other terms for policy, administrative, and legislative purposes, there remain questions as to whether intellectual disability is a disability or a health condition. As a health condition, intellectual disability can be coded as a disorder in the International Classification of Diseases [8]. The WPA Section on Psychiatry of Intellectual Disability agrees that intellectual disability is a health condition and notes that is "a syndromic grouping or meta-syndrome analogous to the construct of dementia, which is characterized by a deficit in cognitive functioning prior to the acquisition of skills through learning... the intensity of the deficit is such that it interferes in a significant way with individual normal functioning as expressed in limitations in activities and restriction in participation (disabilities)" [8, 9]. However, the impairments in intellectual functioning central to intellectual disability are also classified within WHO's International Classification of Functioning, Disability and Health (ICF) in disability rather than health terms. The American Association on Intellectual and Developmental Disabilities (AAIDD) by focusing mainly on functioning, adaptive behavior, and support needs which correspond with the ICF conceptual model; it also sees intellectual disability as a disability with "significant limitations both in intellectual functioning and in adaptive behavior as expressed in conceptual, social, and practical adaptive skills", with the disability originating before age 18 [10].

In the United States, intellectual disability is considered a subset of developmental disabilities (DD), which is defined in federal statute [11] as:

- (a) a severe, chronic disability in an individual 5 years of age or older,
- (b) with onset before 22 years of age,
- (c) which results in substantial functional limitations in three or more areas of life activity (self-care, receptive and expressive language, learning, mobility, self-direction, capacity for independent learning, economic self-sufficiency).

These varying definitions illustrate one of the significant epidemiological challenges in intellectual disability—who represents a "case." The picture is further complicated by continued use in other jurisdictions of the term "learning disabilities," which the UK National Health Service defines as a condition that affects the way a person learns new things in any area of life, affects the way a person understands information, and how he or she communicates. This means they can have difficulty understanding new or complex information, learning new skills, and coping independently. Learning disabilities can be mild, moderate or severe and profound and someone is described as a person with profound and multiple learning disabilities (PMLD) when there is more than one disability, with the most significant being learning disabilities. Often this means there is also a sensory or physical disability, complex health needs, or mental health difficulties, and the persons needs help from someone else with most daily living skills areas [12].

Levels of disability are also a consideration in intellectual disability. Severity levels (mild, moderate, severe, and profound) in the U.S., as defined in *DSM-5*, are based on adaptive functioning in the conceptual, social, and practical domains. Both in the U.S. and in European countries severity of intellectual disability is also defined on the basis of cognitive skills and the distribution of IQ scores as used in the International Statistical Classification of Diseases and Related Health Problems (ICD-10) [13]. However, in the dataset available for epidemiological analysis there is rarely reporting of independently established levels of intellectual disability, information on assessments used or if classification is based on historical report and/or clinical impression. Both historical reports and clinical impression may utilize different scoring criteria or none and are more likely in data on older adults with intellectual disability.

Incidence of intellectual disability refers to the number of new cases identified in a specified time period. Prevalence of intellectual disability refers to the number of people who are living with the condition in a given time period. The determination of incidence and prevalence of intellectual disability is complicated then when available reports do not use the same operational definitions when selecting and identifying individuals with intellectual disability. Further variations in study design and terminology, different sample size and sample characteristics (including varying interest in representativeness), and choices made among diagnostic tools also affect reported incidence and prevalence data.

Terminology is beginning to become more standardized with movement from "mental retardation"[1] and developmental disability in the U.S, and from learning disability in the U.K. and several other countries to more general adoption of the term intellectual disability. There continues to be a lack of consensus on whether all developmental disabilities and all learning disabilities "fit" within intellectual disability but some studies report as if this is accepted practice. Further concerns in the U.S. have arisen with respect to population surveys as there is a requirement to use six functional questions from the American Community Survey to capture disability status in vision, hearing, mobility, cognition, independent living, and societal participation [14]. The question "Because of a physical, mental, or emotional condition, does anyone (in your household) have serious difficulty concentrating, remembering, or making decisions?", includes people with intellectual disability, but also many others with both life-long and late-onset conditions. This means the item is not a good proxy question for intellectual disability and offers no information on level of intellectual disability. Few population surveys therefore contain the necessary questions to establish a person with intellectual disability in epidemiological terms as a "case" and the exclusion in many of those surveys of people living in out-of-home placements also means that there are fewer "cases" to find.

---

[1] "Mental retardation" is now considered a pejorative term and its use is generally avoided.

An illustration of the challenge these barriers represent can be found in estimates of the incidence of intellectual disability. In a 2011 meta-analysis of international studies of intellectual disability prevalence for individuals across the life span was estimated at 10.37/1000 or 1.04% [15] and a further meta-analysis found prevalence for the same life-span group to range from .05% to 1.55% [4]. For adults (not just those who are aging) this translates to prevalence for adults at 4.94/1000 or .49% [15], or ranging from .05 to .08% [4]. This means that in a U.S. Census Bureau study that approximately 1.2 million (0.5%) of civilian, noninstitutionalized adults had an ID in 2010 [14]. Yet there are still popular estimates of 3% [1].

Despite these definitional and methodological limitations, much can be gleaned from existing datasets about the health, well-being and healthcare utilization of adults, particularly aging adults who have been identified in various countries and jurisdictions as having intellectual disability.

2.3 The Changing Aging Lives of People with Intellectual Disability

There is evidence from national databases that the numbers of individuals older than 35 and older than 60 have steadily risen [16, 17]. In the U.S., on the basis of estimates, life expectancy for persons with intellectual disability has been reported to have increased from an average 18.5 years in the 1930s, to 59.1 years in the 1970s, and to an estimated 66.2 years in 1993 [18] with projections that by 2020 the number of those aged over 65 will have doubled [19]. There are similar projections in the UK, other European countries, and in Australia [20]. However, recent discussions related to data in The Lancet [21, 22], and data drawn from several countries have highlighted that continued growth in longevity may have stalled, despite there being more absolute numbers of older adults with intellectual disability [23, 24]. These findings based largely on reviews of administrative datasets illustrate the power of epidemiological approaches to challenge the power of "popular wisdom" about a population. What remains to be done is to use data available in a similar way to understand the reasons for this change in longevity and the potential to initiate again changes likely to begin moving people with intellectual disability toward enjoying quality lives as long as the general population.

The needs of all older adults are similar: good management of age-related chronic conditions, housing that accommodates changing abilities with age, adequate nutrition, access to timely and appropriate health care, and opportunities for positive social engagement [25]. However, due to their life-long disability, older adults with intellectual disability also have unique life experiences and perceptions compared with age peers in the general population that must also be considered [17, 26]. It is perhaps the data that is emerging on the disproportionately high levels of avoidable or treatable causes of premature death among people with intellectual disability [22] that points up the opportunity in epidemiological research to identify variables in health and well-being that are amenable to change.

2.4   Chronic Conditions and the Aging Years

Sustained efforts of families, providers, communities, and professionals have improved lives as people with intellectual disability have aged but aging also presents challenges. Holland [27] speculated that people with intellectual disability who survived into old age were probably healthier and hardier than those who did not [27, 28]. However, he was also concerned at the potential of additional age-related disabilities and with the lack of preparedness of service networks. Findings from census data in Scotland appear to support both these speculations and conclusions. Scottish rates of illness and death were higher for people with intellectual disability under age 34 years as compared to the general population of the same age, but the rates were similar between ages 35–44 years. But comparatively, health became progressively poorer as people with intellectual disability aged beyond 45 years [29]. In other words, it does appear that survivors with intellectual disability in their younger years do in their older years present with a rate of health concerns that is different from their own middle years, is more severe than is seen in the general population, and potentially will challenge service system responses.

In a number of investigations of chronic illness among people with intellectual disability, similarities and dissimilarities with the general population have been highlighted and a higher prevalence noted of disorders, as well as a higher level of diagnoses that go unrecognized and untreated [30–33]. The problems with definitions, timeframes, and sources of data notwithstanding, there is support across studies for a greater prevalence among aging adults with intellectual disability, as compared to the general population and their own younger years, of gastrointestinal disorders, respiratory disorders (such as pneumonia), epilepsy, sensory impairments, dental disease, osteoporosis, dementia, mental illness, and behavioral challenges [33–36]. People with intellectual disability, as they age, have been shown to become high and frequent users of primary health care services—both general population health professionals and intellectual disability specialists. In addition, there are data emerging of different patterns and combinations of morbidities, less focus on preventive interventions, and inattention to population health among people with intellectual disability. Taken together the utilization data particularly suggest a lack of preparedness for aging people with intellectual disability in general population health delivery [37, 38].

The impact of such differences has been found to be further compounded by lack of surveillance and by inequalities in access to health services [39, 40]. Many health professionals are unfamiliar with and have received little training in the typical health and functioning issues in older adults with intellectual disability [41], meaning they may miss underlying health problems [38] increasing the potential for under-reporting of conditions. There are also reports that communication barriers [42], higher and different comorbidity, poorer management of health conditions, and minimal emphasis on prevention mean poorer care and that significant physical health-related burdens fall upon caregivers [20, 38, 43]. For these reasons there are growing recommendations for the development and use of health indicator surveys to better document inequalities, highlight differences in health and health needs and track improvement over time.

2.5   Health Indicators

There have been several developments with respect to health indicators. In the U.S. the National Core Indicators Project addresses individual outcomes; health, welfare, and rights; system performance; staff stability; and family indicators. More specifically, the health, welfare, and rights domain targets healthcare services, health behaviors, medication rates, safety considerations, rights protection and use of restraints [40, 44]. Data gathered periodically from volunteer states provides the opportunity to compare across States and time, and with similarly available data on the general population.

In Europe, the Pomona project built upon the generic European Community Health Indicators effort by establishing 18 health indicators for people with intellectual disability: demographics (prevalence of intellectual disability, living arrangements, daily occupation, income/SES, life expectancy); health status (epilepsy, oral health, body mass index, mental health/psychiatric disorder, sensory capacities, mobility); determinants of health (physical activity, challenging behaviors, psychotropic medications); and health systems (hospitalization and contact with healthcare professionals, health checks, health promotion, specific training for physicians) and identified potential sources for the related data [32, 45, 46].

An Irish-centered project focusses on health indicators for older people with intellectual disability that directly links with Ireland's National Indicators on Positive Ageing (NIPA). The NIPA established a series of indicators and mapped them onto available databases so that routine measurements were possible of progress in achieving positive ageing with the following four goals:

1. Removing barriers to participation and provide more opportunities for the continued involvement of people as they age in all aspects of cultural, economic and social life in their communities according to their needs, preferences and capacities.
2. Supporting people as they age to maintain, improve or manage their physical and mental health and wellbeing.
3. Enabling people to age with confidence, security and dignity in their own homes and communities for as long as possible.
4. Support and use research about people as they age to better inform policy responses to population ageing in Ireland.

Much of these data are drawn from the on-going Irish Longitudinal Study on Ageing. Funding provided for the establishment of the National Indicators for Positive Ageing for People with Intellectual Disabilities (NIPAPID) project will map data from the

Intellectual Disability Supplement to The Irish Longitudinal Study on Ageing onto the same indicators [47]. Next steps will also support the development of additional intellectual disability-specific indicators in pursuit of a fifth goal:

5. Understanding how additional supports and education may mitigate additional challenges to positive ageing resulting from differences in disease patterns and in family and community supports.

Consistent with [48], by being embedded in the indicators for the general population, NIPAPID will be able to highlight where health disparities exist and over time how well they are being addressed.

2.6 Enhancing Surveillance: Special Disability Surveys— Inclusion in Public Health Surveys

A number of countries have initiated population level surveys specific to disabilities. These surveys include in the USA, the 1994–1995 National Health Interview Survey—Disability Supplement; in Australia, the Survey of Disability, Ageing and Carers in 1998 and 2003; in China, the National Sample Survey on Disability in 2006; in the UK Life Opportunities Survey begun in 2009 and is continuing; and in Ireland, the National Disability Survey in 2006 [48]. These surveys tend to be one-time or occasional and use varying definitions of disability. This is also true where efforts have been made to include disability and intellectual disability identifiers in public health surveys [48]. As noted by Fujiura et al. [49] in a review of surveys in 131 national systems from 12 countries in eight global regions, some 25% of the data systems coded for intellectual disability, but there were concerns about both the quality of the data and variations in definitions [48].

Seeking to respond to these concerns, the Intellectual Disability Supplement to The Irish Longitudinal Study on Ageing, established in 2006, has completed three waves of comprehensive data collection. It selects its nationally representative sample from Ireland's National Intellectual Disability Database, collects a full range of demographic, social engagement, living situation, health and healthcare utilization data and draws out of home placement, community, family care and independent living participants, collects data every 3 years, at every other data collection completes physical measures to confirm self-report data and matches its questions and approaches as closely as possible to the general population Irish Longitudinal Study on Ageing to ensure its ability to support comparisons. Other countries have not yet replicated this approach; however, increasingly there are administrative datasets in the health and healthcare utilization arena that have a similar attention to validity of questions and confirmation of reports and the ability to directly compare with the general population.

2.7   Physical Health

When using both administrative datasets and population surveys aging people with intellectual disability are compared with older adults in the general population, they have been found to have:

– Higher rates of unhealthy lifestyles [38, 41] with the highest rates of unhealthy weight gain, obesity, cardiovascular disease (CVD), and CVD-related mortality among those living independently [50].
– Higher levels of medication use and excess polypharmacy [51, 52]
– Poor dental hygiene and an elevated level of missing teeth with little replacement e.g., with dentures [53].
– Higher rates of females having poorer health than males as they age [29]
– Sedentary lifestyles that mean they are less likely than the general population to achieve levels of physical activity that would positively affect health [54]
– Higher rates of chronic conditions, such as dementia [55, 56]
– Earlier onset of menopause for women with intellectual disability increasing their risks for dementia and early mortality [57]
– Increased pain levels, sarcopenia, osteoporosis, and arthritis particularly for those who have neuromuscular disorders (e.g., cerebral palsy) [58, 59].
– Different patterns of co-occurring conditions with greater levels of co-occurring mental health concerns [38]

These findings again highlight the need to gather variables across a range of life areas, not simply health and healthcare utilization, and also to have the ability to compare with general population findings. Healthcare and resource planning which considers populations which exclude persons with intellectual disability will necessarily neglect the needs of this group.

2.8   Mental Health

Health concerns also include psychosocial or mental health issues. A summation of available studies of mental health and behavioral concern prevalence suggested total rates of mental health concerns range from 20% to 40% of assessed older people with intellectual disability and that psychiatric disorders, including dementia, increase as people with intellectual disability age (for a review, see [60]). Other reviews argue that the picture is more complex, with most mental health concerns appearing to decline with age, except for dementia, which increases [61]. Regardless, behavioral phenotypes (particularly for dementia); side effects of medications that they may metabolize differently from others; higher rates of sensory impairments that increase communication difficulties; aging-specific disorders (such as

Alzheimer's disease) may predispose persons with intellectual disability to depression and anxiety; as may life events such as bereavements and abuse [62]. Large datasets targeting people with intellectual disability, if they are to provide needed insights must therefore collect data not simply on mental health diagnoses, but also on the co-occurring concerns including life events. Findings, for example, from the Intellectual Disability Supplement to the Irish Longitudinal Study on Ageing confirm what has been highlighted by Dodd et al. [62], but note more specifically that epilepsy, unaddressed pain, comorbidity, life events and the consequences of polypharmacy appear of most concern [63, 64]. Here too a greater understanding of both the additional mental health needs and differences in contributing factors for people with intellectual disability must be part of policy and resource planning. This is more likely to occur if there is comparable data available to general population data currently informing decisions.

2.9   Frailty

Another relevant concept that is increasingly influencing health care for older adults in the general population is frailty. Large, particularly longitudinal, datasets are now permitting greater exploration of underlying influences in health for aging persons with intellectual disability, and this includes attention to frailty. Evenhuis et al. [65], using a standard general population definition of frailty (i.e., high vulnerability to adverse health conditions), measured frailty in people with intellectual disability in a longitudinal dataset of persons with intellectual disability drawn largely from out-of-home placements. Using five criteria: weight loss, poor grip strength, slow walking speed, low physical activity, and poor endurance or exhaustion, they found that people with intellectual disability at ages 50–64 had a prevalence of frailty (11%) that was similar to that of the general population at ages 65 and older (7–9%). Age, Down syndrome, dementia, motor disability, and severe intellectual impairment were found to be associated with frailty, but statistically only explained 25% of the variance.

Using an alternative Frailty Index and using data from the same large intellectual disability-specific dataset, the researchers found that people with intellectual disability older than age 50 had frailty scores similar to most elderly people older than 75 [66]. The index comprised 50 health-related deficits, including physical, social, and medical problems, and established that high levels of frailty among people with intellectual disability were associated with potentially preventable and reversible factors including very low levels of physical activity, social relationships, and community participation [67]. Such findings are encouraging further exploration of frailty in other large datasets, greater attention to the variables that are likely to be most relevant for the measurement of frailty in persons with intellectual disability, and the emergence of variables where prevention and treatment may reduce impact, supporting the testing of interventions focused upon health promotion as well as condition treatment.

2.10   Health Maintenance and Improvement as People Age

Access and support are critical to health maintenance and improvement, including access to appropriate foods and health screening, participation in physical activity and follow-up preventive care, and support from social networks [63, 68, 69]. People with intellectual disability embark on life from a particularly disadvantaged, even impoverished, position [30]. As a range of studies in several countries relying on record reviews and self-reported data have demonstrated, they are more likely to have lived in poverty; have poorer physical and mental health; have higher levels of obesity [70]; are more likely to lead sedentary lifestyles [71]; tend to have nutritionally poor diets [72, 73]; participate less than the general population in physical activity [74]; and are less likely to have benefitted from preventive health screening and health promotion [20, 31, 33, 36]. Higher rates have also been found of obesity and cholesterol which with lower rates found for physical activity increase the potential for diabetes, hypertension, heart disease, and arthritis late in life [20, 63, 75, 76].

There are also findings emerging that suggest that health supportive screenings are under-utilized. In Samele et al. [77], for example, uptake of cervical cancer screening in the UK was 84–89% overall, but only 13–47% in the population of people with intellectual disability. There are similar findings for vision and hearing impairment and for dental care [30, 78]. Yet systematic review evidence [79] suggests that screening for people with intellectual disability is so beneficial that specifically designed health checks should become a routine part of primary care. These findings are helpful to informing policymakers and decision-makers, but they also present a challenge to researchers and practitioners to develop, test, and advance interventions that are likely to be responsive.

2.11   Dementia

Dementia in people with Down syndrome exceeds that of the general population; one study reported a prevalence of 2% in people ages 30–39 years, 9.4% in people ages 40–49 years, 36.1% in people ages 50–59 years, and 54.5% in people ages 60–69 years [80], as compared with general population rates of between 4.3% and 10% in people ages 65 years and older. Reports of the prevalence of dementia for other people with intellectual disability (who do not have Down syndrome) are more equivocal, with both findings of rates similar to the general population [19] and also of higher rates [81]. People with Down syndrome and dementia experience an early and precipitous but then extended decline; pose care concerns given wandering, sleep disturbance, and incontinence; and in some instances, experience auditory and visual hallucinations [56, 82]. In addition, depression and other mental health symptoms are sometimes mistaken for dementia or may co-occur with dementia [83]. Data from a longitudinal follow-up of a group of women with Down syndrome confirmed that when dementia symptoms were present, that there is also increased incidence of health conditions such as hearing, vision, and mobility impairments, depression, epilepsy, and lung disease [35, 47].

Dementia is an example of a health condition where incidence, prevalence and needed responses among adults with intellectual disability have been different from those of the general population. If policy and decision-makers assume that incidence of dementia prior to age 65 is exceptional, as much general population data suggests, then services designed will fail to be responsive to the actual needs of people with intellectual disability and dementia. Epidemiological studies with the same methodological rigor as those available for the general population will help to highlight these differences in ways in which they are more likely to be heard.

Other chapters address each of these and additional health issues in more detail. What is important here is that epidemiological approaches to the aging and health of people with intellectual disability are gaining attention and are providing new insights, confirming the overall picture that had previously emerged from smaller, less stringently designed studies. Epidemiological findings are also offering new ideas and explanations for what is different in aging for people with intellectual disability even as they also confirm what is similar; thanks to built-in capacity in many of the datasets used to compare to the general population. All of this is happening, despite the limitations noted in available datasets.

2.12 Improving Epidemiological Research

For epidemiological research to best realize its potential for understanding and supporting the lives of people with intellectual disability, it is important that greater standardization occur in the definition of intellectual disability. Given the continuing disability versus health condition divide, the need to further reconcile developmental disabilities and learning disabilities with intellectual disability, as well as continuing concerns about standardization of interpretations of levels of disability, this will be difficult. It would also be helpful if identifiers for intellectual disability were added to more national datasets and if samples selected more likely included people with intellectual disability living in out-of-home settings. Perhaps the pending move to ICD-11 classifications will help advance such standardization [8]. The greatest opportunity for such standardization is in administrative datasets and in disability population surveys [3]. At the very least researchers and administrators of these resources must take the responsibility of routinely and consistently providing in their studies and reports the definition of intellectual disability utilized as well as definitions of levels of ID, if reported. This should extend to also reporting data by sex and age preferably using consistent or easily converted categories of age [3]. Efforts to facilitate making datasets publicly available, in formats that are easily analyzed and with codes to easily identify subpopulations will increase the ability to use such data effectively and for the benefit of people with intellectual disability [48, 84].

A long-standing concern in all data related to people with intellectual disability is the potential for bias resulting from use of self-reported and proxy provided data [85]. There are examples of researchers relying on epidemiological data who have included and reported on tests of the validity of proxy provided data (see [86]). However, there are inherent assumptions in many datasets that participants have the ability to understand and answer questions which instead may be challenging for some individuals with intellectual disability with the level of challenge untested and not ascertained. Equally, there are assumptions that proxies have the ability to answer all questions when particularly for questions addressing subjective appraisals, there is available evidence of differences between the person themselves and their proxies in such appraisals [6]. Better reporting in datasets of how proxies are chosen and for which questions will increase confidence in the data. Finally, there is the concern that self-report data whether from people with intellectual disability or from the general population is simply wrong or misremembered. This is particularly of concern with diagnostic, healthcare utilization and medication data. The greater availability to researchers of electronic case/health records, administrative datasets and medication records already occurring for epidemiological investigations for the general population is more slowly occurring for the population with ID. Progress is needed as it will make available more complete data and in formats that will likely better support comparisons with the general population.

In the meantime, data collections for people with intellectual disability that include review of case records and/or where periodically there are physical measures (for example, of blood pressure and body mass index) help to measure the reliability of these and other self-reports relied upon. More intrusive measures such as the collection of bloods present consent and feasibility challenges, but they may also confirm what is self-reported and provide new variables that help in our understanding of disease development, progress and impact on daily life.

2.13   Conclusion

Much work is still needed to better understand the prevalence, incidence and contributors to chronic health conditions in people with intellectual disability as they age. Fortunately, the field has moved beyond small exploratory studies and is making greater use of existing datasets and opportunities to compare with the general population. There remain considerable challenges in utilizing existing datasets to track people with intellectual disability as they age, given differences in definitions of intellectual disability and quality issues in terms of how data is gathered. Nevertheless, such studies by offering up a fuller range of variables to consider in understanding the health, healthcare utilization, and aspects of daily lives of people with intellectual disability are helping to increase understanding of opportunities for beneficial intervention. Where there is an opportunity to compare findings with the general population, as is increasingly occurring, this provides an additional window to highlight what is the same and what sometimes is dramatically different for people with intellectual disability.

References

1. Prasher VP, Madhavan GP. Epidemiology of intellectual disability and comorbid conditions. Intellectual Disability and Health. 2017. Accessed from: http://www.intellectualdisability.info/mental-health/articles/epidemiology-of-intellectual-disability-and-comorbid-conditions.
2. Hodapp RM, Goldman SE, Urbano RC. Using secondary datasets in disability research: special issues, special promise. Int Rev Res Dev Disabil. 2013;45:1–33.
3. Friedman DJ, Parrish RG, Fox MH. A review of global literature on using administrative data to estimate prevalence of intellectual and developmental disabilities. J Pol Pract Intellect Disabil. 2018;15:43–62.
4. McKensie K, Milton M, Smith G, Ouellette-Kuntz H. Systematic review of the prevalence and incidence of intellectual disabilities: current trends and issues. Curr Dev Disord Rep. 2016;3:104–15.
5. Urbano RC. Large scale datasets referenced in Volume 45 of the International Review of Research in Developmental Disabilities. Int Rev Res Dev Disabil. 2013;45:329–41.
6. Emerson E, Felce D, Stancliffe RJ. Issues concerning self-report data and population-based data sets involving people with intellectual disabilities. Intellect Dev Disabil. 2013;51:333–48.
7. World Health Organization. Definition: intellectual disability. 2010. Accessed from: http://www.euro.who.int/en/health-topics/noncommunicable-diseases/mental-health/news/news/2010/15/childrens-right-to-family-life/definition-intellectual-disability.
8. Salvador-Carulla L, Reed GM, Vaez-Azizi LM, Cooper SA, Martinez-Leal R, Bertelli M, Adnams C, Cooray S, Deb S, Akoury-Dirani L, Girimaji SC, Katz G, Kwok H, Luckasson R, Simeonsson R, Walsh C, Munir K, Saxena S. Intellectual developmental disorders: towards a new name, definition and framework for "mental retardation/intellectual disability" in ICD-11. World Psychiatry. 2011;10:175–80.
9. Salvador-Carulla L, Bertelli M. Mental retardation' or 'intellectual disability': time for a conceptual change. Psychopathology. 2008;41:10–6.
10. Schalock RL, Borthwick-Duffy SA, Bradley M, editors. Intellectual disability: definition, classification, and systems of supports. 11th ed. Washington, DC: American Association on Intellectual and Developmental Disabilities; 2010.
11. Developmental Disabilities Assistance and Bill of Rights Act. 2000 The Administration on Developmental Disabilities: The Developmental Disabilities Assistance and Bill of Rights Act of 2000. Retrieved on 17 Jan 2018.
12. National Health Service. Learning disabilities. 2018. Accessed from: https://www.nhs.uk/conditions/learning-disabilities/.
13. Van Bakel M, Einarsson I, Arnaud C, Craig S, Michelsen SI, Pildava S, Uldall P, Cans C. Monitoring the prevalence of severe intellectual disability in children across Europe: feasibility of a common database. Dev Med Child Neurol. 2013; https://doi.org/10.1111/dmcn.12281.
14. Brault MW. Americans with disabilities: 2010, Current population reports, P70-131, U.S. Census Bureau. Washington, DC: U.S. Government Printing Office; 2012.
15. Maulik PK, Mascarenhas MN, Mathers CD, Dua T, Saxena S. Prevalence of intellectual disability: a meta-analysis of population-based studies. Res Dev Disabil. 2011;32:419–36.
16. Kelly C, O'Donohoe A. HRB statistics series 24. Annual report of the National Intellectual Disability Database Committee 2013. Main findings. Dublin: Health Research Board; 2014.
17. McCallion P, McCarron M. People with disabilities entering the third age. In: McConkey R, Gilligan R, Iriarte EG, editors. Disability in a global age: a human rights based approach. London: Palgrave McMillan; 2015.
18. Braddock D. Aging and developmental disabilities: demographic and policy issues affecting American families. Ment Retard. 1999;37:155–61.
19. Janicki MP, Dalton AJ. Prevalence of dementia and impact on intellectual disability services. Ment Retard. 2000;38:277–89.
20. Bigby C, McCallion P, McCarron M. Serving an elderly population. In: Agran M, Brown F, Hughes C, Quirk C, Ryndak D, editors. Equality and full participation for individuals with severe disabilities: a vision for the future. Baltimore, MD: Paul H. Brookes; 2014. p. 319–48.

21. McCallion P, McCarron M. Death of people with intellectual disabilities in the UK. Lancet. 2014;383(9920):853–5.
22. Heslop P, Blair PS, Fleming PJ, Hoghton MA, Marriott AM, Russ LS. The Confidential Inquiry into premature deaths of people with intellectual disabilities in the UK: a population-based study. Lancet. 2014;383(9920):889–95.
23. Lauer E, McCallion P. Mortality of people with intellectual and developmental disabilities from select U.S. States. J Appl Res Intellect Disabil. 2015;28:394–405.
24. McCarron M, Gill M, McCallion P, Begley C. Health Co-morbidities in ageing Persons with Down syndrome and Alzheimer's dementia. J Intellect Disabil Res. 2005;49(7):560–6.
25. McCallion P. Aging in place. In: Whitfield K, Baker T, editors. Handbook of minority aging. New York, NY: Springer; 2014. p. 277–90.
26. Kåhlin I, Kjellberg A, Nord C, Hagberg J-E. Lived experiences of ageing and later life in older people with intellectual disabilities. Ageing Soc. 2015;35:602–28.
27. Holland AJ. Ageing and learning disability. Br J Psychiatry. 2000;176:26–31.
28. Holland AJ, Hon J, Huppert FA, Stevens F. Incidence and course of dementia in people with Down's syndrome: findings from a population-based study. J Intellect Disabil Res. 2000;44:138–46.
29. Hughes-McCormack LA, Rydzewska E, Henderson A, MacIntyre C, Rinoul J, Cooper S-A. Prevalence and general health status of people with intellectual disabilities in Scotland: a total population study. J Epidemiol Community Health. 2018;72:78–85.
30. Emerson E, Baines S. Health inequalities and people with learning disabilities in the UK. Tizard Learn Disabil Rev. 2011;16:42–8.
31. Emerson E. Health status and health risks of the "hidden majority" of adults with intellectual disability. Intellect Dev Disabil. 2011;49:155–65.
32. Van Schrojenstein Lantman-De Valk HM, Metsemakers JF, Haveman MJ, Crebolder HF. Health problems in people with intellectual disability in general practice: a comparative study. Fam Pract. 2000;17:405–7.
33. McCarron M, Swinburne J, Burke E, McGlinchey E, Mulryan N, Andrews V, Foran S, McCallion P. Growing older with an intellectual disability in Ireland 2011: first results from the intellectual disability supplement of the irish longitudinal study on ageing. Dublin: School of Nursing & Midwifery, Trinity College Dublin; 2011a. http://nursing-midwifery.tcd.ie/assets/research/doc/ids_tilda_2011/ids_tilda_report_2011.pdf
34. Cooper SA, Smiley E, Morrison J, Williamson A, Allan L. Mental ill-health in adults with intellectual disabilities: prevalence and associated factors. Br J Psychiatry. 2007;190:27–35.
35. McCarron M, McCallion P, Reilly E, Mulryan N. A prospective 14-year longitudinal follow-up of dementia in persons with Down syndrome. J Intellect Disabil Res. 2014a;58:61–70.
36. McCarron M, McCallion P, Fahey-McCarthy E, Connaire K. The role and timing of palliative care in supporting persons with intellectual disability and advanced dementia. J Appl Res Intellect Disabil. 2011b;24(3):189–98.
37. McCallion P, Swinburne J, Burke E, McGlinchey E, McCarron M. Understanding the similarities and differences in aging with an intellectual disability: linking Irish general population and intellectual disability datasets. In: Urbano R, editor. Using secondary datasets to understand persons with developmental disabilities and their families (IRRDD-45). New York, NY: Academic Press; 2013a.
38. McCarron M, Swinburne J, Burke E, McGlinchey E, Carroll R, McCallion P. Patterns of multimorbidity in an older population of persons with an intellectual disability: results from the intellectual disability supplement to the irish longitudinal study on ageing (IDS-TILDA). Res Dev Disabil. 2013;34:521–7.
39. Anderson LL, Humphries K, McDermott S, Marks B, Sisarack J, Larson C. The state of the science of health and wellness for adults with intellectual and developmental disabilities. Intellect Dev Disabil. 2013;51:385–98.
40. Krahn GL, Fox MH. Health disparities of adults with intellectual disabilities: what do we know? What do we do. J Appl Res Intellect Disabil. 2014;27:431–46.
41. Haveman M, Heller T, Lee L, Maaskant M, Shooshtari S, Strydom A. Major health risks in aging persons with intellectual disabilities: an overview of recent studies. J Pol Pract Intellect Disabil. 2010;7:59–69.

42. Scheepers M, Kerr M, O'Hara D, Bainbridge D, Cooper S, Davis R, Wehmeyer M. Reducing health disparity in intellectual disabilities: a report from the Health Issues Special Interest Research Group of the International Association for the Scientific Study of Intellectual Disabilities. J Pol Pract Intellect Disabil. 2005;2:249–55.

43. Lightfoot E, McCallion P. Older adults and developmental disabilities. In: Berkman B, Kaplan D, editors. Handbook of social work in health & aging. 2nd ed. New York, NY: Oxford University Press; 2015.

44. Smith G, Ashbaugh J. National core indicators project: phase II consumer survey technical report. 2001. Accessed on April 15th 2018. Available at: http://www.hsri.org.

45. Haveman M, Perry J, Salvador-Carulla L, Walsh PN, Kerr M, Van Schrojenstein Lantman-de Valk H, Van Hove G, Berger DM, Azema B, Buono S, Cara AC, Germanavicius A, Linehan C, Määttä T, Tossebro J, Weber G. Ageing and health status in adults with intellectual disabilities: results of the European POMONA II study. J Intellect Dev Disabil. 2011;36:49–60.

46. Walsh PN. Health indicators and intellectual disability. Curr Opin Psychiatry. 2008;21(5):474–8.

47. McCarron M, Carroll R, McCallion P. A prospective 20-year longitudinal follow-up of dementia in persons with Down syndrome. J Intellect Disabil Res. 2017b;61(9):843–52. https://doi.org/10.1111/jir.12390.

48. Krahn GL, Fox MH. Health disparities in people with intellectual disabilities: What do we know? J Appl Res Intellect Disabil. 2014;27(5):431–46.

49. Fujiura GT, Rutkowski-Kmitta V, Owen R. Make measurable what is not so: national monitoring of the status of persons with intellectual disability. Am J Intellect Dev Disabil. 2010;35:244–58.

50. Tyler CV, Schramm SC, Karafa M, Tang AS, Jain AK. Electronic health record analysis of the primary care of adults with intellectual and other developmental disabilities. J Pol Pract Intellect Disabil. 2010;7:204–10.

51. O'Dwyer M, Pekler J, McCallion P, McCarron M, Henman M. Factors associated with polypharmacy and excessive polypharmacy in older people with Intellectual Disability differ from the general population; a cross-sectional observational nationwide study. BMJ Open. 2016;6:e010505. https://doi.org/10.1136/bmjopen-2015-010505.

52. Raghavan R, Pater P. Ethical issues of psychotropic medication for people with intellectual disabilities. Adv Ment Health Intellect Disabil. 2010;4(3):34–8.

53. MacGiolla Phadraig C, McCarron M, Burke E, Cleary E, McGlinchey E, McCallion P, Nunn J. Total tooth loss and complete denture use in older adults with intellectual disabilities in Ireland. J Public Health Dent. 2015;75:101–8.

54. Mann J, Zhou H, McDermott S, Poston MB. Healthy behavior change of adults with mental retardation: attendance in a health promotion program. Am J Ment Retard. 2006;111:62–73.

55. Jokinen N, Janicki MP, Keller S, McCallion P, Force LT. Guidelines for structuring community care and supports for people with intellectual disabilities affected by dementia. J Pol Pract Intellect Disabil. 2013;10:1–24.

56. McCarron M, Haigh M, McCallion P. Health, Wellbeing and Social Inclusion: Ageing with an Intellectual Disability in Ireland. Wave 3 IDS-TILDA. Dublin: School of Nursing & Midwifery, Trinity College Dublin; 2017. https://www.tcd.ie/tcaid/assets/pdf/wave3report.pdf

57. Coppus AM, Schuur M, Vergeer J, Janssens AC, Oostra BA, Verbeek MM, van Duijn CM. Plasma β amyloid and the risk of Alzheimer's disease in Down syndrome. Neurobiol Aging. 2012;33:1988–94.

58. Burke E, McCallion P, Carroll R, Walsh JB, McCarron M. An exploration of the bone health of older adults with an intellectual disability in Ireland. J Intellect Disabil Res. 2017;61:99–114.

59. Strax TE, Luciano L, Dunn AM, Quevedo JP. Aging and developmental disabilities. Phys Med Rehabil Clin N Am. 2010;21:419–27.

60. Tyrrell J, Dodd P. Psychopathology in older age. In: Davidson PW, Prasher VP, Janicki MP, editors. Mental health, intellectual disabilities and the aging process. Oxford: Blackwell Publishing; 2003. p. 22–37.

61. Jacobson J. Prevalence of mental and behavioural disorders. In: Davidson PW, Prasher VP, Janicki MP, editors. Mental health, intellectual disabilities and the aging process. Oxford: Blackwell Publishing; 2003. p. 9–21.

62. Dodd P, Guerin S, McEvoy J, Buckley S, Tyrrell J, Hillery J. A study of complicated grief symptoms in people with intellectual disabilities. J Intellect Disabil Res. 2008;52:415–25.
63. McCallion P, Burke E, Swinburne J, McGlinchey E, Carrol R, McCarron M. Influence of environment, predisposing, enabling and need variables on personal health choices of adults with intellectual disability. Health. 2013;5:749–56.
64. McCarron M, O'Dwyer M, Burke E, McGlinchey E, McCallion P. Epidemiology of epilepsy in older adults with an intellectual disability in Ireland: associations and service implications. Am J Intellect Dev Disabil. 2014c;119:253–60.
65. Evenhuis HM, Hermans H, Hilgenkamp TI, Bastiaanse LP, Echteld MA. Frailty and disability in older adults with intellectual disabilities: results from the healthy ageing and intellectual disability study. J Am Geriatr Soc. 2012;60:934–8.
66. Schoufour J, Mitnitski A, Rockwood K, Evenhuis HM, Eckteld M. Development of a frailty index for older people with intellectual disabilities: results from the HA-ID study. Res Dev Disabil. 2013;34:1541–55.
67. Hilgencamp TI, van Wijck R, Evenhuis HM. Low physical fitness levels in older adults with ID: results of the HA-ID study. Res Dev Disabil. 2012;33:1048–58.
68. Taggart L, Coates V, Truesdale-Kennedy M. Management and quality indicators of diabetes mellitus in people with intellectual disability. J Intellect Disabil Res. 2013;57:1152–63.
69. McCallion P, Jokinen N, Janicki MP. Aging. In: Wehmeyer ML, Brown I, Percey M, Shogren KA, Fung M, editors. A Comprehensive Guide to Intellectual and Developmental Disabilities. Baltimore, MD: Paul Brookes Press; 2017b.
70. Lennox N, Bain C, Rey-Conde T. Effects of a comprehensive health assessment programme for Australian adults with intellectual disability: a cluster randomized trial. Int J Epidemiol. 2007;36:139–46.
71. McGuire BE, Daly P, Smyth F. Lifestyle and health behaviours of adults with an intellectual disability. J Intellect Disabil Res. 2007;51:497–510.
72. Ewing G, McDermott S, Thomas-Koger M, Whitner W, Pierce K. Evaluation of a cardiovascular health program for participants with mental retardation and normal learners. Health Educ Behav. 2004;31:77–87.
73. Humphries K, Traci MA, Pepper AC, Seekins T. Nutrition education and support program for community-dwelling adults with intellectual disabilities. Intellect Dev Disabil. 2008;46:335–45.
74. Temple VA, Walkley JW. Physical activity of adults with intellectual disability. J Intellect Dev Disabil. 2003;28:323–34.
75. Evenhuis HM, Theunissen M, Denkers I, Verschuure H, Kemme H. Prevalence of visual and hearing impairment in a Dutch institutionalized population with ID. Journal of Intellectual Disability. Research. 2001;45:457–64.
76. McCallion P, Hogan M, Santos FH, McCarron M, Service K, Stemp S, Keller S, Fortea J, Bishop K, Watchman K, Janicki MP. Consensus Statement of the International Summit on Intellectual Disability and Dementia related to end-of-life care in advanced dementia. J Appl Res Intellect Disabil. 2017a;30(6):1160–4.
77. Samele C, Seymour L, Morrid B, Central England People First, Cohen A, Ericson E. A formal investigation into health inequalities experienced by people with learning difficulties and people with mental health problems. London: Sainsbury Centre for Mental Health; 2006.
78. MacGiolla Phadraig C, Nunn J, McCarron M, McCallion P. Why do edentulous adults with intellectual disabilities not wear dentures? Wave 2 of the IDS TILDA cohort study. J Prosthodont Res. 2017;61:61–6.
79. Robertson J, Roberts H, Emerson E, Turner S, Greig R. The impact of health checks for people with intellectual disabilities: a systematic review of evidence. J Intellect Disabil Res. 2011;55:1009–19.
80. Prasher VP. End-stage dementia in adults with Down syndrome. Int J Geriatr Psychiatry. 1995;10:1067–9.
81. Cooper SA. Epidemiology of psychiatric disorders in elderly compared to younger adults with learning disabilities. Br J Psychiatry. 1997;170:375–80.

82. McCarron M, Carroll R, Kelly C, McCallion P. To understand differing patterns of age of death by gender and level of ID, for people with ID in Ireland. J Appl Res Intellect Disabil. 2014b;27:314.
83. McCarron M, Griffiths C. Nurses roles in supporting aging persons with intellectual disability and mental health problems: challenges and opportunities for care. In: Davidson P, Prasher V, Janicki MP, editors. Mental health, intellectual disabilities and the aging process. London: Blackwell; 2003. p. 223–37.
84. Ad Hoc IASSID Working Group on Demographic Studies Data Standardization. Need for demographic data standardization: report of the Ad Hoc IASSID Working Group on Aging-Related Demographic Studies Data Standardization. J Pol Pract Intellect Disabil. 2005;2:57–9. https://doi.org/10.1111/j.1741-1130.2005.00008.x.
85. Perry J, Felce D. Factors associated with outcome in community group homes. Am J Ment Retard. 2005;110:121–35.
86. Foran S, McCarron M, McCallion P. Expanding assessment of Fear of Falling among older adults with an intellectual disability: a pilot study to assess the value of proxy responses. ISRN Geriatr. 2013;2013:493042. https://doi.org/10.1155/2013/493042.

Overview of the Important Physical Health Concerns

3

Éilish Burke, Márie O'Dwyer, Eimear McGlinchey,
Sinéad Foran, Caoimhin MacGiolla Phadraig,
Rachael Carroll, Philip McCallion, and Mary McCarron

3.1 Introduction

As we celebrate the longer life expectancy of people with intellectual disability, prospects around better health outcomes are expected. However poor health continues to be reported for people with an intellectual disability who have higher levels of chronic conditions multi-morbidity and greater complexity identified in health needs

É. Burke (✉)
School of Nursing and Midwifery and Trinity Centre of Ageing and Intellectual Disability,
Trinity College, The University of Dublin, Dublin, Ireland
e-mail: eburke7@tcd.ie

M. O'Dwyer
School of Pharmacy and Pharmaceutical Science, Trinity College, The University of Dublin,
Dublin, Ireland

E. McGlinchey
Global Brain Health Institute and Trinity Centre for Ageing and Intellectual Disability,
Trinity College, The University of Dublin, Dublin, Ireland

S. Foran
Health Sciences Nursing and Health Care, School of Nursing and Health Care, Waterford
Institute of Technology, Waterford, Ireland

C. M. Phadraig
Special Care Dentistry, School of Dental Science, Trinity College, The University of Dublin,
Dublin, Ireland

R. Carroll
School of Nursing and Midwifery, and The Trinity Centre for Ageing and Intellectual
Disability, Trinity College, The University of Dublin, Dublin, Ireland

P. McCallion
School of Social Work, College of Public Health, Temple University, Philadelphia, PA, USA

M. McCarron
Faculty of Health Sciences and The Trinity Centre for Ageing and Intellectual Disability,
Trinity College, The University of Dublin, Dublin, Ireland

© Springer Nature Switzerland AG 2019
V. P. Prasher, M. P. Janicki (eds.), *Physical Health of Adults with Intellectual and
Developmental Disabilities*, https://doi.org/10.1007/978-3-319-90083-4_3

and earlier mortality as compared to their peers without identified life-long disabili-ties [1–5]. Among the conditions and contributing factors to the disparities are, obe-sity, metabolic risk factors and poor cardiovascular health, osteoporosis, falls and fractures, gastrointestinal conditions such as reflux and constipation, sensory impair-ment (especially eye disease), oral health, increased dementia prevalence and notable levels of polypharmacy. This chapter gives an overview of these commonly reported health conditions and identifies the continuing health disparities that exists for people with intellectual disability with suggestions for prevention and support.

3.2 People with Intellectual Disability and Self-perception of Health

The World Health Organization (WHO) suggests that how people approach and experience their later years is very much influenced by how they perceive their own ageing and notes that these perceptions are a major determinant of ageing in good health [6]. All dimensions of health and well-being from physical, psychological and social factors, are considered when a person rates their own perception of health; yet there is substantial evidence of a relationship between current self-perception of health and future health and well-being [7]. Burke and colleagues demonstrated that whilst people with intellectual disability identify aging with decline and, despite high levels of chronic conditions, they rated their overall health as good, had a positive appraisal of aging, and overall demonstrated their readiness to embrace an active long life [8, 9]. The Intellectual Disability Supplement to The Irish Longitudinal Study on Ageing (IDS-TILDA) continues to report the positive ratings people have of their own health, especially those in older age. Most recently, 46% of those aged 65 years and over rated their health as very good to excellent [1]. These findings are consistent with those of Gibbons et al. [10] who reported that generally participants in their study perceived themselves in good health. Notwithstanding the high prevalence of chronic health conditions identified among people with intellectual disability, such positive assessment of their own health bodes well for promoting active involvement in positive aging.

3.3 Sensory Impairment

Eye disease is one of the most common conditions identified among those with intellectual disability [5, 11] and is more prevalent than that found in the general population. Evenhuis et al. [11] reported the prevalence of both eye and hearing impairment at greater levels than the general population, also confirmed by Burke et al. [1]. Increases in prevalence of eye disease are associated with particular phe-notypes especially Down syndrome [12]. In their study, conditions such as cata-racts, blepharitis and conjunctivitis, and inflammatory conditions of the eye, were found to be the most common conditions. Similarly, auditory impairment is more prevalent in people with Down syndrome and at a younger age due to structural anomalies, such as a narrow ear canal [13]. See Chaps. 7 and 8.

McCarron et al. [5] reported a prevalence of over 70% of those over the age of 40 years being multi-morbid, defined as the presence of two or more chronic health conditions. Notable in this study was that eye disease was the most common co-occurring chronic condition noted. The high prevalence of sensory impairment highlights the need for regular sensory screening [14] reports that many cases of vision problems, such as poor distance vision, were treatable by glasses, but few people with intellectual disability had such prescriptions. McCarron et al. [3, 15] have persistently identified low uptake of sensory screening, for example almost 40% of participants had not had a hearing test in more than 3 years.

Visual and auditory impairment is challenging to detect, however, with planned ophthalmological and auditory care impairment can be detected and treated and these debilitating conditions ameliorated [14]. The International Association for the Scientific Study of Intellectual disability [16] has published guidelines recommending specialist screening for age-related visual and hearing impairment among people with intellectual disability, which should commence at the age of 45 years and earlier at age 30 years for those with Down syndrome.

3.4   Obesity, Waist Circumference, and the Weight Paradox

Overweight and obesity is commonly measured by Body Mass Index (BMI) which is calculated using height and weight producing a figure in kilograms per meter squared (kg/m^2). A range from 25 to 29.9 kg/m^2 indicates an individual is overweight, and a BMI greater than 30 kg/m^2 indicates a state of obesity. Increased weight presents the most prominent contemporary global health care challenge [17] with obesity, a modifiable health condition, being the fifth principal cause of death globally [18]. Obesity contributes to increased prevalence of chronic disease and increased healthcare costs [19]. Of particular concern is that obesity is reported as being more pervasive among adults with intellectual disability [20], with research consistently reporting higher rates especially among females and those adults with Down syndrome [21]. Similarly, Burke et al. [1] reported higher rates of obesity among women, with overall prevalence higher than that identified among the general population, a finding replicated in many countries [1, 22, 23].

Obesity in people with intellectual disability may contribute to increased dependency in activities of daily living, and reduce community participation and, may be a major determinant of chronic ill health with increasing age [24]. This will lead to increasing risk for secondary health conditions, lifelong chronic ill health and impaired quality of life. Additionally people with intellectual disability can present with non-modifiable factors such as medication use, mobility limitation or particular phenotype that will further increase the chronic health risks. Additionally, disparity in relation to access to appropriate health promotion, barriers to physical activity, sedentary lifestyles, poor motivation or dependency on caregivers, may further influence weight management, increasing the individual's susceptibility to obesity and subsequently, risk of poor health.

Table 3.1 World Health Organization indicators and cut-off points (WHO, 2011) [29]

Indicator	Cut-off points		Risk of metabolic complications
	Male	Female	
Waist circumference	>94 cm	>80 cm	Increased
Waist circumference	>102 cm	>88 cm	Substantially increased

It is claimed that one of the single most influential factors in tackling the weight problem among people with intellectual disability would be increasing levels of moderate or vigorous physical activity [25]. However, for example, there are reports from Ireland that a sedentary lifestyle or inactivity exists for almost three quarters of the older population of adults with intellectual disability [1, 3]. Weight management is complex and physical activity alone will not tackle this growing problem. An overall approach to healthy lifestyle behaviour is necessary. The pervasive nature of obesity among adults with intellectual disability is also influenced by medication used for secondary conditions and choice and control issues [17, 26]. There is a paucity of evidence on lifestyle behavioural programmes that have proven successful in weight reduction for people with intellectual disaiblity, and it is an area that warrants further investigation [27].

Waist circumference, an indicator of the visceral fat that exist within the abdomen and surrounding vital organs, or central obesity is now considered a more accurate measure of overall body fat and is commonly utilized as an indicator of risk for cardiovascular events [28]. The World Health Organization have presented cut-off points for waist measurement which are sex specific, and the greater the circumference the higher the risk for metabolic complications that exist (see Table 3.1).

In the general population there is a direct correlation between central obesity and cardiovascular conditions, such as hypertension [1, 30], With respect to adults with intellectual disability, Burke and colleagues [1], using objective measurement of waist circumference, found that most adults (91.7%) were at substantial risk of metabolic complications, with females at greater risk than males. Burke et al. [1] further compared these findings with those of the general population and noted that fewer adults with intellectual disability were within the normal waist circumference ranges (11.6% versus 21% respectively)—with the vast majority (74.9%) indicating substantially increased risk compared to the general population (54.0%). Education of caregivers, healthcare professionals, and the adults themselves should be undertaken to address these rates of overweight and obesity. More support will mean that the inevitable chronic ill health and negative social consequences of obesity can be prevented and avoided.

Lynch et al. [31] noted that those adults who perceive themselves the correct weight are more likely to maintain a healthy weight. Being told by your physician that you are overweight or obese is associated with the adult forming a more realistic self-perception of weight and an increased likelihood of the desire to lose weight [32]. Healthcare professionals are uniquely positioned to support individuals with weight management; however, they often fail to do so. Healthcare professionals need to diagnose obesity, educate support workers and individuals with intellectual disability of weight status and promote weight management programmes. As life expectancy increases for people with intellectual disability, as well as opportunities to choose one's own lifestyle, the impact of poor choices affecting health will become more observable. If left unchecked, obesity related conditions will emerge with significant implications on quality life years lived, healthcare costs, and overall quality of life for people with intellectual disability as they age. Even a modest weight loss can mitigate against the occurrence of cardiovascular diseases, neuro-cognitive decline, and other serious complications.

3.5   Musculoskeletal Health, Osteoporosis and Osteopenia

The World Health Organization has identified musculoskeletal conditions as a leading contributor to years lived with disability worldwide, with 10% of the world's population over the age of 60 years having significant clinical problems that can be attributed to osteoarthritis [33]. As noted by the WHO Director General:

> "Perhaps the most fundamental difficulty in regard to rheumatic diseases is that the problem is insufficiently appreciated and understood. Critical to this lack of appreciation is an information deficit." ([33]: p. 2).

Osteoporosis is one of the most prevalent musculoskeletal conditions and is directly associated with ageing [34]. The WHO definition is based on bone mineral density (BMD) measured by dual-emission X-ray absorptiometry scanning (DXA) which results in a t-score. There are three categories, normal BMD (T-score of -0.999 and above); osteopenia (t-score of -1.0 to -2.499); osteoporosis (T-score $\leq$ -2.5) [35]. This low bone mass results in micro-architectural deterioration with a resulting increased susceptibility to fracture due to the increase in bone fragility. These fractures are most common on the vertebral body, the proximal femur and distal forearm. They are mainly associated with and commonly occur in postmenopausal women and older aged adults; this type of osteoporosis is known as primary osteoporosis and is directly associated with advancing age [36].

However, having BMD central to an operational definition poses problems because although there is a well-established relationship between fracture risk and low t-score, the problem that arises is that the risk is a continuous one and if the cut off of -2.5 is only considered, those with a t-score greater than this are left untreated and it is known that many fractures occur among the cohort with greater t-scores [37]. Therefore, defining osteoporosis and osteopenia cannot be dependent on BMD alone; a holistic approach must be adopted and include the multitude of risk factors that contribute to the disorder. Several studies report a varied prevalence of osteoporosis among individuals with intellectual disability. One factor is that when intellectual disability present, there is difficulty conducting DXA screening due to access issues, anxiety, non-compliance or mobility issues, therefore measurement of risk is compromised. Lin et al. [38] reported a prevalence of 26.1% among a cohort of institutionalized residents with intellectual disability in Taiwan, whereas

Schmidt et al. [39] and Leslie et al. [40] reported prevalence of osteoporosis at 67.6% and 78.5%, respectively. In Ireland, McCarron et al. [41] reported a prevalence of doctor's diagnosed osteoporosis at 8%, then at 16% 3 years later [3], and at 21% three more years later of the same persons [1]. However, this differed considerably from the objectively measured rates of 41% for osteoporosis and 33% for osteopenia found in the study's objective health assessments [8, 9]. Both these data elements indicate that there is an alarmingly high percentage of people with intellectual disability with compromised bone integrity, placing them at risk of fracture.

Apart from net bone loss, non-modifiable and modifiable risk factors contribute to the development of osteoporosis and osteopenia. Non-modifiable risks include female sex, increased age, family history of osteoporosis, being Caucasian and a history of prior fracture. Late menarche, early menopause, and low endogenous estrogen levels are also associated with low bone mineral density [33, 37]. The modifiable risks include sedentary lifestyle, smoking, poor dietary habits, lack of exposure to sunlight, and estrogen deficiency. Certain medications are also indicated as risk factors; for example, anticonvulsants and glucocorticoids [42].

People with intellectual disability have an increased loading of risks that predispose them to developing osteopenia and osteoporosis [43]. These increased risks are reported to be outside the common accepted risk factors, such as smoking, increased alcohol consumption, parental history, and specific corticosteroid use—as seen for the general population. For people with intellectual disability, areas such as polypharmacy and poorer lifestyle choices put this population at increased risk of suboptimal bone health. In addition, people with intellectual disability face additional challenges in maintaining their own health and accessing healthcare screenings.

Good musculoskeletal health means that joint's, muscle and bone work well without pain. Those with good musculoskeletal health can carry out activities with ease and without pain, but most importantly good musculoskeletal health means that a person can live quite independently. As the population of people with intellectual disability ages, it is becoming more important for people to invest in musculoskeletal health so they can maintain stability, strength, co-ordination, avoid falls and be pain free, as they age. People increasingly want to live active later lives and, with many health policies placing the onus on the individual to maintain their own health, optimizing bone health is a goal which requires a multifactorial approach to provide needed support and education.

3.6   Oral Health Amongst Adults with Intellectual Disability

Oral health is of considerable concern in adults with intellectual disability; particularly as they grow older. The impact of aging includes normal structural change and processes, such as tooth wear and gingival recession and often irreversible impact of diseases, mainly dental caries, periodontal disease and traumatic injury across the life-course (See Table 3.2) [44]. See Chap. 11.

Table 3.2 Summary of common physiological and pathological processes affecting the oral cavity and surrounding structures with increasing age

Tissue	Common aging physiological processes relating to oral health	Common aging pathological processes relating to oral health
Neuromuscular	Reduction in muscle mass, fibres and tone and declining neural function due to reduction in neurons and changes to neurotransmitter function lead to reduced masticatory forces	Impaired chewing, especially with accumulative tooth loss.
Joint	Remodelling of the articular surfaces and disc following tooth loss.	Anterior disc displacement; Osteoarthritis
Mucosa	Thinning squamous epithelium, with loss of elasticity and atrophy, diminution of taste and smell	Increasing risk of infection such as candidiasis; increasing frequency of oral cancer and precancerous lesions
Gingivae and periodontium	Gingival recession	Increasing prevalence and severity of periodontal disease.
Pulp	Loss of vascularity and reduced nerve supply	Accumulative impact of pulpal infection and its treatment.
Salivary gland	Reduced salivary flow due to medications or a sensation of dry mouth (xerostomia).	Reduced salivary flow secondary to radiotherapy or medical conditions such as Sjogreen's disease and Diabetes Mellitus. Dry mouth related caries, dysphagia, mucositis, candidiasis, dysarthria, halitosis and difficulty wearing denture
Teeth	Tissue surface loss due to abrasion, abfraction, erosion and attrition. Thickening of dentine due to dentinal sclerosis and secondary dentine deposition +/− thinning of enamel	Root surface caries; Accumulative impact of dental caries and its treatment; Dental trauma leading to fracture amongst other dentoalveolar injuries.
Bone	Atrophy of alveolar bone mainly due to tooth loss.	Osteoporosis

Systemic cell types and tissues, such as immune cells are omitted from the above diagram, though changes to these and their cytokines (immune senescence) and other local tissues such as cementum have obvious impact on the oral environment in aging

Over the life course of an individual with intellectual disability, the changes summarized in Table 3.2 challenge the maintenance of oral health, which has significance for the ability to speak, smile, smell, taste, touch, chew, swallow and convey a range of emotions through facial expressions with confidence and without pain, discomfort and disease of the craniofacial complex [45]. The conceptual complexity of oral health is matched by the difficulties in agreeing what this phenomenon actually looks like. While it is impossible to set a cut off for what constitutes a healthy mouth or "functional" dentition, much research suggests that we need the front 20 teeth, or thereabouts, present, disease free and fairly intact for aesthetics, chewing and biting, that is comfortable and socially acceptable [46]. The aim of modern oral healthcare then, is to maintain 20 healthy front teeth throughout life, comfortably and happily.

For people with intellectual disability, good oral health can be difficult to achieve. Firstly, oral disease is often more common and has poorer outcomes for people with intellectual disability. Dental caries, which often occurs at similar rates to the general population, tend to be untreated or treated by extraction rather than conservative options like fillings or root canal treatments. Research suggests that periodontal disease can be up to nine times more prevalent among middle-aged adults with intellectual disability, compared to the general population [47, 48]. As such, periodontitis is an even greater contributor to tooth loss for adults with intellectual disability than caries [49]. Combined, as compared to the general population, the increased prevalence and unfavorable management of these diseases lead to greater levels of and ultimately, complete tooth loss (edentulism) in adults with intellectual disability. In Ireland, for example, older adults are over twice as likely to be edentulous, the oral equivalent to mortality, if they have intellectual disability [50]. Figure 3.1 demonstrates the frequent finding of tooth loss and untreated edentulism in a national population [15].

Secondly, the impact of oral disease is magnified for people with intellectual disability because of the interrelation of oral and general health. For example, poor oral hygiene and periodontitis are associated with increased risk of pneumonia, cardiovascular disease, and diabetes [51, 52] and oral Streptococcus Viridans are associated with infection of the heart and heart valves [53]. Dental pain can also go

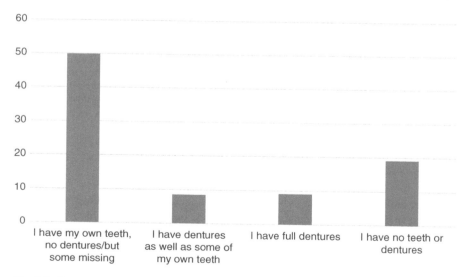

Fig. 3.1 Dentate status of older adults with ID in Ireland in 2017. Note: Data from the IDS-TILDA Study Report retrieved from https://www.tcd.ie/tcaid/assets/pdf/wave3report.pdf

undiagnosed and present as behaviors may be problematic [54, 55]. Treatment by the dental team can often necessitate restrictive supports such as anesthesia, sedation or clinical holding, which do make the treatment of oral disease possible, but also add complexity, waiting times, and increase severity of treatment [56]. For adults with intellectual disability, especially as they age, the above is often compounded by multi-morbidity, polypharmacy, high dependency, and probable frailty [5, 57, 58].

Total tooth loss is associated with poorer nutritional health, dementia, some cancers, and even death [59–61]. For people with intellectual disability, edentulism is a common phenomenon, which is seldom treated using dentures or implants, reducing ability to chew most foods, and probably contributing to chronic constipation. Greater emphasis needs to be placed upon the importance of maintaining the natural dentition in populations with intellectual disability for as long as possible [62]. Table 3.3 highlights this potential impact.

The accumulative and irreversible nature of oral diseases means that lifelong measures to promote oral health are needed. The responsibility to achieve this outcome lies as much on the shoulders of policy makers and dentists as it does on the individual and often his or her family and caregivers. The multifactorial nature of oral disease places an onus on family and healthcare professionals, as much as on policy makers and practitioners, to facilitate healthful behaviors. From birth, health and social policies are needed to ensure that oral health is prioritized as an integral component of general health. In this way families can be empowered, for example through education in oral care and nutrition, or, by having access to appropriate supports. These supports can only flourish in an environment where oral health is simply as important as any other form of health. People with intellectual disability can achieve oral health through increased awareness, skills and motivation to remove plaque and maintain a healthy diet and, by visiting dental services according to their individual risk of oral disease.

Given the above, it may be surprising to note that people with intellectual disability are actually very "good attenders" at dental services across the world, often attending dentists far more often than the general population. Owens and colleagues

Table 3.3 Potential Impact of oral diseases on the health and well-being of adults with intellectual disability

Oral disease	Increased risk
Poor oral hygiene and periodontal disease	Pneumonia Cardiovascular disease
Dental caries	Pulpal pain Odontogenic infection, facial swelling and cellulitis
Tooth loss and Edentulism	Difficulty eating Constipation Aesthetic insufficiency Oral disability
Anxiety, discomfort and pain	Challenging behaviour Avoidance of necessary care Need for restrictive supports

highlight that oral healthcare services are perhaps inappropriate rather than inaccessible for many with intellectual disability [63]. This means that there is a need for access, but only if oral healthcare services are structured, staffed, and financed to promote risk assessment, prevention, and conservative treatment of the main oral diseases in a way that meets the needs people with intellectual disability.

The oral health of adults with intellectual disability is poorer than that of the general population. This leads to "oral disability" for adults with intellectual disability. There is a need for a paradigm shift politically, socially, and personally at home and at the dentist office to achieve better oral health for subsequent generations of adults with intellectual disability.

3.7   Gastrointestinal Conditions and Adults with Intellectual Disability

Frequently, many health conditions go unrecognized and unmet in people with intellectual disability [64] adding to concerns about multi-morbidity rates [2, 5]. Multi-morbidity is complex yet many healthcare pathways are focused on the management of single diseases. Gastrointestinal (GI) problems are among the most prevalent conditions that often go undiagnosed [65]. It is known that gastrointestinal diseases are one of the greatest contributors of ill health and a contributor to death among people with intellectual disability [66]. The rates are 2.5 times greater in people with intellectual disability as compared with the general population. Kuhlmann et al. [65] also found that 25% of these deaths among people with intellectual disability were due to bowel obstructions, and 13% to perforated ulcers. Complicating the issue is that for those adults with severe to profound intellectual disability, communication difficulties or difficulties expressing their own health needs, adds to the likelihood that their health problems go undiagnosed and subsequently untreated, thus reducing life expectancy [64, 67].

Helicobacter pylori infections are also highly prevalent among people with intellectual disability, with reported prevalence rates between 22% and 84%, especially for those living longer than 4 years in an institutional setting [68]. What is concerning about these high rates is that Helicobacter pylori is a contributing factor in conditions such as peptic ulceration and gastrointestinal cancers. In a study in the UK, Duff and colleagues identified that 48% of deaths were as a result of stomach cancers, something not previously reported [69].

Gastroesophageal reflux disease (GERD) is another condition of the GI that frequently goes untreated and overlooked among people with intellectual disability. GERD can lead to esophagitis, gastritis, and intestinal perforation and is a major clinical problem, especially for those adults with severe to profound levels of intellectual disability. Other contributing risks include medication use, particularly anti-epileptic medicines and, the presence of cerebral palsy [70]. Clinical manifestations include hematemesis, anemia, rumination and regurgitation, with some studies associating aspirate pneumonia [71] with GERD.

At minimum, gastric reflux causes abdominal and esophageal discomfort and irritability [70]. However, some individuals with intellectual disability may have aberrant nociceptive processing whereby their ability to interpret and distinguish pain is impaired and may require an exaggerated painful response to engage descending anti-nociceptive signals, meaning a cycle of self-injurious behavior may be initiated. One condition that causes severe visceral pain is GERD. Visceral structures are highly sensitive to inflammation and distention contributing to the severe pain associated with GERD; individuals affected by this pain may engage in self-injurious behavior in order to suppress their pain [72]. Greater surveillance, physical activity and positioning especially for those with compromised mobility and posture, as well as pharmacological treatment, needs to be considered when devising care plans for those at risk.

Constipation, another highly prevalent GI chronic condition, is one of the most difficult to define. Generally speaking constipation is a highly prevalent gastrointestinal motility disorder classified by infrequent bowel movements, the passage of hard stool, and difficulty passing stool. It is highly symptomatic and individual to each person [73, 74]. Böhmer et al. [75] noted a prevalence of 69% among people with intellectual disability. Similarly, McCarron and colleagues have seen a considerable rise in diagnosed prevalence over the 10 years of their study, from 16.3% in the first wave (2011) to 43.5% in the third wave [15].

Risk factors for constipation are multifactorial and include gastrointestinal problems, neurological disease, cancer, polypharmacy, mobility challenges, and level of intellectual disability, older age, female sex, cerebral palsy, Down syndrome, and level of physical activity regardless of functional status. Gastrointestinal conditions as a direct cause of constipation or a symptom of constipation are common and may often be dismissed as minor; however constipation can cause considerable distress and anxiety [75]. Kinnear et al. [2] identify constipation as the fourth highest occurring chronic condition among people with intellectual disability especially females; yet it is one of the most treatable co-morbidities. People living in institutional settings are also more likely to present with constipation [76]. In a study by McDermott [77] people with intellectual disability were 2.7 times more likely to suffer from constipation and individuals presenting with concomitant mental health conditions similarly were over twice as likely to suffer. The anticholinergic burden associated with the medication treatment of these conditions is a major contributing factor in these cases [57, 58].

Constipation is often treatable through non-pharmacological means. The inclusion of adequate dietary fiber and fluid intake is essential; however, since nutritional imbalance leading to constipation is highly prevalent among people with intellectual disability [78] what is prominently identified as the treatment of constipation is the continuous and permanent use of laxatives. For example, Evenhuis [79] reported a 58% permanent use of laxatives, with McCarron et al. [15, 80] reporting that 40% of their cohort were taking laxatives (with 42% taking two or more agents). Diet and lifestyle changes should be the treatment of choice for this debilitating and life threatening condition. Constipation is reversible. Fiber, fluids and physical activity are required as part of the overall management programme for constipation, however people with intellectual disability require support to achieve this goal.

3.8 Falls in Adults with Intellectual Disability

A serious fall can be the beginning of a path to dependence and poorer quality of life. Across the world, falls are considered to be on the most significant health issues facing adults as they age and are often described as one of the 'geriatric giants' of ageing. Falls in adults with intellectual disability are very often the result of the physiological changes that occur as a direct result of getting older. Loss of lean muscle mass, changes in gait pattern, balance impairment, sensory, neuromuscular changes, and increasing co-morbidities all influence falling. The consequences of a fall can be profound; resulting in significantly reduced quality of life due to increased injury, increased hospitalization, reduced mobility, prolonged recovery time, and in some cases, even death [81–83]. This issue is even more serious for adults with intellectual disability who experience higher rates of falls and falls related injuries than those in the general population.

It is well-established that one in three older adults in the general population will experience a fall each year [84, 85], with increasing age considered the most significant risk factor to increase the likelihood of a fall. Studies have shown that 28–35% of community dwelling adults over 64 years of age fall each year. This increases to 32–42% of adults over 70 years of age, rising to 58% in adults aged between 91 and 105 years of age [86, 87]. McCarron et al. [15] reported a prevalence of falls at 27.2% among those adults in an Irish population (Table 3.4).

Other studies, such as Cox et al. [88] and Hsieh et al. [89] have recorded somewhat similar prevalence data, 30% and 24.6% respectively; again, their data is derived from younger study cohorts meaning younger individuals with intellectual disability may have a similar prevalence rate for falls as a much older cohort in the general population. Furthermore, the risk for falls related injuries may also be higher with over 12% experiencing a serious falls-related injury [90] compared with 5% in the general population [91].

The resulting economic burden to health services is well documented by Gannon et al. [92], Hartholt et al. [93] and Burns et al. [94], as well as the personal consequences to the individual including hospitalization, further disability, and loss of confidence in performing everyday activities.

Table 3.4 Prevalence of falls in the Intellectual Disability Supplement to the Irish Longitudinal Study on Ageing from Wave 1 (2011) to Wave 3 (2017) [15, 41]

	IDS TILDA wave 1	IDS-TILDA wave 3
N	753	608
Any fall (%)	26.7	27.2
Recurrent fall (%)	14.6	15.9
Injurious fall (%)	13.2	12.5

What is most concerning among this population is the occurrence of recurrent falls. Recurrent falls are generally defined as two or more falls in the previous 12 months and can present with a different set of risk factors [95]. One off or single falls are more likely to be due to environmental causes, whereas recurrent fallers are more likely to present with co-morbid, chronic conditions. Recurrent falls are very high among people with intellectual disability, with the IDS TILDA study reporting a 15.9% prevalence rate [15] (see Table 3.4). This figure is much greater when compared to older adults in the general population; practitioners should be surveillant and identify those at risk of falling multiple times.

Todd and Skelton [96] classify risk factors for falls as either intrinsic (factors related to the individual) or extrinsic (factors external to the individual), however, a fall may occur as a result of an interaction between both intrinsic and extrinsic factors, increasing risk of falling and falls related injuries. Extrinsic factors generally refer to environmental hazards, such as floor surfaces, lighting, use of steps and stairs in the everyday living environment, and the inappropriate use of equipment for the assistance with activities of daily living (ADLs). The intrinsic risk factors vary among people with intellectual disability and tend to be slightly different than those observed in the general population. Additionally, many of these factors are present over the lifespan of the individual. A comparison between the intrinsic factors in the general population and people with intellectual disability that may increase the risk for falling can be found in Table 3.5.

Many people with intellectual disability rely on others to recall and record their fall. This is important because poor recollection of the fall can lead to under-reporting and inadequate recognition of those individuals who may be at increased risk of falling. There is currently no specific falls risk assessment tool validated for use in

Table 3.5 Comparison of intrinsic risk factors for falls between adults in the general population and adults with intellectual disability

Intrinsic factors present in the general population	Intrinsic factors present in people with intellectual/developmental disabilities
Previous falls history	Previous falls history
Age	Living circumstances
Sex	Disorders of gait and balance
Living circumstances	History of fracture
Disorders of gait and balance	Physical inactivity
Physical inactivity	Presence of seizure disorder
History of fracture	Difficulty performing ADLs
Sarcopenia	Vision impairment
Vision impairment/disease	Fear of falling
Urinary incontinence	Use of AEDs
Cerebrovascular disease	Excessive Polypharmacy (10 or more medications)
Dementia	
Fear of falling	
Medication use	
Polypharmacy	

an older population of people with intellectual disability (see [97], for instrumentation applicable to adults), therefore, the presence and application of a falls policy in clinical practice is essential for the safe monitoring and management of falls.

In keeping with best practice guidelines, people with intellectual disability should be asked/reviewed for any fall in the previous 12 months when they present for routine health assessments by health/social care practitioners [98]. Individuals who have fallen in the previous year should be asked about the frequency and circumstances of falls. Any falls assessment must be multifactorial in nature, taking into account the many risk factors that may contribute to the likelihood of falling. Clinical practitioners must be familiar with the local pathways for referral if there is concern regarding the type and nature of the falls.

Frontline practitioners must realize that falls intervention is integral to their roles and responsibilities. Van Hanegem et al. [99] established a statistically significant reduction in falls in a group of 39 people with intellectual disability following a 10-week exercise programme focusing on balance and gait abilities. Likewise, Crockett et al. [100], also found a reduction in falls and improvements in balance and mobility over an 18 month period in a group of 50 adults with intellectual disability, following a specifically tailored exercise programme. Interventions aimed at reducing falls should therefore focus on physical activity levels as well as physical health, medication use, and history of falling. Any physical activity programme must include elements of strength and balance training. With timely assessment of risk, application of a falls policy and appropriately designed falls intervention programmes, the risk of falls can be significantly reduced in this population.

3.9 Dementia and Adults with Down Syndrome

A clear link between Down syndrome and Alzheimer's disease (AD) has long been established in the literature, in terms of neuropathology, histology, and clinically, with difficulties in timely diagnosis recognized as a challenge [101]. Individuals with Down syndrome have four to five times an overexpression of the amyloid precursor protein (APP) due to a triple copy of chromosome 21 [102]. This overexpression of APP leads to deposition of amyloid ß. The amyloid cascade hypothesis suggests that the deposition of amyloid ß plays a critical role in the development of Alzheimer's disease, and thus can explain the high risk of Alzheimer's disease for those adults with Down syndrome. It is accepted that by age 40, practically all individuals with Down syndrome will show neuropathological and neuro-imaging features of Alzheimer's disease [103–105], even if associated dementia is not evident.

In the general population, prevalence rates of dementia in those aged 60 and over are between 5% and 7% [106]. Early onset dementia is the term given to those where onset of dementia is below 65 years of age, and young onset dementia for those under the age of 45 [107]. The greatest prevalence of early onset dementia is found in those with Down syndrome [108]. This is confirmed in several population-based prevalence studies [80, 101, 109–114], with consensus findings that AD is far more prevalent in individuals with Down syndrome than those adults with

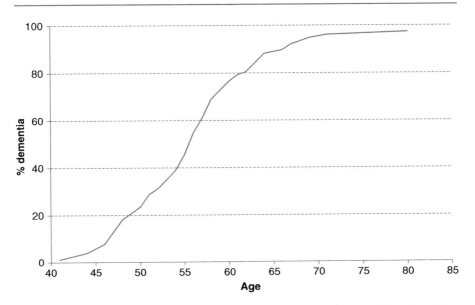

Fig. 3.2 Cumulative risk of developing dementia by age [80]. Note: Data from [80] retrieved from
https://www.ncbi.nlm.nih.gov/labs/articles/28664561/

intellectual disability from other etiologies or those adults in the general population.
Studies looking at age specific prevalence have found a sharp increase in AD from
age 40–60 [80, 101, 110, 111]. Coppus et al. [110] reported that, from the age of 45,
dementia prevalence doubled with each 5 year interval, up to the age of 60, after
which prevalence declined, which would most likely be explained by higher mortality rates in this age group, as there was no decrease in incidence of dementia over
the age of 60.

In a recent longitudinal study following 77 adults with Down syndrome over a
20 year period, it was found that 97.4% developed dementia. The risk for developing dementia for people with Down syndrome was calculated at 23.1% in people
aged 50, 45% in those aged 55, and 88% by age 65 [15, 80]; see Fig. 3.2. Mean age
of onset for people with Down syndrome in this study was 55 years with a median
survival of 7 years [80]. This was slightly higher than the 51.7 years reported in
previous studies [115].

McCarron et al. [80] reported that in Wave 3 of the IDS-TILDA longitudinal
study, 35.5% (n = 38) of adults with Down syndrome had a doctor's diagnosis of
dementia, which rose from 15.6% found in Wave 1 (McCarron et al., 2011). This
compared to 3.4% (n = 17) of those with intellectual disability from other etiologies
who reported a diagnosis of dementia. What is of concern, however, is that, of those
who did not have a diagnosis of dementia, 47.5% had never had a dementia assessment. This raises the important issue of the need for consistent and standardized
assessment of people with Down syndrome.

Table 3.6 Prevalence of difficulties in activities of daily living

	Wave 1	Wave 2	Wave 3
Dressing	44.4	52.6	73
Bathing	72.2	71.1	78.4
Eating	35.1	55.3	70.3
In and out of bed	15.8	10.5	54.1
Toileting	8.3	23.7	48.6

Diagnoses of epilepsy and dementia are highly associated, where one study found that a diagnosis of epilepsy came on average 0.57 years after a dementia diagnosis [80]. In the IDS-TILDA study noted above, 35.7% (n = 215) of the sample reported epilepsy in Wave 3. For individuals with Down syndrome, it was found that 30% of those with a new diagnosis of dementia also had a new diagnosis of epilepsy. This supports previous research where new onset seizures in later life for adults with Down syndrome are associated with the onset of dementia. For those with Down syndrome, prevalence of epilepsy without dementia was low at 13.7%, however among people with Down syndrome with dementia, the prevalence of epilepsy rose to 54.8%. Of those with a new diagnosis of epilepsy in Wave 3 (n = 15), 66.7% (n = 10) had Down syndrome. Diagnoses of dementia by Wave 3, was also associated with increasing difficulties in activities of daily living (ADLs), such as dressing, bathing, eating, getting in and out of bed, and toileting (see Table 3.6).

The data from IDS-TILDA builds upon the prior studies noted to further highlight the need for a baseline and annual follow-up assessment for symptoms of dementia for people with Down syndrome, as has been recommended by Burt and Aylward [116] and continues to be recommended by the British Psychological Association [117]. Difficulties in assessment of people with Down syndrome despite validation of informant-based measures and objective assessments, reinforce the value of regular and standardized approaches by health care professionals.

3.10 Medication Use and Adults with Intellectual Disability

Among adults the prevalence of polypharmacy and the risks of potentially inappropriate prescribing (PIP) increases with advancing age and morbidity. There are several definitions of polypharmacy, but it is generally understood to refer to the concurrent use of multiple medicines by one individual [118]. Medications play a critical role in maintaining health in older adults [119], and in many circumstances polypharmacy may be therapeutically beneficial [118]. However, polypharmacy is associated with increased prescribing errors, high risk prescribing and a higher prevalence of associated adverse drug reactions (ADRs). Poor health outcomes with the use of ten or more medicines (excessive polypharmacy) has been identified to carry particular risk [118, 120, 121]. See Chap. 15.

A large proportion of adults with intellectual disability are exposed to polypharmacy and have been identified as among "the most medicated groups in society", with rates of polypharmacy exceeding those of the general population [122–124].

There is a limited evidence base underpinning the safety of polypharmacy in adults with intellectual disability and multi-morbidity. While polypharmacy may be therapeutically beneficial in the treatment of multiple chronic conditions, difficulties with consent to treatments, poor evidence bases (having an intellectual disability is an exclusion criteria from randomized controlled trials), difficulties in communication of symptoms and side effects of medicines, and increased sensitivity and adverse effects associated with medicines due to the presence of organic dysfunction associated with the intellectual disability [125] make polypharmacy even more challenging. Older adults with intellectual disability are at additional risk of experiencing the "prescribing cascade", where the side effects of medicines are misdiagnosed as symptoms of another problem, or symptoms are misattributed to the underlying intellectual disability resulting in further medications prescribed and further risk of side effects and interactions [126]. One example is the prescribing of anticholinergic medications for movement disorders to treat extrapyramidal symptoms associated with antipsychotic agents, a practice no longer recommended in older adults [57, 58, 127].

Rates of reported polypharmacy in adults with intellectual disability have differed based on methodological issues and samples. A study in Victoria, Australia included 897 adults with intellectual disability aged from 18 to 82 years (over 90% were under 60), and all levels of intellectual disability, and reported that over 20% used 5–9 medicines [128]. In Ontario, Canada, medication use patterns were explored among 52,404 adults aged 18–64 years with intellectual disability receiving primary care services and support from the Ontario Disability Support Group [129]. This study had a prevalence rate of 42.1% in those aged 55–64 years for polypharmacy (≥5 medicines), and 3% for 11 or more medicines. Both the Australian and Canadian studies selected their cohorts from those using health services which may mean that reported rates were inflated because those with no medicines or chronic conditions were under-represented or absent [128, 129].

Polypharmacy was identified as an independent factor associated with prescription errors in a study of 600 randomly selected individuals with intellectual disability age 50 years and over who reported medicine use in the Healthy Ageing Intellectual Disabilities Study (HA-ID) in the Netherlands [130]. Participants were from independent and residential settings. Most prescription errors detected related to drugs acting on the central nervous system (43.2%).

In a Dutch national survey of general practice differences between 712 individuals with intellectual disability and controls (patients with no intellectual disability who were matched on age and sex), those with intellectual disability received four times more repeat prescriptions compared to controls [124]. In an Irish cross-sectional study of 736 older adults with intellectual disability (Wave 1 of IDS-TILDA), 21% of adults were identified taking ten or more medicines (excessive polypharmacy) on a regular basis and 35% took 5–9 medicines [57, 58]. This was much higher than the general older population in Ireland, where 2% were exposed to excessive polypharmacy (ten or more medicines) [131].

Studies in the intellectual disabled population have also identified a different pattern of frequently reported medicine classes implicated in polypharmacy compared to the older general population reflecting the different patterns of multi-morbidity, with higher levels of neurological, mental health and gastro-intestinal conditions for older adults with intellectual disability. O'Dwyer and colleagues noted antipsychotics, antiepileptics and laxatives represented the most frequently reported therapeutic drug class, with over four in ten older adults with intellectual disability exposed to antipsychotics [57, 58] These findings contrast with those reported in literature for the general older population, where cardiac therapies, analgesics, gastrointestinal agents, and antithrombotic represent therapeutic classes that are the most frequently reported [131–133].

There has been significant research carried out in the older population examining risks associated with cumulative sedative and anticholinergic medicines and associations with cognitive decline and mortality [134, 135]. Findings from Wave 1 and 2 of the IDS-TILDA study have revealed that older adults with intellectual disability in Ireland were significantly more likely to have a high sedative and anticholinergic burden, which was significantly associated with side effects, for example, constipation and daytime sedation [57, 58, 136].

Further research is needed on the long term effects of medicine use in older adults with intellectual disability, particularly psychotropic medicines and sedative and anticholinergic medicines (which may adversely affect physical and cognitive outcomes). More specific prescribing criteria developed for people with intellectual disability may guide identification of potentially inappropriate prescribing at a population level and associated adverse outcomes which consider the most commonly utilized medicine combinations and classes. In the absence of such research, practitioners must be particularly vigilant about the consequences of their prescribing practices.

3.11   Conclusion

The preparedness of healthcare professionals and health services to support, care, and treat adults with intellectual disability should be questioned. The challenges identified in this chapter must be priorities for service providers and healthcare services alike. It is a success story that people with intellectual disability are living longer, but it is a story that brings with it particular challenges. As research studies explore and discover new and emerging bodies of evidence of the health challenges facing people with intellectual disability transferring this knowledge to practice becomes increasingly essential. Intellectual disability is not universally part of the core training of healthcare professionals—a concern that as only through awareness and knowledge can healthcare for people with intellectual disability improve. Policy makers too need to pay attention. People with intellectual disability need equity with reasonable adjustments to ensure they receive their health services equally. Services of excellence will result when they build upon a body of knowledge of contributors to appropriate healthcare services that meet individual needs and maximize health and wellbeing. Such research and resulting evidence should also be the basis for education of health practitioners and improvements in health services delivery to support a life-course model of care and spotlight on health disparities to better improve the overall well-being of people with intellectual disability.

References

1. Burke E, McGlinchey E, O'Dwyer M, Foran S, Mac Giolla Phadraig C, O'Connell J, McCarron M. Physical health, prevalence and incidence of chronic health conditions across 10 years. 2017. Accessed from: https://www.tcd.ie/tcaid/assets/pdf/wave3report.pdf.
2. Kinnear D, Morrison J, Allan L, Henderson A, Smiley E, Cooper S-A. Prevalence of physical conditions and multimorbidity in a cohort of adults with intellectual disabilities with and without down syndrome: cross-sectional study. BMJ Open. 2018;8:e018292.
3. McCarron M, Burke E, Cleary E, Carroll R, McGlinchey E, McCallion P. Changes in physical and behavioural health of older adults with intellectual disability. Advancing years, different challenges: wave, 2. In: Burke E, McCallion P, McCarron M, editors. Advancing years, different challenges: wave 2 IDS-TILDA: findings on the ageing of people with an intellectual disability: an Intellectual Disability Supplement to The Irish Longitudinal Study on Ageing. Dublin: Irish Longitudinal Study on Ageing; 2014. p. 79.
4. McCarron M, Carroll R, Kelly C, McCallion P. Mortality rates in the general Irish population compared to those with an intellectual disability from 2003 to 2012. J Appl Res Intellect Disabil. 2015;28:406–13.
5. McCarron M, Swinburne J, Burke E, McGlinchey E, Carroll R, McCallion P. Patterns of multimorbidity in an older population of persons with an intellectual disability: results from the intellectual disability supplement to the Irish longitudinal study on aging (IDS-TILDA). Res Dev Disabil. 2013;34:521–7.
6. World Health Organization. Active ageing: a policy framework. Geneva: World Health Organisation; 2002.
7. Riise HKR, Riise T, Natvig GK, Daltveit AK. Poor self-rated health associated with an increased risk of subsequent development of lung cancer. Qual Life Res. 2014;23:145–53.
8. Burke E, McCarron M, Carroll R, McGlinchey E, McCallion P. What it's like to grow older: the aging perceptions of people with an intellectual disability in Ireland. Ment Retard. 2014a;52:205–19.
9. Burke EA, McCallion P, McCarron ME. Advancing years, different challenges: wave 2 IDS-TILDA. Findings on the ageing of people with an intellectual disability. Dublin: Trinity College Dublin; 2014b.
10. Gibbons HM, Owen R, Heller T. Perceptions of health and healthcare of people with intellectual and developmental disabilities in Medicaid managed care. Intellect Dev Disabil. 2016;54:94–105.
11. Evenhuis H, Theunissen M, Denkers I, Verschuure H, Kemme H. Prevalence of visual and hearing impairment in a Dutch institutionalized population with intellectual disability. J Intellect Disabil Res. 2001;45:457–64.
12. Krinsky-McHale SJ, Jenkins EC, Zigman WB, Silverman W. Ophthalmic disorders in adults with Down syndrome. Curr Gerontol Geriatr Res. 2012;2012:974253. https://doi.org/10.1155/2012/974253.
13. Kiani R, Miller H. Sensory impairment and intellectual disability. Adv Psychiatr Treat. 2010;16:228–35.
14. Warburg M. Visual impairment in adult people with moderate, severe, and profound intellectual disability. Acta Ophthalmol Scand. 2001;79:450–4.
15. McCarron M, Haigh M, McCallion P. Health, wellbeing and social inclusion: ageing with an intellectual disability in Ireland evidence from the first ten years of the intellectual disability supplement to the Irish Longitudinal Study on Ageing (IDS-TILDA) Wave 3 IDS TILDA. Dublin: Irish Longitudinal Study on Ageing; 2017a. Accessed from: https://www.tcd.ie/tcaid/assets/pdf/wave3report.pdf.

16. Santos-Teachout R, Evenhuis H, Stewart L, Kerr M, McElduff A, Böhmer CJM, Davis R, Beange H, Lennox N, Turner G. Health Guideline for Adults with an Intellectual Disability. The International Association for the Scientific Study of Intellectual Disabilities. 2002. Accessed from https://www.iassidd.org/uploads/legacy/pdf/healthguidelines.pdf.

17. Grondhuis S, Aman M. Overweight and obesity in youth with developmental disabilities: a call to action. J Intellect Disabil Res. 2014;58:787–99.

18. World Health Organisation. Global health risks – mortality and burden of diseases attributable to selected major risks. Geneva: World Health Organisation; 2009.

19. Kearns K, Dee A, Fitzgerald AP, Doherty E, Perry IJ. Chronic disease burden associated with overweight and obesity in Ireland: the effects of a small BMI reduction at population level. BMC Public Health. 2014;14:143. https://doi.org/10.1186/1471-2458-14-143.

20. Bradley S. Tracking obesity in people with learning disability. Learn Disabil Pract. 2005;8:10–4.

21. Hsieh K, Rimmer JH, Heller T. Obesity and associated factors in adults with intellectual disability. J Intellect Disabil Res. 2014;58:851–63. https://doi.org/10.1111/jir.12100.

22. Flegal KM, Carroll MD, Ogden CL, Curtin LR. Prevalence and trends in obesity among us adults, 1999-2008. JAMA. 2010;303:235–41.

23. Leahy S, Nolan A, O'Connell J, Kenny RA. Obesity in an ageing society: implications for health, physical function and health service utilisation The Irish Longitudinal Study on Ageing 2014. Dublin: The Irish Longitudinal Study on Ageing; 2014.

24. Patterson PD, Moore CG, Probst JC, Shinogle JA. Obesity and physical inactivity in rural America. J Rural Health. 2004;20:151–9.

25. Emerson E. Underweight, obesity and exercise among adults with intellectual disabilities in supported accommodation in northern England. J Intellect Disabil Res. 2005;49:134–43.

26. Wansink B, Hanks AS, Kaipainen K. Slim by design: Kitchen counter correlates of obesity. Health Educ Behav. 2016;43:552–8.

27. Rimmer JH, Yamaki K. Obesity and intellectual disability. Dev Disabil Res Rev. 2006;12:22–7.

28. Lee JJ, Ho C, Chen H-J, Huang N, Yeh JC. Is the 90th percentile adequate? The optimal waist circumference cutoff points for predicting cardiovascular risks in 124,643 15-year-old Taiwanese adolescents. PLoS One. 2016;11:e0158818.

29. World Health Organization. Waist circumference and waist-hip ratio: report of a WHO expert consultation, Geneva; 2011. 8–11 Dec 2008.

30. Lin L-P, Liu C-T, Liou S-W, Hsu S-W, Lin J-D. High blood pressure in adults with disabilities: influence of gender, body weight and health behaviors. Res Dev Disabil. 2012;33:1508–15.

31. Lynch E, Liu K, Wei GS, Spring B, Kiefe C, Greenland P. The relation between body size perception and change in body mass index over 13 years: the coronary artery risk development in young adults (cardia) study. Am J Epidemiol. 2009;169:857–66.

32. Mueller KG, Hurt RT, Abu-Lebdeh HS, Mueller PS. Self-perceived vs actual and desired weight and body mass index in adult ambulatory general internal medicine patients: a cross sectional study. BMC Obes. 2014;1:26.

33. World Health Organization. Prevention and management of osteoporosis: report of a WHO scientific group: World Health Organization. Diamond Pocket Books (P) Ltd. Geneva: World Health Organization; 2003. Accessed from: http://apps.who.int/iris/bitstream/10665/42841/1/WHO_TRS_921.pdf.

34. Department of Health and Children (DOHC). Tackling chronic disease. A policy framework for the management of chronic diseases. Dublin: Department of Health and Children, Hawkins House; 2005.

35. Genant HK, Cooper C, Poor G, Reid I, Ehrlich G, Kanis J, Nordin BC, Barrett-Connor E, Black D, Bonjour J-P. Interim report and recommendations of the World Health Organization task-force for osteoporosis. Osteoporos Int. 1999;10:259–64.

36. Siris ES, Miller PD, Barrett-Connor E, Faulkner KG, Wehren LE, Abbott TA, Sherwood LM. Identification and fracture outcomes of undiagnosed low bone mineral density in postmenopausal women: results from the national osteoporosis risk assessment. JAMA. 2001;286:2815–22.

37. Kanis J, McCloskey E, Johansson H, Cooper C, Rizzoli R, Reginster J-Y. European guidance for the diagnosis and management of osteoporosis in postmenopausal women. Osteoporos Int. 2013;24:23–57.
38. Lin L-P, Hsu S-W, Yao C-H, Lai W-J, Hsu P-J, Wu J-L, Chu CM, Lin J-D. Risk for osteopenia and osteoporosis in institution-dwelling individuals with intellectual and/or developmental disabilities. Res Dev Disabil. 2015;36:108–13.
39. Schmidt EV, Byars JR, Flamuth DH, Schott JJS, M C. Prevalence of low bone-mineral density among mentally retarded and developmentally disabled residents in intermediate care. Consult Pharm. 2004;19:45–51.
40. Leslie WD, Pahlavan PS, Roe EB, Dittberner K. Bone density and fragility fractures in patients with developmental disabilities. Osteoporos Int. 2009;20:379–83.
41. McCarron M, Swinburne J, Burke E, McGlinchey E, Andrews V, Mulryan N, Foran S, McCallion P. Growing older with an intellectual disability in Ireland 2011: first results from the intellectual disability supplement to the irish longitudinal study on ageing (IDS-TILDA). Dublin: School of Nursing and Midwifery, Trinity College Dublin; 2011.
42. Beerhorst K, de Krom M, Aldenkamp B, Tan F. Severe early onset osteoporosis in five young men with an intellectual disability, epilepsy and long-term antiepileptic drug use. Epilepsia. 2009;50:77.
43. Center J, Beange H, McElduff A. People with mental retardation have an increased prevalence of osteoporosis: a population study. Am J Ment Retard. 1998;103:19–28.
44. McKenna G, Burke FM. Age-related oral changes. Dent Update. 2010;37:519–23.
45. Glick M, Williams DM, Kleinman DV, Vujicic M, Watt RG, Weyant RJ. A new definition for oral health developed by the FDI World Dental Federation opens the door to a universal definition of oral health. Br Dent J. 2016;221:792–3. https://doi.org/10.1038/sj.bdj.2016.953.
46. Kanno T, Carlsson GE. A review of the shortened dental arch concept focusing on the work by the Kayser/Nijmegen group. J Oral Rehabil. 2006;33:850–62. https://doi.org/10.1111/j.1365-2842.2006.01625.x.
47. Crowley E, Whelton H, Murphy A, Kelleher V, Cronin M, Flannery E, Nunn J. Oral health of adults with an intellectual disability in residential care in Ireland 2003. Galway: Department of Health and Children; 2005.
48. Scott A, March L, Stokes ML. A survey of oral health in a population of adults with developmental disabilities: comparison with a national oral health survey of the general population. Aust Dent J. 1998;43:257–61.
49. Gabre P, Martinsson T, Gahnberg L. Incidence of, and reasons for, tooth mortality among mentally retarded adults during a 10-year period. Acta Odontol Scand. 1999;57:55–61.
50. Mac Giolla Phadraig C, McCallion P, Cleary E, McGlinchey E, Burke E, McCarron M, Nunn J. Total tooth loss and complete denture use in older adults with intellectual disabilities in Ireland. J Public Health Dent. 2015;75:101–8. https://doi.org/10.1111/jphd.12077.
51. Kinane D, Bouchard P. Periodontal diseases and health: consensus report of the Sixth European Workshop on Periodontology. J Clin Periodontol. 2008;35(8 Suppl):333–7. https://doi.org/10.1111/j.1600-051X.2008.01278.x.
52. Scannapieco FA, Rethman MP. The relationship between periodontal diseases and respiratory diseases. Dent Today. 2003;22:79–83.
53. NICE. NICE Short Clinical Guidelines Technical Team. Prophylaxis against infective endocarditis: antimicrobial prophylaxis against infective endocarditis in adults and children undergoing interventional procedures. London: National Institute for Health and Clinical Excellence; 2008.
54. Mason J, Scior K. Diagnostic overshadowing' amongst clinicians working with people with intellectual disabilities in the UK. J Appl Res Intellect Disabil. 2004;17:85–90.
55. McKenzie K, Smith M, Purcell AM. The reported expression of pain and distress by people with an intellectual disability. J Clin Nurs. 2013;22:1833–42.
56. Mac Giolla Phadraig C, Griffiths C, McCallion P, McCarron M, Donnelly-Swift E, Nunn J. Pharmacological behaviour support for adults with intellectual disabilities: frequency and predictors in a national cross-sectional survey. Community Dent Oral Epidemiol. 2018;46:231–7. https://doi.org/10.1111/cdoe.12365.

57. O'Dwyer M, Maidment ID, Bennett K, Peklar J, Mulryan N, McCallion P, Henman MC. Association of anticholinergic burden with adverse effects in older people with intellectual disabilities: an observational cross-sectional study. Br J Psychiatry. 2016a;209:504–10. https://doi.org/10.1192/bjp.bp.115.173971.

58. O'Dwyer M, Peklar J, McCallion P, McCarron M, Henman MC. Factors associated with polypharmacy and excessive polypharmacy in older people with intellectual disability differ from the general population: a cross-sectional observational nationwide study. BMJ Open. 2016b;6:e010505. https://doi.org/10.1136/bmjopen-2015-010505.

59. Emami E, de Souza RF, Kabawat M, Feine JS. The impact of edentulism on oral and general health. Int J Dent. 2013;2013:498305. https://doi.org/10.1155/2013/498305.

60. Felton DA. Complete edentulism and comorbid diseases: an update. J Prosthodont. 2015;25:5–20. https://doi.org/10.1111/jopr.12350.

61. Polzer I, Schimmel M, Muller F, Biffar R. Edentulism as part of the general health problems of elderly adults. Int Dent J. 2010;60:143–55.

62. Shapira J, Efrat J, Berkey D, Mann J. Dental health profile of a population with mental retardation in Israel. Special Care Dent. 1998;18:149–55.

63. Owens J. Access to dental services for people with learning disabilities: quality care? J Disabil Oral Health. 2011;12:17–27.

64. Cooper S-A, Melville C, Morrison J. People with intellectual disabilities: their health needs differ and need to be recognised and met. Br Med J. 2004;329:414–5.

65. Kuhlmann L, Joensson IM, Froekjaer JB, Krogh K, Farholt S. A descriptive study of colorectal function in adults with Prader-Willi Syndrome: high prevalence of constipation. BMC Gastroenterol. 2014;14:63. https://doi.org/10.1186/1471-230X-14-63.

66. Patja K, Mölsä P, Iivanainen M. Cause-specific mortality of people with intellectual disability in a population-based, 35-year follow-up study. J Intellect Disabil Res. 2001;45:30–40.

67. Symons FJ, Harper VN, McGrath PJ, Breau LM, Bodfish JW. Evidence of increased nonverbal behavioral signs of pain in adults with neurodevelopmental disorders and chronic self-injury. Res Dev Disabil. 2009;30:521–8.

68. Morad M, Merrick J, Nasri Y. Prevalence of helicobacter pylori in people with intellectual disability in a residential care centre in Israel. J Intellect Disabil Res. 2002;46:141–3.

69. Duff M, Scheepers M, Cooper M, Hoghton M, Baddeley P. Helicobacter pylori: has the killer escaped from the institution? A possible cause of increased stomach cancer in a population with intellectual disability. J Intellect Disabil Res. 2001;45:219–25.

70. Böhmer C, Niezen-de Boer M, Klinkenberg-Knol E, Nadorp J, Meuwissen S. Gastro-oesophageal reflux disease in institutionalised intellectually disabled individuals. Neth J Med. 1997;51:134–9.

71. Hsu W-T, Lai C-C, Wang Y-H, Tseng P-H, Wang K, Wang C-Y, Chen L. Risk of pneumonia in patients with gastroesophageal reflux disease: a population-based cohort study. PLoS One. 2017;12:e0183808.

72. Peebles KA, Price TJ. Self-injurious behaviour in intellectual disability syndromes: evidence for aberrant pain signalling as a contributing factor. J Intellect Disabil Res. 2012;56:441–52. https://doi.org/10.1111/j.1365-2788.2011.01484.x.

73. Cockburn-Wells H. Managing constipation in adults with severe learning disabilities. Learn Disabil Pract. 2014;17(9):16–22. https://doi.org/10.7748/ldp.17.9.16.e1582.

74. Morad M, Nelson NP, Merrick J, Davidson PW, Carmeli E. Prevalence and risk factors of constipation in adults with intellectual disability in residential care centers in Israel. Res Dev Disabil. 2007;28:580–6.

75. Böhmer C, Taminiau J, Klinkenberg-Knol E, Meuwissen S. The prevalence of constipation in institutionalized people with intellectual disability. J Intellect Disabil Res. 2001;45:212–8.

76. Salvador-Carulla L, Martínez-Leal R, Heyler C, Alvarez-Galvez J, Veenstra MY, García-Ibáñez J, Carpenter S, Bertelli M, Munir K, Torr J. Training on intellectual disability in health sciences: the European perspective. Int J Dev Disabil. 2015;61:20–31.

77. McDermott A. A descriptive quantitative study examining the prevalence of constipation among older adults with an intellectual disability in Ireland. (Masters by Research), University of Dublin Trinity College, Trinity College Dublin. (TX-2-205). 2016.

78. Stewart KJ. Speech and swallowing rehabilitation in the home: a comparison of two service delivery models for stroke survivors. Thesis. Edith Cowan University. 2014. Accessed from: http://ro.ecu.edu.au/theses/1579/.
79. Evenhuis HM. Medical aspects of ageing in a population with intellectual disability: III. Mobility, internal conditions and cancer. J Intellect Disabil Res. 1997;41:8–18.
80. McCarron M, McCallion P, Reilly E, Dunne P, Carroll R, Mulryan N. A prospective 20-year longitudinal follow-up of dementia in persons with Down syndrome. J Intellect Disabil Res. 2017b;61:843–52.
81. Pin S, Spini D. Impact of falling on social participation and social support trajectories in a middle-aged and elderly European sample. SSM Popul Health. 2016;2:382–9. https://doi.org/10.1016/j.ssmph.2016.05.004.
82. Stevens JA, Mack KA, Paulozzi LJ, Ballesteros MF. Self-reported falls and fall-related injuries among persons aged 65 years in the United States, 2006. J Safety Res. 2008;39:345–000.
83. Terroso M, Rosa N, Torres Marques A, Simoes R. Physical consequences of falls in the elderly: a literature review from 1995 to 2010. Eur Rev Aging Phys Act. 2014;11:51–9. https://doi.org/10.1007/s11556-013-0134-8.
84. Orces CH. Emergency department visits for fall-related fractures among older adults in the USA: a retrospective cross-sectional analysis of the National Electronic Injury Surveillance System All Injury Program, 2001–2008. BMJ Open. 2013;3:e001722. https://doi.org/10.1136/bmjopen-2012-001722.
85. Tinnetti ME, Speechley M, Ginter SF. Risk factors for falls among elderly persons living in the community. N Engl J Med. 1988;319:1701–7.
86. Fleming J, Matthews FE, Brayne C. Falls in advanced old age: recalled falls and prospective follow-up of over-90-year-olds in the Cambridge city over-75s cohort study. BMC Geriatr. 2008;8:6.
87. Talbot LA, Musiol RJ, Witham EK, Metter EJ. Falls in young, middle-aged and older community dwelling adults: perceived cause, environmental factors and injury. BMC Public Health. 2005;18(5):86.
88. Cox CR, Clemson L, Stancliffe RJ, Durvasula S, Sherrington C. Incidence of and risk factors for falls among adults with an intellectual disability. J Intellect Disabil Res. 2010;54:1045–57.
89. Hsieh K, Rimmer J, Heller T. Prevalence of falls and risk factors in adults with intellectual disability. Am J Intellect Dev Disabil. 2012;117:442–54. https://doi.org/10.1352/1944-7558-117.6.442.
90. Finlayson J, Morrison J, Jackson A, Mantry D, Cooper SA. Injuries, falls and accidents among adults with intellectual disabilities. Prospective cohort study. J Intellect Disabil Res. 2010;54:966–80.
91. Hartholt KA, van Beeck EF, Polinder S, van der Velde N, van Lieshout EM, Panneman MJ, Patka P. Societal consequences of falls in the older population: injuries, healthcare costs, and long-term reduced quality of life. J Trauma Acute Care Surg. 2011;71(3):748–53.
92. Gannon B, Shea O, Hudson E. The economic cost of falls and fractures in people aged 65 and over in Ireland: technical report to NCAOP/HSE/DOHC. Galway: National University Ireland; 2007.
93. Hartholt KA, Polinder S, Van der Cammen TJ, Panneman MJ, Van der Velde N, Van Lieshout EM, Van Beeck EF. Costs of falls in an ageing population: a nationwide study from the Netherlands (2007-2009). Injury. 2012;43:1199–203. https://doi.org/10.1016/j.injury.2012.03.033.
94. Burns ER, Stevens JA, Lee R. The direct costs of fatal and non-fatal falls among older adults - United States. J Safety Res. 2016;58:99–103. https://doi.org/10.1016/j.jsr.2016.05.001.
95. Lord S, Sherrington C, Menz H, Close C. Falls in older people: risk factors and strategies for prevention. 2nd ed. Cambridge: Cambridge University Press; 2007.
96. Todd C, Skelton DA. What are the main risk factors for falls among older people and what are the most effective interventions to prevent these falls? Health Evidence Network report. Copenhagen: WHO Regional Office for Europe; 2004. Accessed from: www.euro.who.int/document/E82552.pdf.

97. Chiba Y, Shimada A, Yoshida F, Keino H, Hasegawa M, Ikari H, Miyake S, Hosokawa M. Risk of fall for individuals with intellectual disability. Am J Intellect Dev Disabil. 2009;114:225–36.
98. National Institute for Healthcare and Clinical Excellence. NICE clinical guideline: falls in older people. 2015. reter: https://www.nice.org.uk/guidance/qs86.
99. Van Hanegem E, Enkelaar L, Smulders E, Weerdesteyn V. Obstacle course training can improve mobility and prevent falls in people with intellectual disabilities. J Intellect Disabil Res. 2014;58:485–92. https://doi.org/10.1111/jir.12045.
100. Crockett J, Finlayson J, Skelton DA, Miller G. Promoting exercise as part of a physiotherapy-led falls pathway service for adults with intellectual disabilities: a service evaluation. J Appl Res Intellect Disabil. 2015;28:257–64.
101. Tyrrell J, Cosgrave M, Mccarron M, McPherson J, Calvert J, Kelly A, McLaughlin M, Gill M, Lawlor B. Dementia in people with Down's syndrome. Int J Geriatr Psychiatry. 2001;16:1168–74.
102. Jennings D, Seibyl J, Sabbagh M, Lai F, Hopkins W, Bullich S, Gimenez M, Reininger C, Putz B, Stephens A, Catafau AM, Marek K. Age dependence of brain β-amyloid deposition in Down syndrome: an [^{18}F]florbetaben PET study. Neurology. 2015;84:500–7.
103. Lamar M, Foy CM, Beacher F, Daly E, Poppe M, Archer N, Prasher V, Murphy KC, Morris RG, Simmons A, Lovestone S, Murphy DG. Down syndrome with and without dementia: an in vivo proton Magnetic Resonance Spectroscopy study with implications for Alzheimer's disease. Neuroimage. 2011;57:63–8.
104. Roizen NJ, Patterson D. Down's syndrome. Lancet. 2003;361:1281–9.
105. Schupf N, Zigman WB, Tang MX, Pang D, Mayeux R, Mehta P, Silverman W. Change in plasma Aβ peptides and onset of dementia in adults with Down syndrome. Neurology. 2010;75:1639–44.
106. World Health Organization. Dementia: a public health priority. Geneva: World Health Organization; 2012.
107. Masellis M, Sherborn K, Neto PR, Sadovnick DA, Hsiung G-YR, Black SE, Prasad s, Williams M. Early-onset dementias: diagnostic and etiological considerations. Alzheimers Res Ther. 2013;5(Suppl 1):S7.
108. Hartley D, Blumenthal T, Carrillo M, Dipaolo G, Esralew L, Gardiner K, Granholm C, Iqbal K, Krams M, Lemere C, Lott I, Mobley W, Ness S, Nixon R, Potter H, Reeves R, Sabbagh M, Silverman W, Tycko B, Whitten M, Wisniewski T. Down syndrome and Alzheimer's disease: common pathways, common goals. Alzheimers Dement. 2015;11:700–9.
109. Cooper SA. High prevalence of dementia among people with learning disabilities not attributable to Down's syndrome. Psychol Med. 1997;27:609–16.
110. Coppus A, Evenhuis H, Verberne G, Visser F, Van Gool P, Eikelenboom P, Van Duijin C. Dementia and mortality in persons with Down's syndrome. J Intellect Disabil Res. 2006;50:768–77.
111. Holland AJ, Hon J, Huppert FA, Stevens F, Watson P. Population-based study of the prevalence and presentation of dementia in adults with Down's syndrome. Br J Psychiatry. 1998;172:493–8.
112. Sekijima Y, Ikeda S-I, Tokuda T, Satoh S-I, Hidaka H, Hidaka E, Ishikawa M, Yanagisawa N. Prevalence of dementia of Alzheimer type and apolipoprotein E phenotypes in aged patients with Down's syndrome. Eur Neurol. 1998;39:234–7.
113. Strydom A, Livingston G, King M, Hassiotis A. Prevalence of dementia in intellectual disability using different diagnostic criteria. Br J Psychiatry. 2007;191:150–7.
114. Strydom A, Shooshtari S, Lee L, Raykar V, Torr J, Tsiouris J, Jokinen N, Courtenay K, Bass N, Sinnema M, Maaskant M. Dementia in older adults with intellectual disabilities— Epidemiology, presentation, and diagnosis. J Pol Pract Intellect Disabil. 2010;7:96–110.
115. Prasher VP, Kirshnan VH. Age of onset and duration of dementia in people with Down syndrome: integration of 98 reported cases in the literature. Int J Geriatr Psychiatry. 1993;8:915–22.

116. Burt D, Aylward EH. Test battery for the diagnosis of demntia in individuals with intellectual disability. J Intellect Disabil Res. 2000;44:175–80.
117. The British Psychological Society & Royal College of Psychiatrists. Dementia and people with intellectual disabilities: guidance on the assessment, diagnosis, interventions and support of people with intellectual disabilities who develop dementia. UK: British Psychological Society Leicester; 2015.
118. Duerden M, Avery T, Payne R. Polypharmacy and medicines optimisation: making it safe and sound. London: King's Fund; 2013.
119. Thompson R, Linehan C, Glynn M, Kerr M. A qualitative study of carers' and professionals' views on the management of people with intellectual disability and epilepsy: a neglected population. Epilepsy Behav. 2013;28:379–85.
120. Gnjidic D, Hilmer SN, Blyth FM, Naganathan V, Waite L, Seibel MJ, Le Couteur DG. Polypharmacy cutoff and outcomes: five or more medicines were used to identify community-dwelling older men at risk of different adverse outcomes. J Clin Epidemiol. 2012;65:989–95.
121. Guthrie B, McCowan C, Davey P, Simpson CR, Dreischulte T, Barnett K. High risk prescribing in primary care patients particularly vulnerable to adverse drug events: cross sectional population database analysis in Scottish general practice. BMJ. 2011;342:d3514. https://doi.org/10.1136/bmj.d351410.1136/bmj.d3514.
122. Häßler F, Thome J, Reis O. Polypharmacy in the treatment of subjects with intellectual disability. J Neural Transm. 2015;122(Suppl 1):S93–100. https://doi.org/10.1007/s00702-014-1219-x.
123. Peklar J, Kos M, O'Dwyer M, McCarron M, McCallion P, Kenny RA, Henman MC. Medication and supplement use in older people with and without intellectual disability: an observational, cross-sectional study. PLoS One. 2017;12:e0184390.
124. Straetmans JM, van Schrojenstein Lantman-de HM, Schellevis FG, Dinant G-J. Health problems of people with intellectual disabilities: the impact for general practice. Br J Gen Pract. 2007;57:64–6.
125. Taylor D, Paton C, Kapur S. The Maudsley prescribing guidelines in psychiatry. New York, NY: John Wiley & Sons; 2015.
126. Rochon PA, Gurwitz JH. Optimising drug treatment for elderly people: the prescribing cascade. Br Med J. 1997;315:1096.
127. O'Mahony D, O'Sullivan D, Byrne S, O'Connor MN, Ryan C, Gallagher P. STOPP/START criteria for potentially inappropriate prescribing in older people: version 2. Age Ageing. 2014;44:213–8.
128. Haider SI, Ansari Z, Vaughan L, Matters H, Emerson E. Prevalence and factors associated with polypharmacy in Victorian adults with intellectual disability. Res Dev Disabil. 2014;35:3071–80.
129. Ouellette-Kuntz HM, Lake JK, Wilton AS. Chapter 6, Medication use. Atlas on the primary care of adults with developmental disabilities in Ontario. 2013. Accessed from: http://www.ices.on.ca/~/media/Files/Atlases-Reports/2013/Atlas-on-developmental-disabilities/Full-Report.ashx.
130. Zaal RJ, van der Kaaij AD, Evenhuis HM, van den Bemt PM. Prescription errors in older individuals with an intellectual disability: prevalence and risk factors in the Healthy Ageing and Intellectual Disability Study. Res Dev Disabil. 2013;34:1656–62.
131. Richardson K, Moore P, Peklar J, Galvin R, Kenny RA. Polypharmacy in adults over 50 in Ireland: opportunities for cost saving and improved healthcare. Dublin: The Irish Longitudinal Study on Ageing, Lincoln Place, Trinity College Dublin; 2012.
132. Barat I, Andreasen F, Damsgaard EMS. The consumption of drugs by 75 year-old individuals living in their own homes. Eur J Clin Pharmacol. 2000;56:501–9.
133. Haider SI, Johnell K, Thorslund M, Fastbom J. Analysis of the association between polypharmacy and socioeconomic position among elderly aged ≥77 years in Sweden. Clin Ther. 2008;30:419–27.

134. Hilmer SN, Mager DE, Simonsick EM, Cao Y, Ling SM, Windham BG, Shorr RI. A drug burden index to define the functional burden of medications in older people. Arch Intern Med. 2007;167:781–7.
135. Ruxton K, Woodman RJ, Mangoni AA. Drugs with anticholinergic effects and cognitive impairment, falls and all-cause mortality in older adults: a systematic review and meta-analysis. Br J Clin Pharmacol. 2015;80:209–20.
136. O'Connell J, Burke E, Mulryan N, O'Dwyer C, Donegan C, McCallion P, O'Dwyer M. Drug burden index to define the burden of medicines in older adults with intellectual disabilities: an observational cross-sectional study. Br J Clin Pharmacol. 2017;84:553–67.

Assessing Physical Health

4

Gerard J. Kerins and Ilana Stol

4.1   Introduction

The assessment of physical health in adults with intellectual disability is both rewarding and challenging. Real opportunities exist to improve the physical health of this group through early identification of health problems and psychosocial issues to reduce future morbidity and mortality and to provide anticipatory guidance and support for adults with intellectual disability and their caregivers as they navigate each stage of life. The clinical care of this group is provided by a variety of professionals; thus, standards of care must continue to be developed and disseminated in order to ensure that minimum levels of care are applied to all groups. The appropriate history taking, physical examination, and assessment of health in adults with intellectual disability will continue to become more important as this group ages, and as with the general population, with increasing age often comes increasing disease burden, making the assessment all the more crucial. One important aspect of the care of those adults with intellectual disability is the false notion that they may not want to pursue or may not benefit from the same diagnostic or therapeutic approaches as other adults in the general population. Those who care for adults with intellectual disability this population must always ensure that those with intellectual disability receive the most appropriate care. As more data regarding the care of this unique but heterogeneous group emerges, it is clear that those adults with intellectual disability respond no less optimally as do adults in the general population in terms of morbidity and mortality, to standard and accepted treatments. While this is true, clinicians must also maintain a constant sense of flexibility and adaptability in order to appropriately modify their care to fully explore patients' medical problems and formulate treatment plans.

G. J. Kerins (✉) · I. Stol
Section of Geriatrics, Department of Internal Medicine, Yale University School of Medicine, Yale New Haven Health System, New Haven, CT, USA
e-mail: Gerard.Kerins@ynhh.org

© Springer Nature Switzerland AG 2019
V. P. Prasher, M. P. Janicki (eds.), *Physical Health of Adults with Intellectual and Developmental Disabilities*, https://doi.org/10.1007/978-3-319-90083-4_4

This chapter reviews appropriate history taking mechanisms as well as physical examination approaches to adults with intellectual disability. Emphasis is placed on those common conditions which affect these adults and the relevant ways to make such diagnoses in an early and appropriate manner. First, a summary of history taking will be reviewed with attention being paid to how such a process can be completed using surrogate informants and functional status to compile a detailed and relevant history. In addition, focusing on certain historical factors for specific conditions that may affect this group of adults more commonly should foster early diagnosis and treatment. The history, especially in this population, may be the most appropriate and accurate way to assess current health status and enable appropriate decisions regarding diagnostic testing and treatment strategies. Second, the physical assessment and evaluation of this group will be reviewed, noting that modification of the typical physical examination procedure may at times be needed in order to obtain the most relevant clinical information. The logical use of laboratory data and other ancillary testing can serve to further improve the diagnostic accuracy and foster early identification of potentially serious health problems. Certainly, the efficient and effective use of diagnostic testing such as blood tests, X-ray examination and scans, for example, in this group may be difficult because of certain physical and intellectual limitations which may impact the ability to complete them. One should be assured that if indicated, such tests are completed, even if additional measures are required to help during the diagnostic process.

4.2 History Taking

The process of obtaining a detailed history from adults with intellectual disability is a complex task which often depends on the availability of surrogate informants and focusing on subtle nonverbal information. How such persons and their caregivers perceive wellness or healthiness can impact this history taking process. While numerous tools have been validated to assess perceived health and quality of life in adults without lifelong disabilities, there is generally a paucity of such research for adults with intellectual disability, which has largely been limited by lack of appropriate methods and measures for objective assessment for health perception among these adults who often articulate their feelings and needs differently. More recently, however, there is a growing body of research aimed at formulating a tool combining both closed and open responses for perceived health assessment for adults with intellectual disability, though none has yet been validated [1, 2].

History taking should always be completed in a quiet, well-lit environment with appropriate surrogates present and interviewed in advance, as needed. Because of communication difficulties—whether it be inability to see, speak, hear, or otherwise express oneself effectively—adults with intellectual disability may not be able to articulate even in simple terms what might be their health concern(s). Inability to communicate should not be mistaken for a lack of health problems, pain, disability, or illness. Particular attention must be paid to alternative expression of a chief medical complaint that has prompted an adult with intellectual disability to seek medical attention. Caregivers may be, and often are, the only other means of eliciting such information. The chief concern, which is in the adult's own words or actions as to why he or she is seeking medical care, should be the first step in the process; every attempt should be made to obtain history from both the patient and surrogate prior to formulating a treatment plan. Health care providers should always respect the autonomy of those with intellectual disability, and never by appearance alone assume that one is unable or unwilling to provide an accurate or detailed history. Asking the patient about his or her health, even if the patient may not fully understand, should precede any attempt to obtain history from caregivers. Many times, caregivers or other informants are crucial to this data-gathering process, particularly with reference to type of medication prescribed and information regarding any changes in function or previous hospital admissions.

If possible, providing a physically separate space from patient and caregiver when performing the interview is an important means by which providers can obtain history which each party may wish to keep private or feel uncomfortable sharing in the presence of the other. Caregivers may, for example, wish to discuss separately future changes in living situation or disruptive behaviors exhibited by the patient. This encounter could also serve as an appropriate time for providers to screen for caregiver burden issues [3], especially as caregivers of adult children age they often become particularly vulnerable to stressors of caregiving [3, 4] which could have significant impact on their mental and physical wellbeing [5, 6]. One may consider utilizing a caregiver burden assessment tool such as the Family Quality of Life Scale [7]. Screening for caregiver burnout and connecting caregivers with appropriate resources and services is essential for continued stability of both the caregiver and patients' health. Persons with intellectual disability may also wish to discuss certain issues, such as sexuality or interpersonal concerns, separately from caregivers. This encounter could also serve as an appropriate time for providers to screen for abuse [8] (which is particularly important given that, as of 2012, violent crime and sexual assault has occurred against people with intellectual and developmental disabilities at much higher rates than the general population) [9]. It is also important to obtain a sexual history not only because of the import of providing counseling on safe sexual practices (and potential need for other screening, such as sexually transmitted infections) and contraception, but also as a means of screening for partner or caregiver violence/abuse.

Cooperation, or lack thereof, of an adult during the history and physical exam should never be a barrier to appropriate care and treatment, but data suggest that negative patient behaviors in adults with intellectual disability can and does impact health care for certain types of conditions and treatments, particularly surrounding sensitive care, such as gynecologic examinations [10]. Furthermore, these behaviors may, in fact, be further exacerbated by the health conditions themselves [11], leading to potentially worse outcomes if the underlying health problems leading to problem behaviors are not identified early (for example, agitation due to pain from underlying medical condition, or excessive itching due to underlying allergy).

Adults with intellectual disability, similar to age peers in general, may have nonspecific presentations of specific illnesses or atypical presentations of common diseases where certain symptoms may be altered or absent. In addition, acute diseases in many adults with intellectual disability are often manifested by changes in activities of daily living (changes in ability to dress, feed, bathe, or toilet oneself). Functional changes from baseline may be the only indicator of underlying disease [12]. Thus, a keen knowledge of baseline function is crucial in assessing any changes in a patient's health. Even those adults with marked physical and functional deficits at baseline may exhibit further, more accelerated decline as the only sign of a new or progressing illness. Focus on functional change in obtaining history will then be an effective manner to enhance early identification of developing morbidity in this group. Although a variety of functional assessment tools have been validated and are widely used with older adults in general [13], to a lesser extent these tools may be relevant and useful in measuring functional status in this group [14–16] Just asking directly about any change or alteration from baseline regarding self-care (dressing, feeding, bathing, sleeping) may be an adequate way to assess functional change. Asking the patient and caregiver in an open-ended manner to describe daily routine is one practical method to accomplish this task. Looking for any change manifested by altered daily routine may be another way to help identify a developing illness or disease.

4.3   Review of Systems

A typical review of systems should be completed with attention being paid to those conditions which are more common in this group, including but not limited to Alzheimer's-related dementia, thyroid disease, seizure disorder, cataracts, congenital heart disease, sleep apnea, fungal and nail infections, and osteoporosis [17, 18]. Each patient on a routine basis should be asked about the following areas when conducting a review of the following systems.

4.3.1   Skin

The skin history should specifically include questions about any nail or related fungal infections or atopic dermatitis [19]. Although such skin conditions may at times appear to be trivial, they can significantly impact function and quality of life. In addition, it is important to specifically ask about any new or changing skin patterns or moles, recognizing that many adults with intellectual disability are at the same risk as age-peers for the development of skin cancers.

4.3.2   Neurologic

A review as it relates to the head and related structures should specifically focus on any recent, new, or different character or nature of seizure disorders. Recent studies suggest that slightly more than 20% of adults with Down syndrome experience seizures, with seizure occurrence increasing significantly in older age [20] Although this high rate of occurrence of seizures has been recognized for years, data analyses suggest that late onset seizures may accompany the aging process in general [21], and thus any new neurological changes should be discussed at all ages when examining adults with Down syndrome. Any abnormal movements should not be dismissed, for they may be atypical seizures. An examiner should specifically ask about any new tics, neurological deficits, or repetitive motions which may, in fact, represent atypical seizures in this population. Given the high rate and earlier age of onset of dementia of the Alzheimer's type in adults with Down syndrome, as well as more generally in adults with other forms of intellectual disability, it is important to inquire about any cognitive changes noted, while recognizing that the first signs of dementia are often reflected by subtle functional changes, which may not be routinely picked up by caregivers.

4.3.3 Eyes/Ears/Nose/Throat

The eye review must include any information concerning changes in vision or visual status, particularly any evidence of cataracts, which might be impacting on function but might not be readily apparent. Adults with intellectual disability experience visual impairments at a significantly higher rate than age peers in general [22] One should not be discouraged from asking about such visual changes, even if there has been a full ophthalmologic evaluation within the past year, recognizing that among some adults with intellectual disability cataracts and visual disturbance may progress very rapidly and present even at an earlier age.

Any evidence of recent or recurrent ear infections or tendency toward impacted cerumen should be asked about specifically. The mouth and throat examination is important with regard to any changes or new difficulty in swallowing, any recent or prior history of aspiration, or any tendency to choke while eating certain types of foods, especially in adults in whom dementia has been diagnosed or is suspected. Extensive dental caries or related dental diseases should always be reviewed.

4.3.4 Breast

With respect to the history of breast disease, the review of systems among female adults should include asking specifically about any prior history of lumps or masses; asking such history of male individuals is also appropriate. Prior history or routine use of mammography should also be reviewed. There is no evidence to suggest that the use of screening mammography is any less effective among women with intellectual disability [23], but may be more problematic—particularly among adults with aversion to screening devices.

4.3.5 Respiratory

The respiratory review of systems should focus on any evidence of recurrent infections, such as pneumonia, or any new or changing breathing patterns, including new or worsening exertional dyspnea which may signal pulmonary or cardiac dysfunction. Recent studies have suggested that adults with intellectual disability are more likely to have more frequent, longer, and recurrent hospital admissions for respiratory disease [24] Detailed questioning about sleep should also include any evidence of snoring, frequent awakening, or any other signs or symptoms of sleep apnea.

4.3.6 Cardiovascular

The heart review of systems should focus on diseases associated with metabolic syndrome, such as hypertension, coronary artery disease, and diabetes [25] given that coronary disease is a leading cause of death in adults with intellectual disability [26]. Thus, not surprisingly, obesity and morbid obesity also have a higher prevalence in this group [27], and any weight gain should be discussed in particular detail, as it may uncover underlying metabolic disease or be the first sign of underlying heart failure. It is also important to ask about and look for evidence of congenital heart disease, which is common among adults with Down syndrome and may be present from birth (many are undiagnosed), may be only first diagnosed with the development of obvious symptoms as these adults age [28]. It is important to note, that unlike in adults with intellectual disability, while persons with Down syndrome have increased prevalence of congenital cardiac conditions, interestingly, there is a low percentage of atherosclerotic complications in this group, including coronary artery disease [20] and vascular dementia [29].

4.3.7 Gastrointestinal

The gastrointestinal review of systems should focus on any history or signs and symptoms of gastro-esophageal reflux disease (GERD), which is quite prevalent in this group [30, 31], and can cause discomfort, sleep disturbances, and cough. Asking about malabsorption syndromes in general, and celiac disease in particular, is recommended given its high association with Down syndrome, though there currently there is not an uniform recommendation regarding screening in these group [32]. Constipation has an increased prevalence in some people with intellectual disability [33], perhaps due to other underlying diseases (thyroid dysfunction), immobility, or diet [34]. Any change in character or nature of bowel habits should be fully explored. A review of the patient's diet for extent of fiber and healthy nutrients, and of nature of food intake is also important, recognizing that a change in eating habits may be a marker for a developing illness or disease, including cognitive decline. As with the general population, any significant weight gain or loss should be a red flag and explored in greater detail.

4.3.8 Genitourinary

The urological review of systems should include any new incontinence or any new symptoms of dysuria, polyuria or inability to complete normal self-toileting. Incontinence may be a major urological issue among certain adults with intellectual disability; thus, detailed a history should be obtained in an attempt to uncover the type, nature, and character of the incontinence. Often such a detailed history can reveal environmental and behavioral factors which can be modified to reduce incontinence or at least improve episodes so as to decrease caregiver burden.

A detailed sexual history is also important to obtain, with particular attention being paid to any signs or symptoms by history of sexual abuse, mistreatment, or any evidence of sexually transmitted diseases [35], which affect persons with intellectual and developmental disabilities disproportionately than from the general population. In women, presence of menstruation and related history and menopausal symptoms should be asked about, especially since women with Down syndrome generally experience an early menopause and may be predisposed to early osteoporosis [36].

4.3.9 Endocrine

Particular attention should be paid to signs and symptoms of hypothyroidism, especially as over 40% of older adults with Down syndrome experience hypothyroidism [20] Questions should include review of symptoms of both underactive or overactive thyroid and whether it is related to constipation, cold intolerance, weight loss or gain, palpitations, or related complaints. However, often such traditional symptoms may be lacking or may not be reportable and, therefore, the examiner must be careful to elicit detailed evidence of thyroid disease. Screening for Type II diabetes is indicated in patients with specific risk factors, such as obesity and coronary artery disease, among all adults with intellectual disability, although in Down syndrome adults due to the higher incidence of autoimmune disorders, Type I diabetes is an important consideration. Chapter 10 reviews endocrinological issues in adults with intellectual disability in greater depth.

4.3.10 Musculoskeletal

Any history of osteoporosis and bone loss should be reviewed, as well as any history of bone density testing and the use of supplemental vitamin D, calcium, estrogen replacement, or other treatments for osteoporosis [37, 38]. Individuals with intellectual disability should be asked about their mobility status and questioned about the presence, frequency, and character of any falls which have occurred.

4.3.11 Psychiatric

The examiner should ask specifically about changes in mood or other signs or symptoms of depression. Many times, as with other older adults, depression may be misdiagnosed as early dementia or some other behavioral disorder. Somatic symptoms in persons with intellectual disability are critical indicators of depression [39]. Depression in these populations may also present as a cognitive deficit, changing behavior, or functional decline. Behavioral changes should also be reviewed, as they could indicate a mood disorder or represent the first sign of dementia or other underlying medical disorder. Furthermore, behavioral disturbances can be a major limiting factor for safe caregiving, and must always be taken seriously and explored.

4.3.12 Medications

A comprehensive review of drug use should include both prescription and non-prescription (over-the-counter) medications. The use of multivitamins and medications, such as pain relievers, prophylactic antibiotics, and topical ointments is common [20]. One helpful approach is the "brown bag" method where caregivers are instructed to place all current medications (including non-prescribed substances) used in a bag and to bring them to the appointment. One other fact to consider is the increasing use in the general population of alternative and herbal therapies and medicines.

Finally, one must be sensitive to the issue of cultural diversity and native language and how such factors may affect history, perception of disease, and reporting of illness in various cultural groups. Differences in primary language usage by caregivers or adults with intellectual disability being examined and that of the examiner may introduce confusion in the value reporting of symptoms and explanations of behavior. Cultural, socio-economic, and environmental differences can impact not only direct care, but also caregiver roles, burden, expectations, and related perceptions [40, 41]. It is therefore important to be sensitive to the impact of cultural differences and their potential implications on patient health. The impact of polypharmacy in the intellectually disabled population is reviewed in Chap. 15.

4.4   Physical Examination

In completing the physical examination with adults with intellectual disability, the examiner should realize that it is important to always be flexible. Although standardized approaches should be used in general, the individual needs and capabilities of each adult require that the examiner be able to modify the general approach at any moment. All relevant symptoms and systems should be examined, but particular attention should be paid to completing as detailed an examination as possible on those specific organs and systems that may yield early diagnosis of conditions known to be common in this group. The associated history may be non-specific and may not point to a particular organ system as the sole source of morbidity. Any change in function, however, which may be the only presenting symptom or sign of a disease process, should prompt a thorough review and physical examination.

Before starting the physical examination, the patient should be made to feel as comfortable as possible in the examination room. If circumstances dictate, the patient should be examined where he or she would be most comfortable (remembering that flexibility is the key to a successful examination). Much of the physical examination can be performed in parts if the patient is unable to cooperate fully with the complete format. For example, observing a patient gait when walking out of the examination room, when rising from a chair, or when situating themselves onto the examination table can provide valuable information without the need for a formal gait assessment. Individuals may also need time to adjust to an unfamiliar environment, and parts of the exam can be revisited at a later time after the patient becomes more acclimated to the situation. Allowing the caregiver, who may have accompanied the adult, to stay with him or her during the examination may make the patient feel more relaxed and comfortable and may enhance the examination process. The examiner should follow an organized systematic format in conducting the physical examination, recognizing that modification and adaptation may be necessary depending on patient cooperation and related circumstances.

In general, observe the patient's overall appearance and presentation. Vital signs should be completed with blood pressure and pulse taken both lying and standing to check for evidence of orthostatic hypotension, which is common among adults with intellectual disability and may be due to medication side effects, and may be under-diagnosed or under-appreciated as the cause of falls, gait disturbance, or functional change in general. A gait assessment is an important step in evaluation, as many adults with intellectual disability have gait disturbances and balance problems which can lead to falls [42, 43], and which can be prevented with assistive devices or environmental adjustments. While there is no easily used office-based tool for gait assessment with this group, some tools taken from the general population may apply for investigating balance [44] For example, the Timed Get Up and Go Test [45] is a simple and efficient tool validated for use with other older adult; it can be considered for use with adults with intellectual disability.

The skin examination should focus on close examination of nails to check for fungal infection, which commonly occurs in persons with Down syndrome. In addition, any evidence of moles or related skin changes deserves a full and aggressive evaluation. Lack of patient cooperation and limited ability to follow certain directions may at times impact the ability to complete a detailed skin examination. However, the face, neck, arms and legs, chest, and back should always be examined for any new rash, moles, or changing character and nature of previously identified lesions.

Examination of the head should include close inspection for any evidence of trauma. Ears should be checked for cerumen impaction, and hearing should be screened as completely and routinely as possible. At times, traditional audioscopic evaluation may not be possible in some adults with intellectual disability due to communication difficulties. Therefore, the examiner may wish to rely on alternative methods to assess hearing. Rubbing the hands together or speaking softly to see if there is any change from either ear may be away to, in a less invasive manner, pick up hearing changes. Observing during the visit that a patient is not reacting to louder stimuli or requires frequent repetition of questions, may also be a rough indicator that hearing is impaired.

Detailed examination of the eyes may be best left to an ophthalmologist, but the primary care provider should complete routine screening for cataracts, which occur more commonly and can progress more quickly in adults with Down syndrome. Every patient should have routine oral and dental examinations not only to look for dental caries, but for any evidence of gingival hyperplasia or underlying gum disease, which may be the result of taking certain medications which are prescribed to people with intellectual disability. If adults have dentures, these should be removed during the oral exams for complete inspection of oral mucosa and to ensure dentures are being regularly cleaned.

The examination of the thyroid gland is extremely important given the high rate of thyroid disease among people with Down syndrome. Both poles of the thyroid should be inspected and palpated to evaluate for any nodules, enlargement, or goiters. Observing how the patient swallows a glass of water may be an additional maneuver which can be completed at the time of the thyroid examination. This may not only enhance the evaluation of the thyroid, but it may also reveal any underlying previously undetermined swallowing disorder or propensity toward aspiration. Even having the patient attempt to swallow various types of fluids may help, in a crude way, to complete a baseline swallowing assessment, which may uncover underlying dysphagia or odynophagia not previously appreciated and is particularly prevalent in this group [46].

A complete respiratory system examination is very important, recognizing that certain adults with intellectual disability have a propensity for recurrent pneumonias and related types of infections, especially as they age and are more prone to aspiration events due to dementia. Auscultation should include all lung fields and assess for any evidence of wheezing, rhonchi, rales, or changing character and nature of breath sounds. The cardiac examination should include a comprehensive auscultatory examination with particular attention to evaluate for any rubs, murmurs, gallops, or extra heartbeats. Special attention should be given to elements of the exam which may suggest cyanosis (such as, digital clubbing) given the prevalence of congenital heart defects in this group. The cardiac examination may reveal underlying disease which warrants further, more invasive, diagnostic testing.

The abdominal, genitalia and rectal examination may best be completed together. A high degree of sensitivity and flexibility will be required. If, for instance, a pelvic examination is absolutely clinically indicated because of vaginal bleeding, general sedation may be required (the use of sedation also may be the safest and most comfortable way to complete a detailed examination). These exams should always be performed with a chaperone and every step should be explained along the way.

All extremities should be checked for edema and peripheral vascular disease, and for any evidence of underlying musculoskeletal disorders. In addition, particular attention must be paid for any evidence of atlantoaxial subluxation syndrome or osteoporosis, which affects select adults with intellectual disability at earlier ages than it does in age-peers. Having the patient place both hands behind his or her head, or the lack of ability to complete this simple maneuver, may also help uncover underlying significant musculoskeletal disease which has a functional impact. The utility of a neurological examination may be limited depending on a patient's ability to follow directions, although any specific neurological deficits may require further detailed examination or additional diagnostic testing (i.e., an electroencephalogram or brain imaging). Such additional testing may be necessary especially if a vascular event or seizure may be a diagnostic consideration.

Finally, all adults with intellectual disability, especially as they age, should have a routine evaluation for cognitive changes. Although no standardized tool may be applicable due to the diversity of capabilities of this group, various screening tools may be useful when placing patient cognition into its appropriate context (i.e., collateral information is obtained regarding patient function over time). How cognitive decline is affecting daily activities and work performance should also be reviewed in detail [47]. Identifying cognitive impairment or dementia in adults with intellectual disability can prove to be particularly challenging, as standard tools for adults in the general population, such as the Mini Mental Status Examination, are likely to produce scores in abnormal range for most individuals with baseline impairment [48]. Although various tools are available to assess cognitive status in adults with intellectual disability, none has been fully validated for all levels of intellectual disability. A wide variation of neuropsychological tests are available [49]. Some can be completed by caregivers but others are by direct interview of the caregivers and/or the person with intellectual disability themselves. A few can be completed in 15–20 min but most tests take considerably longer. Some of the screening tools to consider include: The Dementia Questionnaire for Learning Disability [DLD] (formerly Dementia Questionnaire for Mentally Retarded Persons [DMR]) [50] or the Dementia Screening Questionnaire for Individuals with Intellectual Disabilities [51]. The Down Syndrome Dementia Questionnaire or the Brief Praxis Test [52] can also be used to obtain cognitive baselines and follow individuals over time, but take time as they involve applying measures that test the patient's performance abilities. A simpler measure, The NTG-EDSD [National Task Group-Early Detection and Screen for Dementia], is an early detection screen which incorporates a variant of the DSQIID and has some utility as it captures caregivers' observations of cognitive and functional change that can be followed up within the visit interview [53]. It is important to note that whatever test is chosen, clinicians should generally stick to one to two tools to administer in their practice and become familiar and comfortable with them. As with the general population, no one test will be diagnostic of dementia, but rather, a clinician must take caregiver assessment, changes in function and behaviors, as well objective testing over time, to make an accurate assessment.

A history of declining function, change in mood, memory loss, or related changes in daily activities may provide the first clue to declining cognition. The utility of whichever tools are used will be impacted by the patient's baseline cognitive status and related comorbidity. One important factor is that whatever baseline cognitive assessment is completed, it should be reapplied at various set intervals to pick up on any slight changes which might, otherwise, not be appreciated in the course of daily functioning. It is becoming increasingly clear that early identification, modification, and possible treatment of cognitive changes in adults with intellectual disability may be the best way to delay related morbidity and functional change as it relates to such cognitive decline, as well as to avoid unnecessary treatments and medications. It is important to provide caregivers with practical approaches to manage behaviors in non-pharmacological ways. Furthermore, early diagnosis can help aid families and caregivers in their advanced care planning and anticipate potential needs long before the patient declines.

4.5   Advanced Care Planning

As advances in medical care are leading to longer lifespans of adults with intellectual disability, they and their caregivers face issues of aging and chronic disease much more so than in previous decades. Assessing the physical health of persons with intellectual disability presents an opportunity to discuss advanced care planning, which can be complex and raise a number of ethical issues. Individuals with intellectual disability should not be assumed to lack capacity to make their own medical or end of life decisions. It is important to assess for decisional capacity in all patients, or seek input from a specialist, such as a psychiatrist, should capacity be unclear. If persons are deemed to lack decisional capacity, a surrogate decision-maker should be identified and secured. As these individuals age, often so do their caregivers, which can add an additional layer of complexity when planning for the future, both in terms of surrogate decision making and long term living arrangements. These issues should be identified and discussed as early as possible so that they are able to successfully and safely age with dignity.

4.6   Conclusion

The physical assessment of adults with intellectual disability can be both rewarding and challenging. By following routine and timely practices, many common conditions can be identified at early stages, such that real opportunities exist to minimize morbidity, and ultimately mortality. The history obtaining process may at times rely on surrogates, and thus, the examiner may need to adapt the standardized comprehensive approach in completing this aspect of the evaluation. Seeking out additional sources of information is crucial as an adjunct to that which may be provided by the adult and primary caregiver, or can be found in accompanying medical records. The physical examination should be comprehensive and complete with the realization that many times, because of a variety of factors, the examination may have to be modified or individualized. Ensuring that the person being examined is comfortable should be a high priority. By combining a detailed history with a focused examination, the clinical care of adults with intellectual disability can be optimized in such a way as to ensure the early identification of medical conditions and prompt appropriate treatment tailored to each person's life stage.

References

1. Cocks E, Thomson A, Thoresenm S, et al. Factors that affect the perceived health of adults with intellectual disability: a Western Australian study. J Intellect Dev Disabil. 2017;43:339. https://doi.org/10.3109/13668250.2017.1310816.
2. Ruddick L, Oliver C. The development of a health status measure for self-report by people with intellectual disabilities. J Appl Res Intellect Disabil. 2004;18:143–50. https://doi.org/10.1111/j.1468-3148.2005.00243.
3. Williamson HJ, Perkins EA. Family caregivers of adults with intellectual and developmental disabilities: outcomes associated with U.S. services and supports. J Intellect Dev Disabil. 2014;52:147–59.
4. Piazza VE, Floyd FJ, Mailick MR, Greenberg JS. Coping and psychological health of aging parents of adult children with developmental disabilities. Am J Intellect Dev Disabil. 2014;119:186–98.
5. Chou YC, Lee YC, Lin LC, Kroger T, Chang AN. Older and younger family caregivers of adults with intellectual disability: factors associated with future plans. J Intellect Dev Disabil. 2009;47:282–94.
6. Krauss MW, Seltzer MM, Jacobson HT. Adults with autism living at home or in non-family settings: positive and negative aspects of residential status. J Intellect Disabil Res. 2005;49:111–24.
7. Hu X, Summers JA, Turnbull A, Zuna N. The quantitative measurement of family quality of life: a review of available instruments. J Intellect Disabil Res. 2011;55:1098–114.
8. Thornberry C, Olson K. The abuse of individuals with developmental disabilities. Dev Disabil Bull. 2005;33(1-2):1–19.
9. Bureau of Justice Statistics. 2014. http://www.bjs.gov/index.cfm?ty=pbdetail&iid=5387.
10. Pulcini J, Taylor MO, Patelis T. The relationship between characteristics of women with mental retardation and outcomes of the gynecologic examination. Clin Excell Nurse Pract. 1999;3:221–9.
11. May ME, Kennedy CH. Health and problem behavior among people with intellectual disabilities. Behav Anal Pract. 2010;3:4–12.
12. Lee L, Rianto J, Raykar V, Creasey H, Waite L, Berry A, Chenoweth B, Kavanagh S, Naganathan V. Health and functional status of adults with intellectual disability referred to the specialist health care setting: a five-year experience. Int J Fam Med. 2011;2011:312492. https://doi.org/10.1155/2011/312492.
13. Beaton K, Grimmer K. Tools that assess functional decline: systematic literature review update. Clin Interv Aging. 2013;8:485–94.
14. Hilgenkamp TI, van Wijck R, Evenhuis HM. Instrumental activities of daily living in older adults with intellectual disabilities. Res Dev Disabil. 2011;32:1977–87.
15. McCue M, Chase S, Dowdy C. Functional assessment of individuals with cognitive disabilities: a desk reference for rehabilitation. Pittsburgh, PA: Center for Applied Neuropsychology; 1994.
16. Tasse MJ. Functional behavioural assessment in people with intellectual disabilities. Curr Opin Psychiatry. 2006;19:475–80.
17. Kerins G. Clinical conditions affecting older adults with Down's syndrome. Gerontologist. 1999;39:471.
18. Prater CD, Robert GZ. Medical care of adults with mental retardation. Am Fam Phys J. 2006;73:2175–83.
19. Schepsis C. Prevalence of atopic dermatitis in patients with Down's syndrome. A clinical survey. J Am Acad Dermatol. 1997;6:1019–21.

20. Kerins G, Petrovic K, Bruder M, Gruman C. Medical conditions and medication use in adults with Down syndrome: a descriptive analysis. Down Synd Res Pract. 2007;12:141–7. https://doi.org/10.3104/reports.2009.
21. Waterhouse E, Towne A. Seizures in the elderly: nuances in presentation and treatment. Cleve Clin J Med. 2005;72:S26–37.
22. Carvill S. Review: sensory impairments, intellectual disability and psychiatry. J Intellect Disabil Res. 2001;45:467–83.
23. McIlfatrick S, Taggart L, Truesdale-Kennedy M. Supporting women with intellectual disabilities to access breast cancer screening: a healthcare professional perspective. Eur J Cancer Care (Engl). 2011;20(3):412–20.
24. Chang CK, Chen CY, Broadbent M, Stewart R, O'Hara J. Hospital admissions for respiratory system diseases in adults with intellectual disabilities in Southeast London: a register-based cohort study. Br Med J Open. 2017;7:e014846.
25. de Winter CF, Bastiaanse LP, Hilgenkamp TI, Evenhuis HM, Echteld MA. Cardiovascular risk factors (diabetes, hypertension, hypercholesterolemia and metabolic syndrome) in older people with intellectual disability: results of the HA-ID study. Res Dev Disabil. 2012;33:1722–31.
26. Hollins S, Attard M, van Fraunhofer N, McGuigan SM, Sedgwick P. Mortality in people with learning disability: risks causes, and death certification findings in London. Dev Med Child Neurol. 1998;40:50–6.
27. Hsieh K, Rimmer JH, Heller T. Obesity and associated factors in adults with intellectual disability. J Intellect Disabil Res. 2014;58:851–63.
28. Murdoch J. Congenital heart disease as a significant factor in the morbidity of children with Down's syndrome. J Ment Defic Res. 1984;29:147–51.
29. Lott IT, Doran E, Nguyen VQ, Tournay A, Movsesyan N, Gillen DL. Down syndrome and dementia: seizures and cognitive decline. J Alzheimers Dis. 2012;29:177–85.
30. Bohmer CJ, Niezen-de Boer MC, Klinkenberg-Knol EC, Deville WL, Nadorp JH, Meuwissen SG. The prevalence of gastroesophageal reflux disease in institutionalized intellectually disabled individuals. Am J Gastroenterol. 1999;94:804–10.
31. Macchini F, Leva E, Torricelli M, Valade A. Treating acid reflux disease in patients with Down syndrome: pharmacological and physiological approaches. Clin Exp Gastroenterol. 2011;4:19–22.
32. Pavlovic M, Berenji K, Bukurov M. Screening of celiac disease in Down syndrome - Old and new dilemmas. World J Clin Cases. 2017;5:264–9.
33. Robertson J, Baines S, Emerson E, Hatton C. Constipation management in people with intellectual disability: a systematic review. J Appl Res Intellect Disabil. 2017; https://doi.org/10.1111/jar.12426.
34. Bohmer CJ, Taminiaum JA, Klinkenberg-Knolm EC, Meuwissen SG. The prevalence of constipation in institutionalized people with intellectual disability. J Intellect Disabil Res. 2001;45:212–8.
35. Servais L. Sexual health care in persons with intellectual disabilities. Ment Retard Dev Disabil Res Rev. 2006;12:48–56. https://doi.org/10.1002/mrdd.20093.
36. Schupf N, Zigman W, Kadell D, Lee JH. Early menopause in women with Down's syndrome. J Intellect Disabil Res. 1997;41:264–7.
37. Center J, Beange H, McElduff A. People with mental retardation have an increased prevalence of osteoporosis: a population study. Am J Ment Retard. 1998;103:19–28.
38. Geijer JR, Stanish HI, Draheim CC, Dengel DR. Bone mineral density in adults with Down syndrome, intellectual disability, and nondisabled adults. Am J Intellect Dev Disabil. 2014;119:107–14.
39. Mileviciute I, Hartley SL. Self-reported versus informant-reported depressive symptoms in adults with mild intellectual disability. J Intellect Disabil Res. 2015;59:158–69.
40. Coles S, Scior K. Public attitudes towards people with intellectual disabilities: a qualitative comparison of white British & South Asian people. J Appl Res Intellect Disabil. 2012;25:177–88.

41. Slevin E, McConkey R, Truesdale-Kennedy M, Taggart L. People with learning disabilities admitted to an assessment and treatment unit: impact on challenging behaviours and mental health problems. J Psychiatr Ment Health Nurs. 2008;15:537–46.
42. Chiba Y, Shimada A, Yoshida F, Keino H, Hasegawa M, Ikari H. Risk of fall for individuals with intellectual disability. Am J Intellect Dev Disabil. 2009;114:225–36.
43. Cox CR, Clemson L, Stancliffe RJ, Durvasulam S, Sherringtonm C. Incidence of and risk factors for falls among adults with an intellectual disability. J Intellect Disabil Res. 2010;54:1045–57.
44. Cuesta-Vargas A, Gine-Garriga M. Development of a new index of balance in adults with intellectual and developmental disabilities. PLoS One. 2014;9:e96529.
45. Podsiadlo D, Richardson S. The Timed "Up & Go": a test of basic functional mobility for frail elderly persons. J Am Geriatr Soc. 1991;14:142–8.
46. Chadwick DD, Jolliffe J. A descriptive investigation of dysphagia in adults with intellectual disabilities. J Intellect Disabil Res. 2009;53:29–43.
47. Zigman W, Schupf N, Sersen E, Silverman W. Prevalence of dementia in adults with and without Down's syndrome. Am J Ment Retard. 1996;100:403–12.
48. Deb S, Braganza J. Comparison of rating scales for the diagnosis of dementia in adults with Down's syndrome. J Intellect Disabil Res. 1999;43:400–7.
49. Prasher VP. Alzheimer's disease and dementia in Down syndrome and intellectual disabilities. Oxford: Radcliffe Publishing Limited; 2005.
50. Evenhuis H, Van Der Graaf G, Walinga M, Bindels-de Heus K, Van Genderen M, Verhoeff M, Lantau K, Van Der Meulen-Ennema H, Meester N, Wienen L, Schalij-Delfos N. Detection of childhood visual impairment in at-risk groups. J Pol Pract Intellect Disabil. 2007;4:165–9. https://doi.org/10.1111/j.1741-1130.2007.00114.
51. Deb S, Hare M, Prior L, Bhaumik S. Dementia screening questionnaire for individuals with intellectual disabilities. Br J Psychiatry. 2007;190:440–4.
52. Dalton AJ. Dyspraxia scale for adults with down syndrome. New York, NY: Aging Studies Consortium and Bytecraft Limited; 1996.
53. Esralew L, Janicki MP, Keller SM. National task group early detection screen for dementia (NTG-EDSD) [Chapter 11]. In: Prasher VP, editor. Neurological assessments of dementia in Down syndrome and intellectual disabilities. Appendix I. Basel: Springer; 2017. p. 197–213. https://doi.org/10.1007/978-3-319-61720-6_11.

Part II

Physical Health and Clinical Phenotypes

5

Andre Strydom, Alexander Curmi, and Andrew McQuillin

5.1   Introduction

This chapter explores the various physical health problems associated with specific syndromes, particularly genetic syndromes. These will be illustrated with examples of how various clinical phenotypes manifest in different systems (for example, central nervous system, cardiovascular, or respiratory) within the same and across different syndromes. Noteworthy is how different problems relate to each other— for example, cardiovascular problems associated with many syndromes can limit mobility, which can contribute towards obesity. Obesity can exacerbate hypertension and in turn, worsen cardiovascular problems. Negative or positive feedback loops like these are in many instances typical of pathophysiological processes. The clinician's foresight therefore, and the use of various preventative strategies, are key to managing these potential complications in an adult presenting with a particular clinical phenotype associated with genetic syndromes (see Table 5.1). The prognostic information associated with a syndrome diagnosis is therefore informative and can help to target surveillance and to design care plans.

Treatment and intervention approaches which may be employed are discussed in this chapter as they are critical for optimising quality of life and longevity. Care plans for adults with these complex clinical phenotypes benefit from being

A. Strydom (✉)
Department of Forensic and Neurodevelopmental Science, Institute of Psychiatry, Psychology and Neuroscience, King's College London, London, UK
e-mail: andre.strydom@kcl.ac.uk

A. Curmi
Maudsley Hospital, London, UK
e-mail: alexander.curmi@slam.nhs.uk

A. McQuillin
Molecular Psychiatry Laboratory, Division of Psychiatry, UCL, London, UK
e-mail: a.mcquillin@ucl.ac.uk

© Springer Nature Switzerland AG 2019
V. P. Prasher, M. P. Janicki (eds.), *Physical Health of Adults with Intellectual and Developmental Disabilities*, https://doi.org/10.1007/978-3-319-90083-4_5

Table 5.1 Major specific disorders

Disorder	Approximate incidence	Genetics	Intellectual disability	Major clinical phenotypes
Down syndrome	1:1000	Trisomy 21	Mild to severe	Typical craniofacial features and short stature, congenital cardiac defects, gastro-intestinal malformations, premature aging and Alzheimer's disease
Fragile X syndrome	1:4000	Unstable expansion of a CGG repeat in the *FMR1* gene on chromosome Xq27.3	Mild to moderate	Macro-orchidism, and distinct facial features, including long face, large ears, and prominent jaw. Increased risk of seizures
Angelman syndrome	1:24,000	Maternal Chromosome 15q11.2 deletion	Severe to profound	Motor dysfunction, craniofacial abnormalities, protruding tongue, seizures, hypotonia, absent speech
Cornelia de Lange	1:10,000–1:30,000	Mutation of the NIPBL gene on chromosome 5p13	Moderate to severe	Typical phenotype: small stature, limb abnormalities, characteristic facial features, self-injury, autistic behaviour, eye abnormalities. Mild phenotype also recognised. Associated with frequent infections, vision and hearing problems, GORD, cardiac defects, feeding problems, increased seizure risk
Cri-du-chat syndrome	1:20,000–1:50,000	Chromosome 5p deletion (mostly sporadic)	Mild to severe	Failure to thrive, characteristic facial features with high pitched cry, microcephaly, cardiac and gastrointestinal malformations, frequent infections, psychomotor dysfunction
Lowe syndrome	1–10: 1,000,000 Almost exclusively males	Mutation of *OCRL* gene on Chromosome Xq26	Moderate to severe (75% of cases)	Congenital eye abnormalities (hydrophthalmia), characteristic facial features, infantile hypotonia, renal dysfunction, serum enzyme and musculoskeletal abnormalities.

Syndrome	Prevalence	Genetics	Severity	Clinical features
Myotonic dystrophy	1:8000	Autosomal Dominant Heterozygous CTG repeat expansion in the *DMPK* gene on chromosome 19q13. A second less common form of Myotonic Dystrophy is caused by a tetranucleotide repeat expansion in the *CNBP* gene on chromosome 3q21.3	Mild to moderate (75% of cases)	Facial diplegia, musculoskeletal abnormalities, hypotonia, respiratory problems, feeding difficulties
Neurofibromatosis type 1	1:2600–3000	Autosomal dominant mutation of the *NF1* gene on chromosome 17q11	Borderline to mild	Macrocephaly, short stature, café au lait spots Associated with tumours, neurofibromas, and Lisch nodules in the central nervous system and endocrine disorders
Noonan syndrome	1:1000–1:2500	Heterogeneous, largely autosomal dominant but also sporadic mutations in one of four genes: *PTPN11* (chromosome 12q24.13), *SOS1* (chromosome 2p22.1), *RAF1* (chromosome 3p25.2) and *KRAS* (chromosome 12p12.1)	Mild	Characteristic facial features, short stature, delayed puberty, skeletal and cardio-respiratory abnormalities
Phenylketonuria	1:10,000	Autosomal Recessive mutation of the *PAH* gene on chromosome 12q23.2	Moderate to severe if not treated	Intellectual disability, if not treated
Prader-Willi syndrome	1:15,000	Paternal chromosome 15q11-q13 deletion	Borderline to moderate	Hypotonia, acromicria, failure to thrive, small stature, scoliosis, delayed puberty, skin picking, hyperphagia, obesity.

(continued)

Table 5.1 (continued)

Disorder	Approximate incidence	Genetics	Intellectual disability	Major clinical phenotypes
Rett syndrome	1:10,000 (almost exclusively females)	Mostly sporadic mutations in the *MECP2* on chromosome Xq28	Profound	Initially appear normal with regression at 18 months including physical, social and linguistic problems. Also involves breathing problems, ataxia, abnormal hand movements.
Smith Magenis	1: 25,000	Chromosome 17.p11.2 deletion	Moderate	Characteristic facial features, congenital abnormalities, aggression, scoliosis, sleep disturbance, self-injurious behaviour, hypothyroidism, visual and hearing problems
Tuberous sclerosis	1:7000	Autosomal dominant mutation of the *TSC1* gene on chromosome 9q34.3 or the *TSC2* gene on chromosome 16p13.13	Approximately half with moderate to severe intellectual disability	Behavioural abnormalities, hamartias, hamartomas, skin lesions, neoplasms (brain, renal, pulmonary), autism Increased risk of seizures
22q11.2 Deletion syndrome (Velocardiofacial syndrome or DiGeorge Syndrome)	1:3000	Autosomal dominant hemizygous chromosome 22q11.2 deletion	Mild	Failure to thrive, cleft palate, cerebellar ataxia, feeding problems, hypotonia, hypocalcemia, immune disorders. Raised incidence of respiratory infection and schizophrenia.
Williams syndrome	1:7500	Hemizygous deletion on chromosome 7q11.23 (usually sporadic)	Moderate to severe	Failure to thrive, characteristic faces, feeding problems multi-system abnormalities

formulated in multi-disciplinary settings with regular re-assessments. That being the case, ensuring appropriate access to services with reasonable adjustments made whenever possible is important when working with this group.

5.2 Genetic Concepts

Genetic Mutation—this is a permanent change in the deoxyribonucleic acid (DNA) sequence (this may involve only a single base pair or may include a long sequence of base pairs) such that the DNA sequence is different from that of the rest of the population. Mutations can be broadly divided into *hereditary* or *acquired*. Hereditary mutations (also known as *germ line mutations*) are inherited from the parents and are present in every cell in the individual's body. Conversely, acquired (otherwise known as sporadic or *somatic*) mutations are ones which develop during life. If a somatic mutation occurs very early during life (such as during embryogenesis) then the mutation may still be present in almost all of the cells of that individual's body, however the mutation would still be considered acquired.

Some examples of genetic mutations include insertions (where one or more new base pairs are added to a sequence of DNA), deletions (where one or more base pairs are removed from the sequence), and copy number variations (see below).

CNV (Copy Number Variations)—This is a phenomenon in which a DNA sequence (one kilobase or larger by some definitions) [1] is duplicated or deleted. CNVs are increasingly recognised contributors to genetic diversity within the human genome. Some CNVs may be "pathogenic" and have been linked with altered phenotypes and disease states while others appear to have no particular effect, although this is likely also dependent on other genetic and environmental influences. A recent study conducted in psychiatric clinics in the UK found that potentially pathogenic CNVs were identified in approximately 10–15% of adults with intellectual disability [2].

Tri-nucleotide repeat expansions—This occurs when a tri-nucleotide base sequence is repeated and the number of repeats of that sequence varies between different individuals. Tri-nucleotide repeats are inherited and tend to accumulate from one generation to the next. The number of repeats of the DNA sequence may have an impact on the clinical phenotype observed. A well-known example of this occurs in Fragile X syndrome (FXS) where the number of tri-nucleotide repeats (CGG sequence) on the FMR1 gene may influence the likelihood of developing the disorder and the severity of symptoms.

Pleiotropy—this is when one gene, gene mutation or alteration in chromosomal sequence exerts multiple seemingly unrelated phenotypic effects. This phenomenon explains how a single genetic trait can present clinically in a *syndromic* manner, i.e., with a well-known pattern of correlated signs and symptoms. An example of this is 22q11 deletion syndrome (also known as DiGeorge syndrome or velocardiofacial syndrome), where a deletion on chromosome 22 can cause congenital heart problems, cleft palate, developmental delay, vulnerability to infection as well as predisposition towards schizophrenia (with a prevalence estimated between 22% and 31%) [3] as opposed to 1% in the general population.

Penetrance and variable phenotypes—the penetrance of a particular genotype refers to the proportion of individuals with a particular genetic mutation that actually show clinical signs and symptoms. For example, in a mutation with 80% penetrance, 80% of the individuals with the mutation will develop the related clinical phenotype while 20% will not. Penetrance can be affected by a number of factors including CNVs (see above), environmental modifiers and epigenetic factors. Phenylketonuria is a disorder where inactivating mutations in the PAH gene encoding the enzyme phenylalanine hydroxylase lead to severe intellectual disability if a normal diet is consumed but little to no clinical effect if a phenylalanine restricted diet (*environmental modifier*) is consumed [4].

The pleiotropic effects of genes and variable penetrance of phenotypes explain why different individuals with the same mutation might present with slightly different phenotypic expression. Pleiotropy in combination with common pathways downstream from the genome might also be related to the observation of common phenotypes across some syndromes, for example, congenital heart disease occurring in several syndromes with different genetic mutations.

5.3   Morbidity and Mortality

Over the past 50 years the life expectancy of people with intellectual disability has increased significantly, however such individuals are still much more likely to die before the age of 50 than age peers in the general population [5]. Differences in life expectancy are correlated with the level of intellectual disability, in adults with mild intellectual disability it may in fact be approaching that of the general population [6]. Conversely, adults with moderate to severe intellectual disability have been shown to have all-cause mortality rates which are two or three times higher than the general population [7]. Various phenotypic factors may contribute to increasing morbidity and mortality, and these are noted by system throughout the chapter.

5.3.1   Cardiovascular Problems

Chromosomal abnormalities are often associated with a greater incidence of congenital cardiac malformations (see Table 5.1). Chromosomal disorders which have been associated with cardiac problems include:

5.3.1.1 Down Syndrome (Trisomy 21)

Congenital cardiac malformations are present in approximately 40–60% of individuals born with Down syndrome (DS) and these most commonly include atrioventricular septal defects (45%), ventricular septal defects (35%), secundum atrial septal defects (8%), patent ductus arteriosus (7%) and Teratology of Fallot

(4%). All new-borns with Down syndrome should be screened for these abnormalities at birth and the possibility of a previously undiagnosed malformation should be kept in mind at every medical review.

Surgical correction is now often offered for these malformations, and in general, individuals with DS and congenital cardiac malformations have a good prognosis. Nevertheless, surgical correction can also lead to acquired pathology such as mitral valve prolapse, aortic regurgitation and arrhythmias [8]. Mitral and tricuspid regurgitation is also a possible consequence of surgery [9]. Lastly, as with any individual with a known heart problem or who has undergone a cardiac procedure there is a greater risk of infective endocarditis.

In contrast to an early life risk for congenital heart disease, individuals with DS have a lower incidence of coronary artery disease and hypertension in adulthood, despite a greater incidence of obesity and its complications [10]. The risks of these conditions increases with age and therefore cardiac risk factors should still be monitored on a regular basis as DS individuals age.

5.3.1.2 22q11 Deletion Syndrome (Di George or Velo-Cardio-Facial Syndrome)

There are numerous congenital cardiac defects associated with this condition and they include: tetralogy of Fallot, pulmonary atresia with ventricular septal defect, truncus arteriosus, interrupted aortic arch, isolated anomalies of the aortic arch, and ventricular septal defects [11].

Treatment of these abnormalities typically involves surgical correction, however other presenting features of the disorder (increased vascular reactivity, altered immunological function, tendency towards airway bleeding, laryngeal web and hypocalcaemia) are likely to complicate surgical procedures for these patients. For that reason, specific surgical guidelines are required to manage these adults in the pre, intra and post-operative periods.

5.3.1.3 Turner Syndrome

Congenital cardiac malformations are common in Turner syndrome and are thought to be present in up to one third of adults with this condition [12]. The abnormalities include coarctation of the aorta and a bicuspid aortic valve, although other abnormalities such as hypertension, mitral valve prolapse and conduction defects are also known to occur [13].

Adults with Turner syndrome are also considered to be at increased risk of metabolic syndrome as a whole (hypertension, obesity, type 2 diabetes mellitus, acquired cardiovascular disease).

Cardiovascular problems are a major cause of mortality in Turner syndrome (reducing mortality by at least 10 years as compared to the general population) [14]. Therefore preventative measures such as diet control and management of sedentary lifestyle are essential. Regular cardiology reviews are also important with particular attention paid to cardiac risk factors such as dyslipidaemia and hypertension (even in the absence of congenital cardiac malformations).

5.3.1.4 Prader-Willi Syndrome

Prader-Willi syndrome is generally not associated with clinically significant congenital cardiac malformations. However, because these individuals are known to present with hyperphagia, obesity and type 2 diabetes, the possibility of cardiovascular disease in later life is a cause for concern.

There appears to be an association between Prader-Willi syndrome and sudden death, and there is a suspicion that this could be cardiovascular in origin [15]. Cardiac risk factors should therefore be monitored appropriately throughout life and appropriate preventative measures taken.

5.3.1.5 7q11.23 Deletions (Williams Syndrome)

Williams syndrome results from the deletion of some 26–28 genes, including the *ELN* gene (which codes for the protein Elastin). As a result, individuals with Williams syndrome tend to be hemizygous (only having one copy) of this gene, and this appears to be responsible for the vascular problems which occur in this syndrome [16].

Cardiovascular malformations are very common in adults with Williams syndrome, occurring in up to 80% [17]. A number of different cardiovascular malformations can occur, although the majority of individuals present with some form of aortic stenosis. As previously mentioned this appears to be due to a lack of elastin in these individuals which results in an arterial tree which is less compliant to haemodynamic forces [18]. The lack of elastin also results in unregulated proliferation of smooth muscle in the arterial wall causing occlusion of the lumen. Other cardiovascular abnormalities which tend to occur in Williams syndrome include pulmonary arterial stenosis, coronary artery abnormalities, ventricular septal defects and arrhythmias [19].

As with the other conditions mentioned in this section in-depth cardiovascular screening with regular follow up is essential. Management of these malformations is generally conservative, with approximately 20% requiring a surgical intervention of some kind [17].

Other conditions associated with congenital cardiac malformations include conditions such as Cri du chat and Wolf Hirschhorn syndrome. In conditions such as Fragile X syndrome cardiac malformations (such as dilatation of the aortic root and mitral valve prolapse) [20] tend to become apparent not at birth but in late childhood and adolescence [21]. In conditions such as Edwards syndrome and Patau syndrome where cardiac malformations are also highly prevalent the prognosis is particularly poor.

5.3.2   Respiratory Problems

5.3.2.1 Down Syndrome

Respiratory problems in individuals with DS can range from primary congenital lesions (which tend to be less common) such as narrowed airway or tracheoesophageal fistula to acquired disease such recurrent infection secondary to impaired immunity and/or aspiration. Babies presenting at birth with symptoms suggestive of respiratory problems should be screened appropriately and if necessary the appropriate surgical intervention applied.

It should be noted that throughout life respiratory problems are a major cause of morbidity and mortality, particularly due to infection or if co-morbid with cardiovascular problems. Obstructive sleep apnoea (OSA) is also very common in Down syndrome, and the severity of OSA in these individuals may be related to obesity [22]. Any signs or symptoms suggestive of respiratory de-compensation (related to sleep or otherwise) should therefore be promptly investigated and treated. It may be particularly useful to consider investigation for OSA during childhood as symptoms relating to OSA may not be spontaneously reported to the clinician by individuals or the caregivers and screening approaches may be unreliable.

5.3.2.2 Prader-Willi Syndrome

Individuals with Prader-Willi Syndrome have a primary abnormal respiratory response to hypoxia and hypercapnia, and this is further exacerbated by obesity. As a result, these adults often present with issues such as obstructive sleep apnoea or sleep related alveolar hypoventilation. Adults with Prader-Willi who present with suggestive symptoms (e.g.: excessive daytime sleepiness) should undergo a sleep study. Commonly applied interventions include behavioural management, weight control, a CPAP mask and adenotonsillectomy [23].

5.3.2.3 Other

Respiratory problems can manifest themselves in chromosomal disorders in a variety of other ways. In Rett syndrome (Xq28 mutation) individuals present with breathing problems both during wakefulness and sleep, characterised by periods of hyper and hypoventilation as well as apnoeic episodes [24].

In the mucopolysaccharidoses (such as Hurler and Hunter syndrome) individuals can present with frequent respiratory infections, obstruction of the respiratory tract (as a consequence of enlarged tonsils or adenoids [25], as well as a narrowed trachea, epiglottis and vocal cords [26]).

Cornelia de Lange syndrome (chromosome 5p13 mutation) is associated with a low-pitched "growling" cry during the neonatal period which tends to disappear by late infancy. It is also associated with frequent respiratory infections, particularly aspiration pneumonia as a result of co-morbid gastro-oesophageal reflex disease [27].

Conversely, Cri-du-chat syndrome (partial 5p15.12 deletion) is associated with a high pitched 'cat-like' cry (often due to laryngeal malformation) and a predisposition to respiratory problems which may include neonatal respiratory distress, bronchitis and pneumonia [28].

Chromosomal 4p16.3 deletion (Wolf Hirschhorn Syndrome) is another condition where certain clinical features such as typical facial characteristics and respiratory tract malformations (e.g.: pulmonary stenosis) pre-dispose these individuals to frequent lower respiratory tract infections. These infections represent a major cause of mortality [29] in these individuals who may require frequent treatment with antibiotics.

In 22q11.2 deletion syndrome (di George syndrome) respiratory infections can occur more frequently due to a combination of immunological deficiency, velopharyngeal insufficiency, swallowing difficulties, gastro-oseophaegeal reflux disease and in some cases tracheo-bronchomalacia [30].

It should be self-evident from the content of this section that individuals with chromosomal abnormalities have a predisposition to a variety of respiratory problems. Clinicians should be screening and investigating for these issues routinely, and managing them early and aggressively given their significant contribution to morbidity and mortality.

5.3.3 Gastrointestinal

5.3.3.1 Feeding Difficulties

Feeding difficulties are common in persons with genetic disorders (see Table 5.1) and are a major cause of failure to thrive in these individuals. Feeding difficulties normally arise as a consequence of problems at multiple levels (behaviour, anatomy, physiology) interacting with each other.

For example, conditions such as Down syndrome, Cri du chat, Fragile X, Lesch-Nyhan and Prader-Willi syndromes are associated with hypotonia which can lead to chewing and swallowing difficulties and increase the risk of aspiration pneumonia. In both Down syndrome and Cornelia de Lange syndrome there appears to be a high incidence of gastro-oesophageal reflux disease and its complications (oesophagitis, oesophageal stenosis and aspiration) and interestingly in Cornelia de Lange syndrome these symptoms appear to be associated with behavioural hyperactivity [31].

Noonan's syndrome can present with feeding difficulties in early life in the form of vomiting, abdominal pain, bloating and constipation, and this may be the result of reduced gastric motility (comparable to a pre-term infant) [32].

Assessment of any adult presenting with feeding difficulties should involve a multi-disciplinary approach to formulate a feeding plan which is both safe and realistic [33].

5.3.3.2 Congenital Gastrointestinal Malformations

Some chromosomal disorders are associated with congenital abnormalities of the gastrointestinal tract. One study estimated the incidence of chromosomal abnormalities in individuals presenting with gastrointestinal or abdominal wall malformations at birth to be 29% [34]. The most common chromosomal disorder implicated was Down syndrome.

Based on population surveys done in countries like Sweden and France the incidence of congenital gastrointestinal problems in persons with Down syndrome appears to be approximately 6–7% [35]. A 15-year study analysing data from 1892 individuals identified duodenal stenosis or atresia as the most common GI malformation associated with Down syndrome (3.9%) followed by anal stenosis or atresia (1%), Hirschsprung's disease (0.8%), oesophageal atresia or tracheoesophageal fistula (0.4%) and pyloric stenosis (0.3%) [36].

Conditions such as Edward's syndrome (Trisomy 18) and Patau syndrome (Trisomy 13) also commonly present with gastrointestinal malformations. Edwards syndrome is known to be associated with oesophageal atresia, diaphragmatic hernia, and ophalocoele (when the infant is born with abdominal viscera are outside the abdominal cavity). Patau syndrome is also associated with hernias and ophalocoele as well as exomphalos. As previously mentioned however, these conditions are associated with a very poor prognosis with individuals rarely surviving beyond the first few days of life.

Treatment of gastrointestinal malformations at birth usually necessitate early recognition, stabilisation and surgical correction with appropriate post-operative care.

5.3.3.3 Conditions with Dietary Implications

Phenylketonuria is a condition which results from the deficiency of the enzyme phenylalanine hydroxylase. As a result, adults with this condition require a restricted diet lacking in phenylalanine in order to prevent the most severe clinical manifestations of this disorder, which primarily consist of intellectual disability but may also include eczema, epilepsy and gait abnormalities. Early recognition of the disorder is essential, and current guidelines recommend the restriction of phenylalanine continue lifelong, despite the rigidity of the diet [37]. Generally the prognosis of treated phenylketonuria is considered excellent and life expectancy is normal.

Galactosemia is an autosomal recessive condition which results from the deficiency of the galactose-1-phosphate uridyl transferase (GALT) enzyme. It generally presents shortly after birth with failure to thrive along with a myriad of gastrointestinal symptoms such as vomiting, poor feeding, jaundice, hepatosplenomegaly. It can also present with symptoms such as renotubular dysfunction, cataracts, sepsis and hypotonia. Treatment of this condition generally involves a diet restricted from lactose and galactose, and when left untreated several neuropsychiatric complications occur. These include intellectual disability, and also motor dysfunction (such as cerebellar ataxia), verbal dyspraxia and extra-pyramidal signs [38].

Despite dietary restriction the prognosis in this condition does not appear to be as good as one might expect, with many treated adults still presenting with lower than expected IQ, dyspraxia, cataracts and motor signs. In addition the majority of women with the condition usually present with infertility due to ovarian failure. The reasons for this are as of yet unclear but may include intoxication due to endogenous metabolites of galactose or that the symptoms are a consequence of deficiency of certain glycoproteins or glycolipids found in galactose containing foods [39].

5.3.3.4 Other Gastrointestinal Disorders

Some conditions are associated with gastrointestinal problems which present later in life. Down syndrome appears to be associated with coeliac disease, with studies indicating the prevalence of this condition in adults with Down syndrome to be up to 18% [40]. This is far higher than in the general population in which the prevalence is generally estimated at 1%.

Williams syndrome (7q11.23 deletions) appears to be associated with diverticular disease, constipation as well as cholelithiasis [41]. These issues may partly result from hypercalcemia, which has also been associated with the condition [42].

5.3.4   Metabolic and Endocrine

5.3.4.1 Obesity

Obesity is commonly associated with a number of chromosomal disorders including but not limited to Down syndrome, Angelman syndrome, Turner syndrome, Williams syndrome and Prader-Willi syndrome (see Table 5.1). Obesity is a significant cause of morbidity and mortality in these populations, particularly if co-morbid with hypertension, cardiovascular disease and type 2 diabetes (metabolic syndrome).

Prader-Willi is thought to be most common 'syndromic' cause of obesity and is characterised by hyperphagia secondary to an impaired satiety response. This is likely due to hypothalamic dysregulation and is further complicated by the fact that these individuals tend to have a lower overall calorie requirement than individuals without the disorder [43].

Prevention and management of this problem relies on close monitoring of diet and regular physical exercise, and more severe cases (such as with Prader-Willi syndrome) may necessitate more intensive behavioural strategies and environmental interventions (e.g.: restricting sources of food at home).

5.3.4.2 Other Endocrine Disorders

Chromosomal disorders are associated with a number of different endocrine conditions. For example, Down syndrome appears to confer a predisposition to thyroid disease ranging from congenital hypothyroidism to Grave's disease to Hashimoto's thyroiditis. Studies have estimated the prevalence of thyroid disorders in these individuals to range from between 13% and 63% [44, 45] and a large retrospective cohort study conducted in the UK in 2016 found the incidence rate ratio for hypothyroidism in adults with Down syndrome to be 13.1 (95% CI 11.2–15.2) [46].

Adults with Down syndrome also appear to be at increased risk of developing type 1 diabetes, as indicated by a study in Denmark which found that a population of people with type 1 diabetes have a prevalence of Down syndrome four times greater than would otherwise be expected [47]. In contrast, a UK retrospective cohort study found the incidence rate ratio for diabetes (but not specifically type 1 diabetes) in adults with Down syndrome to be 1.3 [46].

Parathyroid conditions and serum calcium derangement can also be observed in some conditions. 22.q.11 deletion syndrome (velocardiofacial syndrome) is associated with hypoparathyroidism and consequent hypercalcemia. Conversely, Williams syndrome is known to present with infantile hypercalcemia [48].

Chromosomal disorders often present with growth and reproductive problems. For example, Turner syndrome is a known cause of delayed growth and premature ovarian failure [14]. Prader-Willi syndrome generally presents with short stature and can require treatment with exogenous growth hormone. Non-sex linked conditions can also affect reproductive function, as previously mentioned classical galactosemia generally results in infertility in women, and this is likely a result of hypergonadotropic hypogonadism [39].

When dealing with an adult with a particular chromosomal abnormality it is important for clinicians to be aware of the associated endocrine conditions as they can present insidiously and with a wide variety of seemingly unrelated symptoms.

5.3.5 Neurological System

5.3.5.1 Neurodegenerative Diseases

Alzheimer's disease is the most common known neurodegenerative condition, and the cause of the most cases of dementia. Alzheimer's disease is exceedingly common in Down syndrome, with an estimated prevalence of greater than 90% in those over 60 years of age. This is thought to be due to the duplication of the amyloid precursor protein (APP) gene on chromosome 21 [49]. Amyloid precursor protein is the precursor to beta-amyloid which is a protein thought to be central to the pathophysiology of Alzheimer's disease. In contrast to adults in the general population, adults with Down syndrome with emerging dementia may present with behavioural problems (for example irritability, aggression, apathy) prior to overt deficits of memory [50].

Because of the wide variety of possible clinical presentations in these individuals it is crucial that clinicians have a high index of suspicion for the possibility of dementia in ageing adults with Down syndrome and refer them early for cognitive and functional assessment.

5.3.5.2 Epilepsy (Seizures)

Epilepsy (seizure disorders) is commonly encountered in adults with intellectual disability (both those with and without a diagnosed chromosomal abnormality) (see Table 5.1). In addition, the prevalence of epilepsy and seizures in this population appears to be directly proportional to the degree of intellectual disability with an average prevalence of 22.2% [51].

Conditions known to be associated with epilepsy include tuberous sclerosis, Down syndrome, Fragile X syndrome, phenylketonuria (particularly if untreated), Rett syndrome and Wolf-Hirschhorn syndrome.

Epilepsy in individuals with co-morbid intellectual disability represents a significant cause of morbidity and mortality in these individuals, but is under-researched [52]. Nevertheless, clinicians working with these adults should be routinely screening for signs and symptoms which could be suggestive of seizure activity (particularly more subtle presentations, such as absences or behavioural problems) and referring appropriately for neurological investigations, such as EEG.

5.4   Conclusion

As our understanding of the many syndromes which are associated with intellectual disability becomes more sophisticated and our management of these conditions more adept, life expectancy is also increasing. This is obviously desirable, however extended life-span does present challenges to the issue of quality of life, which has a direct relationship to physical health and lifestyle factors.

The role of healthcare providers for this population is gradually changing towards a pattern of preventing and managing chronic illness (as it has for the general population). This new dynamic necessitates an in depth understanding of the particular sets of physical problems commonly encountered in individuals with particular clinical phenotypes. In this chapter we outlined major health co-morbidities associated with some of the more common genetic causes of intellectual disability and commented on how they could be investigated and managed.

References

1. Clancy S. Copy number variation. Nat Educ. 2008;1:95.
2. Wolfe K, Strydom A, Morrogh D, Carter J, Cutajar P, Eyeoyibo M, Hassiotis A, McCarthy J, Mukherjee R, Paschos D, Perumal N, Read S, Shankar R, Sharif S, Thirulokachandran S, Thygesen JH, Patch C, Ogilvie C, Flinter F, McQuillin A, Bass N. Chromosomal microarray testing in adults with intellectual disability presenting with co-morbid psychiatric disorders. Eur J Hum Genet. 2016;25:66–72.
3. Bassett AS. Schizophrenia and 22q11.2 deletion syndrome. Curr Psychiatry Rep. 2008;10:148–57.
4. Cooper DN, Krawxzak M, Polychronakos C, Tyler-Smith C, Kehrer-Sawatzki H. Where genotype is not predictive of phenotype: towards an understanding of the molecular basis of reduced penetrance in human inherited disease. Hum Genet. 2013;132:1077–130.
5. Emerson E, Baines S. Health inequalities and people with learning disabilities in the UK: 2010. Durham: Improving Health & Lives: Learning Disabilities Observatory; 2010.
6. Puri BK, Lekh SK, Langa A, Zaman R, Singh I. Mortality in a hospitalized mentally handicapped population: a 10-year survey. J Intellect Disabil Res. 1995;39:442–6.
7. Tyrer F, McGrother C. Cause-specific mortality and death certificate reporting in adults with moderate to profound intellectual disabilities. J Intellect Disabil Res. 2009;53:898–904.
8. Marder L, Tulloh R, Pascall E. Cardiac disorders in people with Down's syndrome. Paediatr Child Health. 2015;25:23–9.
9. Stos B, Dembour G, Ovaert C, Barrea C, Arape A, Stijns M, Sluysmans T. Risks and benefits of cardiac surgery in Down syndrome with congenital heart disease. Archiv Paediatr. 2004;11:1197–201.
10. Basil JS, Santoro SL, Martin LJ, Healy KW, Chini BA, Saal HM. Retrospective study of obesity in children with down syndrome. J Paediatr. 2016;173:143–8.
11. Carotti A, Digilio MC, Piacentini G, Saffirio C, Di Donato RM, Marino B. Cardiac surgery in 22q11.2 deletion syndrome. Dev Disabil Res Rev. 2008;14:35–42.
12. Dulac Y, Pienkowski C, Abadir S, Tauber M, Acar P. Cardiovascular abnormalities in Turner's syndrome: what prevention? Arch Cardiovasc Dis. 2008;101:485–90.
13. Sybert VP. Cardiovascular malformations and complications in turner syndrome. Pediatrics. 1998;101:e11.
14. Ostberg JE, Conway GS. Adulthood in women with Turner's syndrome. Horm Res. 2003;59:211–21.
15. Patel S, Harmer JA, Loughnan G, Skilton MR, Steinbeck K, Celermajer DS. Characteristics of cardiac and vascular structure and function in Prader-Willi syndrome. Clin Endocrinol (Oxf). 2007;66:771–7.
16. Keating MT. Genetic approaches to cardiovascular disease: supravalvular aortic stenosis, Williams syndrome, and long-QT syndrome. Circulation. 1995;92:142–7.

17. Collins RT II, Kaplan P, Somes GW, Rome JJ. Long-term outcomes of patients with cardiovascular abnormalities and Williams syndrome. Am J Cardiol. 2010;105:874–8.
18. Salaymeh KJ, Banerjee A. Evaluation of arterial stiffness in children with Williams syndrome: does it play a role in evolving hypertension? Am Heart J. 2001;142:549–55.
19. Collins RT. Cardiovascular disease in Williams syndrome. Circulation. 2013;127:2125–34.
20. Sreeram N, Wren C, Bhate M, Roberston P, Hunter S. Cardiac abnormalities in the fragile X syndrome. Br Heart J. 1989;61:289–91.
21. Crabbe LS, Bensky AS, Hornstein L, Schwartz DC. Cardiovascular abnormalities in children with fragile X syndrome. Pediatrics. 1993;91:714–5.
22. Trois MS, Capone GT, Lutz JA, Melendres MC, Schwartz AR, Collop NA, Marcus CL. Obstructive sleep apnea in adults with Down syndrome. J Clin Sleep Med. 2009;5:317–23.
23. Nixon GM, Brouilette RT. Sleep and breathing in Prader-Willi syndrome. Pediatr Pulmonol. 2002;34:209–17.
24. Ramirez JM, Ward CS, Neul JL. Breathing challenges in Rett syndrome: lessons learned from humans and animal models. Respir Physiol Neurobiol. 2013;189:280–7.
25. Shapiro J, Strome M, Crocker AC. Airway obstruction and sleep apnea in Hurler and Hunter syndromes. Ann Otol Rhinol Laryngol. 1985;94:458–61.
26. Peters ME, Arya S, Langer LO, Gilbert EF, Carlson R, Adkins W. Narrow Trachea in mucopolysaccharidoses. Pediatr Radiol. 1985;15:225–8.
27. Chen H. De Lange syndrome. Atlas of genetic diagnosis and counselling. New York, NY: Springer; 2006. p. 276–81.
28. Shapiro AJ, Weck KE, Chao KC, Rosenfeld M, Nygren AOH, Knowles MR. Cri du chat syndrome and primary ciliary dyskinesia. J Pediatr. 2014;165:858–61.
29. Gamble J, Kruian D, Udani A, Greene N. Airway management in a patient with Wolf-Hirschhorn syndrome. Case Rep Paediatr. 2016;2016:7070125.
30. Davies EG. Immunodeficiency in DiGeorge syndrome and options for treating cases with complete athymia. Front Immunol. 2013;4:322.
31. Luzzani S, Macchini F, Valade A, Milani D, Selicorni A. Gastroesophageal reflux and Cornelia de Lange syndrome: typical and atypical symptoms. Am J Med Genet. 2003;119A:283–7.
32. Shah N, Rodriguez M, St. Louis D, Lindley K, Milla PJ. Feeding difficulties and foregut dysmotility in Noonan's syndrome. Arch Dis Child. 1999;81:28–31.
33. Cooper-Brown L, Copeland S, Dailey S, Downey D, Petersen MC, Stimson C, Van Dyke DC. Feeding and swallowing dysfunction in genetic syndromes. Dev Disabil Res Rev. 2008;14:147–57.
34. Nicolaides KH, Snijders RJ, Cheng HH, Gosden C. Fetal gastro-intestinal and abdominal wall defects: associated malformations and chromosomal abnormalities. Fetal Diagn Ther. 1992;7:102–15.
35. Holmes G. Gastrointestinal disorders in Down syndrome. Gastroenterol Hepatol Bed Bench. 2014;7:6–8.
36. Freeman SB, Tofs CP, Romitti PA, Royle MH, Druschel C, Hobbs CA, Sherman SL. Congenital gastrointestinal defects in Down Syndrome: a report from the Atlanta and National Down Syndrome projects. Clin Genet. 2009;75:180–4.
37. Vockley J, Andersson HC, Antshel KM, Braverman NE, Burton BK, Frazier DM, Mitchell J, Smith WE, Thompson BH, Berry SA, American College of Medical Genetics and Genomics Therapeutics Committee. Phenylalanine hydroxylase deficiency: diagnosis and management guideline. ACMG practice guidelines. Genet Med. 2014;16:188–200.
38. Bosch AM. Classical galactosaemia revisited. J Inherit Metab Dis. 2006;29:516–25.
39. Schweitzer S, Shin Y, Jakobs C, Brodehl J. Long-term outcome in 134 patients with galactosaemia. Eur J Paediatr. 1993;152:36–43.
40. Pavlovic M, Berenji K, Bukurov M. Screening of celiac disease in Down syndrome - Old and new dilemmas. World J Clin Cases. 2017;5:264–9.
41. Morris CA, Leonard CO, Ditts C, Demsey SA. Adults with Williams syndrome. Am J Med Genet. 1990;6:102–7.

42. Sangun O, Dundar BN. Severe Hypercalcemia associated with Williams syndrome success-fully treated with pamidronate infusion therapy. J Pediatr Endocrinol Metab. 2011;6:102–7.
43. Swaab DF. Prader-Willi syndrome and the hypothalamus. Acta Paediatr. 1997;423:50–4.
44. Hardy O, Worley G, Lee MM, Chaing S, Mackey J, Crissman B, Kishnani PS. Hypothyroidism in Down syndrome: screening guidelines and testing methodology. Am J Med Genet. 2004;124A:436–7.
45. Lavigne J, Sharr C, Elsharkawi I, Ozonoff A, Baumer N, Brasington C, Cannon S, Crissman B. Thyroid dysfunction in patients with Down Syndrome: results from a multi-institutional registry study. Am J Med Genet. 2017;173:1539–45.
46. Alexander M, Petri H, Ding Y, Wandel C, Khwaja O, Foskett N. Morbidity and medication in a large population of individuals with Down Syndrome compared to the general population. Dev Med Child Neurol. 2016;58:246–54.
47. Bergholdt R, Eising S, Nerup J, Pociot F. Increased prevalence of Down's syndrome in indi-viduals with type 1 diabetes in Denmark: a nationwide population-based study. Diabetologia. 2006;49:1179.
48. Pescovitz OH, Eugster EA. Pediatric endocrinology: mechanisms, manifestations and man-agement. Philadelphia, PA: Lippincott Williams & Wilkins; 2004. p. 9–10.
49. Wiseman FK, Al-Janabi T, Hardy J, Karmiloff-Smith A, Nizetic D, Tybulewicz V, Fisher E, Strydom A. A genetic cause of Alzheimer disease: mechanistic insights from Down Syndrome. Nat Rev Neurosci. 2015;16:564–74.
50. Zis P, Strydom A. Clinical aspects and biomarkers of Alzheimer's disease in Down Syndrome. Free Radic Biol Med. 2018;114:3–9.
51. Robertson J, Hatton C, Emerson E, Baines S. Prevalence of epilepsy among people with intel-lectual disabilities: a systematic review. Seizure. 2015;29:46–62.
52. Lhatoo SD, Sander JWAS. The epidemiology of epilepsy and learning disability. Epilepsia. 2001;1(42):6–9.

Health Status of Adults with Cerebral Palsy

6

Margaret A. Turk and Robert J. Fortuna

6.1 Background

Cerebral Palsy (CP) is among the most common causes for childhood physical disability, with many individuals now living into later adulthood. Although the complex care needs of children with CP are well appreciated, they are frequently less recognized in adults. CP presents as a group of varied conditions, defined by motor dysfunction. These problems with movement and posture are the consequence of an early injury to or anomaly of the developing brain. The injury is permanent and nonprogressive, but the clinical manifestations may change over time through brain maturation and aging. The motor and activity limitations are often accompanied by epilepsy, secondary musculoskeletal problems, and difficulties with sensation, perception, cognition, communication, and behavior [1]. There is no single etiology accountable for CP, but rather a number of possible etiologies, including infection, brain malformations, brain hemorrhage or infarction, prematurity, cerebral hypoxemia, and hyperbilirubinemia. Onset can be pre-natal, natal, or post-natal (insult to an immature brain), with the upper age of onset for inclusion variably described between 2 and 8 years [2]. A diagnosis of CP does not imply an etiology, but rather describes the result of the insult—the motor impairment.

M. A. Turk (✉)
Physical Medicine & Rehabilitation, Pediatrics, and Public Health & Preventive Medicine, SUNY Upstate Medical University, Syracuse, NY, USA
e-mail: turkm@upstate.edu

R. J. Fortuna
Internal Medicine, Pediatrics, and Community Health, University of Rochester School of Medicine and Dentistry, Rochester, NY, USA
e-mail: Robert_Fortuna@URMC.Rochester.edu

© Springer Nature Switzerland AG 2019
V. P. Prasher, M. P. Janicki (eds.), *Physical Health of Adults with Intellectual and Developmental Disabilities*, https://doi.org/10.1007/978-3-319-90083-4_6

6.1.1   Classification Systems

CP is the result of an upper motor neuron insult. There is a range of motor impairment and severity that can be seen, and these are described by measures of motor function and/or activity. Categories of motor abnormalities and topographical patterns of abnormal muscle tone are traditionally used to describe CP. Additionally, function scales are used to define motor severity (see Table 6.1).

There are typically two groups of motor abnormalities described: pyramidal (spastic) and extrapyramidal (ataxic, dyskinetic/athetoid/dystonic). There can also be a mixed presentation of co-existing pyramidal and extrapyramidal signs, although one type usually predominates. At one time, hypotonia was included under the umbrella of CP, but more recently specific etiologies are now able to be diagnosed (e.g., chromosomal abnormalities, autism spectrum disorder); thus, although hypotonia is not consistently included in adults, the identifier may still be present.

Topographical patterns of spasticity describe the number of limbs involved. These include monoplegia (one limb, which may also represent hemiparesis with one limb more significantly involved than the other), hemiplegia/paresis (arm and leg on one side), diplegia (both arms involved more than both leg), triplegia (three limbs, which may represent quadriparesis with one limb having significantly better function compared to the other three), and quadriplegia/paresis (generalized process with all four limbs involved). An alternative approach is to differentiate between unilateral (mono/hemiplegia) and bilateral CP. The Surveillance of Cerebral Palsy in Europe network [3] uses this system to simplify classifications. This language is also used in research to define participants and compare outcomes.

Table 6.1 Classification for adults with cerebral palsy

Motor abnormalities	Topographical patterns	Gross Motor Function Classification System (GMFCS) by level	Manual Ability Classification System (MACS) by level
Pyramidal – Spastic	Topographical patterns	I: Walks without limitations	I: Handles objects easily and successfully
Extrapyramidal – Dyskinetic – Dystonic – Athetoid – Ataxic	– Monoplegia – Hemiplegia – Diplegia – Triplegia – Quadriplegia	II: Walks in most settings; may require assist and may use wheelchair III: Capable of walking using a hand-held assistive mobility device; may also use wheelchair independently for long distances IV: Self-mobility with wheelchair with limitations; may use powered mobility V: Transported in a manual wheelchair	II: Handles most objects but with somewhat reduced quality or speed of achievement III: Handles objects with difficulty; needs help to prepare or modify activities IV: Handles a limited selection of easily managed objects in adapted situations V: Does not handle objects and has severely limited ability to perform even simple actions
Hypotonia			

Severity is defined by motor function scales, which provide objective measures of impairment. The two most widely used measures to quantify motor function, and therefore severity, are the Gross Motor Function Classification System (GMFCS E&R) [4, 5] and the Manual Ability Classification System (MACS) [6]. The GMFCS has been shown to be stable into adulthood, with relatively good prediction of the level of adult gross motor functioning determined by age 12 years [7]. The MACS has not been fully validated for adults; however, stability of assessments [8] and reliability to age 24 years have been established [9]. Oral motor function (including communication, feeding, and swallowing) should also be defined, however no single measurement tool has been accepted as a standard in children or adults. In a comparison study of the GMFCS E&R, MACS, and a communication 5-level scale (Communication Function Classification System) it was noted that the three scales were complementary and helped to provide a useful functional profile of children with CP [10].

6.1.2   Associated Conditions, Secondary Conditions, and Co-morbidities

Associated conditions are those that are commonly seen in people with CP. These conditions are the residual of the underlying pathophysiology and are often present at the time of the diagnosis of CP, although may manifest more over time. Common associated conditions are intellectual disability, seizures, learning disabilities, vision or hearing impairments, and other issues related to poor motor control (e.g., poor oral motor control and feeding resulting in poor weight gain, reflux, development of spasticity, constipation, incontinence). A literature review published in 2006 identified that a large proportion of people with CP had cognitive impairment that varied with the type of CP [11].

Secondary conditions are additional physical or mental health conditions for which the primary disabling condition poses an increased risk for development. There is variability in the timing of presentation, and it is believed that some of these conditions may be preventable. Common secondary conditions for people with CP include fatigue, pain, osteoporosis, and depression.

Comorbid conditions are not known to be causally related to CP, and therefore not associated or secondary conditions. These conditions are those seen in the general population, and adults with CP may be at risk for developing them based on genetic predisposition or the presence of other risk factors. As the linkages between CP and specific health conditions are better understood, conditions now called comorbidities, may in fact be viewed as secondary conditions in the future (e.g., immobility and loss of muscle mass, as a risk for sarcopenia, obesity, malignancy, and vascular disease).

6.2   Epidemiology and Outcomes

There are a variety of strategies world-wide to monitor the prevalence of CP. European and Scandinavian countries provide epidemiologic information from national registries and surveillance systems. Similarly, Canada and Australia have developed national registries. The U.S. monitors through a population-based record-review surveillance system over four regions of the country. Prevalence rates range from 1.5 to 4 per 1000 live births [12–16]), and a pooled overall prevalence of CP is reported at about 2 per 1000 live births [17]. This has been stable over recent years, in the face of improved survival of at-risk premature infants. However, there is no report of the prevalence of CP in an adult population, and all prevalence statistics for adults are usually extrapolated.

6.2.1   Motor Abnormality and Topographical Patterns

In children, the spastic form of CP is the most common. It is commonly believed that this pattern of topographic prevalence persists into adulthood. Bilateral spastic CP is more common than unilateral [3, 18]. Dyskinetic and ataxic forms are usually reported as less than 10%.

6.2.2   Life Expectancy and Mortality

In recent decades, most children with CP survive into adulthood, including those with severe limitations [19–21]. Survival through adulthood appears to be related to the extent of severe impairments. In earlier analyses of U.S. administrative data from the California Department of Developmental Services, survival in high func-tioning adults with CP was more closely aligned with survival in the general popula-tion [22]. In contrast, older subjects with the most severe disabilities rarely survived to age 60 years [23]. More significant impairments and the number of severe impair-ments (usually related to mobility, manual dexterity, feeding, cognition, and/or vision) all affect survival [19–21]. Epilepsy and seizures, commonly associated with CP, especially in those adults with hemiplegia and quadriplegia [11], is associ-ated with an increased risk of death [24]. The need for gastrostomy tube feeding has also consistently been identified as an indicator for increased mortality [25]. In a report on long-term survival of a U.K. cohort born 1940–1950, many of the deaths noted in ages 20–30 years were related to respiratory causes, and deaths in ages 40–50 years were attributable to circulatory conditions and neoplasms [26]. The notion of increased neoplasm as cause for death rates is echoed by the large California database noting a three-times-higher rate for breast cancer in CP than in the general population. This observation may be related to poorer screening and/or treatment [27], or may be related to the hypothesized inflammatory mechanism linkage with chronic neurologic injury and/or obesity [28].

6.2.3   Health Care Utilization

The health care needs of most adults with CP remain complex, involve a variety of clinical resources and medical technologies, and often require specialty services

[29, 30]. A study using data from the Canadian Institute for Health Information, found that utilization rates of outpatient services were 1.9 times higher for adults with CP when compared to age-matched peers [31]. For these same age groups, pneumonia and epilepsy were the most common reasons for hospitalization, followed by mental health issues, infections other than pneumonia, urinary tract infections, lower gastrointestinal problems or constipation, and upper gastrointestinal problems, such as acute gastritis, chronic gastric ulcers, and esophagitis [31]. GMFCS level was also found to be associated with health care utilization [32]. GMFCS III through V were associated with more needs related to mobility aids, orthotics, and therapy and rehabilitation services. Adults with GMFCS IV-V levels showed even greater physician contact and higher usage of some medications (e.g., psychotropics, antiepileptics, laxatives, spasmolytics). Despite increased utilization reported in children, adults with CP, particularly those with lower levels of motor function, had many unmet needs, especially related to support for their mobility needs, and easy access to health services [30].

6.2.4   Performance Changes with Aging

While the insult causing CP is static, the manifestation of secondary conditions and onset of typical aging processes usually result in performance changes and decreasing function over time, often prematurely. The GMFCS scale has allowed researchers to note that level of adult gross motor functioning is usually determined by age 12 years [7]. However, many adults with CP who are able to walk experience decline in walking ability earlier than peers without disability [33]. Therefore, clinicians must be vigilante for health conditions or environmental issues that may influence performance. Adults with CP should not be expected to increase one or two GMFCS levels (i.e., loss of function). If a significant functional decline is noted, an evaluation for etiologies must ensue. Many cross-sectional and convenience samples have identified that there are a variety of reasons for performance change, such as musculoskeletal and cardiovascular issues, obesity, and mental health problems [34–36]. Significant performance change may also increase risk for mortality. A Californian study noted older subjects who lost the ability to walk by age 60 years had poor prognosis for survival [23]. Early recognition of health issues, development of an accessible and appropriate care plan, and continued monitoring are important to assure continued function.

6.2.5   Health-Related Quality of Life and Life Satisfaction

Quality of Life (QOL) remains difficult to measure because of the complex ongoing inter-relationships among function, contextual factors, and individuals' perceptions. Young et al. reported that QOL indicators may vary based on the severity of CP [37]. Although early studies of adults with mild to moderate impairments noted that adults with CP generally reported a good quality of life [38], recent studies that included those with severe CP reported lower health and quality of life scores for youth and young adults than previously reported [37]. Loneliness of older adults with CP has been explored qualitatively. One theme that emerged is common to a typical aging population: importance of social networks. The second relates directly to CP and poor motor control: need to facilitate opportunities for adults with CP to participate in meaningful communication [39]. Given the reports about unmet needs and the need for information and communication support, optimizing any co-occurring medical and functional conditions, addressing mental health concerns, discussing sexual health, and increasing social connectedness may all contribute to improved quality of life for adults with CP.

6.3   Health Conditions

Adults with CP, as they mature and age, usually continue with many of the same conditions they experienced at a younger age. Adults may also develop secondary health conditions related to CP, or other conditions commonly seen in the general population with advancing age. Adults with CP appear to be at greater risk for poorer health and functional outcomes than adults without CP due to sedentary behaviors, sarcopenia, obesity, and cardiometabolic disorders [36, 39]. The most commonly reported conditions in adults with CP are musculoskeletal impairments, fatigue, pain, seizures, intellectual disability, and osteoporosis [28, 36, 40–47]. Obesity status and GMFCS IV-V levels have been found to be associated with multi-morbidity profiles involving prehypertension/hypertension, osteoporosis, osteoarthritis, and asthma [40]. Table 6.2 lists common health conditions for adults with CP.

It is also important to note that conditions that commonly occur in the general population with aging frequently go undetected in many persons with intellectual disability. This is due, in part, to barriers to accessing health care, receiving treatments, and communicating effectively [49–54]. Open communication and clinical recognition of these conditions is vital to providing quality care to adults with CP. Eliciting a typical history and engaging the adult with CP in the process should be undertaken. As well, an appropriate examination is necessary, including examining the person out of the wheelchair. Comprehensive care of adults with CP, therefore, must address conditions associated with CP as well as conditions that are common with aging.

6.4   Musculoskeletal

Musculoskeletal disorders are among the most common complaints of adults in general, especially those over age 65 [55]. A recent analysis of U.S. Medicare claims noted that there was high utilization of care for musculoskeletal disorders among adults with CP, especially among those with athetoid or quadriplegia subgroups (personal communication, D. Thorpe 2018).

Table 6.2 Common health conditions in adults with cerebral palsy[a]

Common related health conditions	Prevention strategies	Treatment strategies
Pain Fatigue	• Routine exercise • Work simplification • Ergonomic evaluations	• Exercise prescription • Encourage good sleep hygiene • Evaluate for pain etiology and treat • Modify equipment or workplace • Evaluate mental health and manage • Progress to pain management program
Musculoskeletal Contractures Hip pathology Knee pathology Foot or ankle pain Back pain	• Monitor and query routinely • Joint protection strategies • Routine exercise • Biomechanic and ergonomic assessments	• Focal musculoskeletal evaluation • Tone management • Modify equipment, workplace, biomechanics of function • Physical therapy prescription • Adjust orthoses and wheelchair
Bone health Osteoporosis Fractures	• Routine exercise, especially weight bearing • Consider calcium/VitD supplement only if osteoporosis and risk factors present • Fracture and fall prevention	• DXA evaluation • Exercise when appropriate
Neurologic Spasticity Seizures Spinal stenosis Nerve entrapments	• Routine monitoring • Adjust medications with reported change • Monitor for changes—high index of suspicion for pathology	• Tone management—medications, botulinumtoxin injections, intrathecal baclofen • Seizure management • Radiologic evaluation • Electrodiagnosis • Surgical referral when appropriate
Genito/urinary conditions Incontinence UTIs	• Monitor and query routinely • Routine gynecologic follow-up for women	• Urodynamic evaluation • Scans/radiographs • Medications and CIC when needed • Urology referral as appropriate
Cardiovascular health	• Monitor blood pressure and typical serum panels • Assess for risk factors	• Treat cardiovascular symptoms and events
Obesity/overweight	• Healthy nutrition and weight management • Measurement of body fat—consider waist circumference, DXA, or BIA • Monitor for metabolic syndrome symptoms/signs	• Manage weight • Promote exercise
Respiratory conditions Infection Sleep apnea	• Routine monitoring • Immunization • Assess sleep hygiene	• Scoliosis evaluation • Sleep study and management • Specialty referral as needed

(continued)

Table 6.2 (continued)

Common related health conditions	Prevention strategies	Treatment strategies
Gastrointestinal Constipation GERD Obstruction Oral-motor problems	• Monitor and query routinely—recognition of severity • Nutritional management • Dental monitoring, hygiene and preventive care	• Adjustment to bowel program regimen • Specialty referral when appropriate • Dental treatment • Botulinum toxin for drooling • ENT referral for drooling management
Deconditioning Falls	• Assess changes in function • Routine exercise • Fall prevention programs	• Therapy prescription—focus on strength and aerobics • Accessible equipment
Mental health	• Routine monitoring, especially for depressive or anxiety symptoms • Assess support, living arrangements	• Specialty referral as appropriate • Referral for psychologic and social support • Use of community resources
Sexual functioning Fertility/ reproduction Emotional/body image	• Provide education about sexuality and function—appropriate for cognition and function • Assure pregnancy high risk needs are met	• Following pregnancy, support may be needed in the home
Health maintenance	Monitoring and Screening—see Table 6.4	

DXA = dual energy X-ray absorptiometry; UTI = urinary tract infection; CIC = clean intermittent catheterization; BIA = bioelectric impedance analysis; ENT = Otolaryngologist
[a]Modified from [48] (Aging with Pediatric Onset Disability and Diseases, Table 21.2 Aging Health and Performance Changes, pp: 567–568)

6.4.1 Evaluation

A comprehensive history and appropriate physical examination must be undertaken to determine the etiology of the musculoskeletal complaint in order to determine appropriate evaluation and treatment. Musculoskeletal physical examination, as in the general population, can direct further evaluation and lead to a differential diagnosis. Understanding the underlying upper motor neuron pathophysiology as it relates to a neuromusculoskeletal examination is important (see Table 6.3). In the presence of spasticity, slow, intermediate, and rapid speeds of stretch can evaluate hypertonicity, passive range limits, and presence of contracture. Other passive maneuvers can identify joint, soft tissue, or neurologic etiologies. When possible, active range and strength testing (assuming there is underlying motor control and not just reflexes or posturing providing movement) are important to document, as well as any movement or activity that elicits pain. Radiographs may be helpful, but the degree of abnormality may not correlate with pain complaints. Osteoporosis may obscure fractures. Computerized axial tomography (CT) may be needed to address concerns not discerned on plain radiograph. Magnetic resonance imaging

Table 6.3 Upper motor neuron syndrome manifestations

Positive signs: abnormal	Negative signs: performance deficits
• Increased tendon reflexes, ± spread	• Weakness
• Clonus	• Paralysis or paresis
• Positive Babinski sign	• Reduced dexterity
• Spasticity	• Fatigue
• Extensor/flexor spasm	
• Mass reflex	
• Dys-synergic patterns with co-contraction with movement	
• Associated reactions and patterns of movement	

(MRI) may be required to evaluate neurologic compromise and certain soft-tissues concerns, such as joint abnormalities. Both may require advanced planning for positioning and ability to maintain a prolonged position to complete the scan. Treatment should be based on diagnosis with cautious and judicious use of medication. Physical medicine and rehabilitation physicians, neurodevelopmentalists, orthopedists, neurologists, and rehabilitation therapists may be helpful for evaluation and treatment. Coordinated care and education is essential and can assist with achieving positive outcomes.

6.4.2 Contractures

The weakness, spasticity, posturing, and immobility seen in CP frequently result in contractures. Muscle imbalances across a joint often result in a tonic contraction. This imbalance can originate from the posturing noted in limbs (preference for flexion in upper limbs and extension in lower limbs) and then poor motor control of muscles that are antagonist to that posture. The degree of contractures is variable, and contractures commonly progress through the lifespan. Soft tissue changes begin very early with this decreased mobility of the joint, including alteration at the structural level including stiffer extracellular matrix, smaller diameter and shorter muscle fibers, and stretched sarcomeres [56]. General loss of flexibility and decreasing activity seen with aging can contribute to progression; however, if there is associated pain or increased spasticity, further evaluation is in order to rule out such etiologies as fracture, neuropathy, arthritis, and cervical myelopathy.

Management of contractures is complex. While the best treatment for contractures is to slow or prevent them, longstanding interventions of daily passive range of motion exercises are now controversial [57] and stretch alone likely does not prevent contractures in neurologically-based etiologies [58]. The goals for treatment should relate to management of pain or improving function, mobility, positioning, or hygiene. Primary spasticity management should also be considered, including spasmolytics, injections, intrathecal baclofen pumps. Maximal prolonged stretching can be accomplished with dynamic bracing or serial casting, often following botulinum toxin injections to agonist muscle groups. Caution must be taken to avoid and watch for pressure points when using immobilizing devices, especially those that remain in place for some days. Active programs involving strengthening of antagonist muscles or aquatic therapies may be useful. Surgical options can be considered if improved range is imperative, including release, tenotomy or tendon lengthening, joint capsule release, or total joint replacement.

6.4.3 Osteoarthritis

Normal joint development requires a complement of mechanical forces and biologic factors. In CP, the presence of abnormal muscle tone, weakness, restricted range of motion with contractures, and resulting abnormal forces and functional load axes may lead to altered joint morphology and remodeling within joints [59]. These alterations, can in turn lead to subluxations, altered cartilage formation, and accelerated degeneration of susceptible joints. Despite this theoretic base, there are no good epidemiologic studies to support this, and often adults with CP are told they have early osteoarthritis without a credible assessment. Therefore, the degree of osteoarthritic changes reported is variable in persons with CP. Although osteoarthritis may be common, the association between osteoarthritic changes and pain is not universal. The degree of radiographic joint degenerative changes does not necessarily correspond to the severity of symptoms. Pain is common in individuals with CP, but the causes are likely multifactorial extending beyond osteoarthritis. Muscle and other soft tissues may contribute to degenerative joint pain. Therefore appropriate evaluation should ensue, including laboratory and imaging studies. Anti-inflammatory medication may be beneficial in select circumstances, but side effects should be considered, especially in the face of other gastrointestinal conditions. Total joint replacements have successfully treated focal joint abnormalities that have been unsuccessfully managed conservatively.

6.4.4 Hip Pathology

Hip pathology is common in persons with CP. Degenerative changes are frequently seen radiographically and are not always related to weight bearing activities [59–61]. Hip subluxation or dislocations occurs when the head of the femur is not fully seated within the acetabulum because of spasticity and contractures; this is more commonly seen in persons who are non-ambulatory or quadriplegic. Usually these changes are noted before adulthood, but may become more painful with age. Multiple treatment options are available. Tone reduction strategies may be beneficial. Persons with more severe symptoms may require surgical treatment. Femoral head resection is an option to control pain in some patients, however, pain often persists or recurs postoperatively [60, 62–64]. Total hip replacements appear to be safe and effective for adults with CP, although implant revision rates appear higher than those in the general population [65].

6.4.5   Knee Pathology

Knee contractures are also common in persons with CP who do not walk, and in those who walk with a crouched gait. Not all knee contractures are painful. There may also be joint laxity or instability, which can be found on examination. Spasticity management, exercise, kinesiotaping, and other interventions may improve range, function, and pain. Surgical treatment options, such as patellar tendon advancement surgeries, may improve pain and improve knee functioning for people with patella alta or chondromalacia patella [66]. In a small cohort from a single center, total knee replacements were reported to be successful, with no increase in revisions and good return to walking status postoperatively [67].

6.4.6   Foot or Ankle Pathology

Ankle and foot contracture are also common, especially in nonambulatory persons with CP. Bracing with ankle and foot orthosis (AFO) or shoe inserts may help. Plantar fasciitis is common, and typical treatments should be considered.

6.4.7   Back Pain and Pathology

The back is among the most common sites of pain for adults with CP, both in those who walk and those who use wheelchairs [36, 44, 68]. Scoliosis and kyphoscoliosis without support can be a source of pain. Higher GMFCS level is a significant risk factor for developing scoliosis; the incidence of scoliosis continues to increase up to the age of 20–25 years [69]. Those with a Cobb angle greater than 40° are at greatest risk for further deterioration, including into adulthood [70]. Scoliosis, in turn, may result in pressure sores, impaired respiratory function, and pain [71]. The evidence for nonsurgical management to correct or halt progression of scoliosis (e.g., modern bracing techniques or optimized seating systems) is mixed [72]. Thus, appropriate examination and evaluation should be documented. In appropriate patients, surgical correction with posterior spinal fusion has been reported to improve the quality of life for those with CP [73].

6.4.8   Osteoporosis and Fractures

Low bone density is found in over 50% of adolescents and adults with cerebral palsy [74, 75]. Multiple factors contribute to the increased prevalence of osteopenia and osteoporosis in adults with cerebral palsy. Altered bone development due to altered weight bearing and mobility impairment likely contributes to limited bone density and accelerated decline. Nutritional status and the potential use of anticonvulsants also influence bone remodeling and the development of osteoporosis.

Assessment of bone mineral density (BMD) in adults with CP can be challenging. The commonly use risk assessment tools, such as the FRAX or SCORE index, have not been adequately studied in adults with CP [76]. In addition, traditional measurement of BMD using dual-energy X-ray absorptiometry (DXA) scans can be limited in adults with CP. Contractures and surgical hardware may limit obtaining DXA scans in the typical locations of the hip and lower spine. Alternative sites for DXA scanning have been developed in children, and replicated in adults, but the data are less robust [77].

A single report notes adults with spastic CP have lower BMD than those with dyskinetic CP [78]. The combination of low bone density, contractures, spasticity, and impaired balance increase the risk of falls and fractures in adults with CP. Fractures are a common reason for hospital admission in young adults [31]. Pathologic fractures typically occur in the long bones [79], but large studies of people with cerebral palsy are limited. Prevention of fractures is critical. Routine exercise and physical activity that emphasizes strength as well as flexibility are critical to decrease risk of falls, however there is no strong evidence that weight bearing or supported weight-bearing are effective to improve bone density [80]. Pharmacotherapy may have a role for some individuals. Much of the therapy for osteoporosis is extrapolated from the general population, especially as a treatment for post-menopausal osteoporosis in women. Studies indicate that bisphosphonates probably increase BMD [79, 80], but the long-term benefits are unknown.

6.5   Pain and Fatigue

Pain and fatigue are among the most noticeable problems in adults with CP, and may be associated with decreases in functional skills [68, 81]. These functional declines do not appear to be related to type of CP [80]. Pain is the one most consistently reported health conditions in adults with cerebral palsy, ranging from 30% to 80% within study groups [36–38, 82–84].

6.5.1   Pain

Pain has consistently been identified as a health condition for adults with CP, and possible sources of pain remain numerous. Women appear to experience more pain than men, and report significantly greater impact on daily life [85]. Careful study of contribution of sources or prevalence of causes for pain has not been undertaken [86]. Etiologies for pain in adults with CP are diverse, and include musculoskeletal conditions (as noted above), neurologic conditions including spasticity, dental conditions, and under- and overweight [36, 86]. Pain can be at multiple sites and etiologies may be overlapping. This complexity along with communication difficulties noted with some adults with CP may delay the recognition and clinical evaluation of pain [36, 86, 87].

A good history and clinical examination can help to direct evaluation, diagnosis, and a management plan. Typical interventions include 1) medications for spasticity (e.g., oral, injection, intrathecal); 2) pain medications and treatments (e.g., acetaminophen, nonsteroidal anti-inflammatories, anticonvulsants, antidepressants, analgesics); 3) physical interventions (e.g., exercise, modalities, regular physical activity, physical/occupational/recreational therapy, aquatic therapy); 4) more aggressive pain management strategies (e.g., trigger point injection, spinal injections, nerve blocks); and 5) alternative treatments (e.g., transcutaneous nerve stimulation, massage, biofeedback, acupuncture, kinesiotaping, counseling, cognitive behavioral approaches, manual medicine) [86, 88]. A recent analysis of U.S. Medical Expenditure Panel Survey data reports that people with longstanding physical disabilities, including adults with CP, use high doses of opioids compared to a mixed non-cancer pain diagnosis group [89]. A cross-sectional survey of adults with CP reported that care for pain management was accessed from a variety of professionals. Physical interventions (e.g., physical therapy, strengthening, modalities) were the most commonly used, and rated as moderately effective [88]. Additional environmental issues to consider are the availability and funding for personal care attendants, frequency of position changes, access to appropriate seating and positioning systems, home accessibility and modification, and worksite arrangements and ergonomics. Poor sleep and limited exercise may also contribute to chronic pain. Good sleep hygiene and adequate activity and exercise should be encouraged. Adults with CP tend to self-manage their pain complaints [90]; those who seek medical care report there are few options offered, usually resulting in minimal improvement [91]. Recommendation is to follow for pain relief, and refer if no improvements noted.

6.5.2   Fatigue

Fatigue is also a common finding in adults with CP, and can be associated with pain, deterioration of skills, depression, and low life satisfaction; there is no reported association with any specific type or severity of CP [30, 36, 92]. Sleep disruption should also be questioned since it is commonly seen with pain and fatigue. This connection between sleep, fatigue, and pain has been not been well described in CP, although recent studies in children with CP have identified sleep disorders are associated with more severe impairments [93, 94]. Anecdotally, the pain/fatigue complex appears to respond positively to directed pain management, good sleep hygiene, medications, and exercise. Appropriate management includes early identification of the problem and its source. Typical management strategies should be offered, and referral for additional sleep therapy, orthopedic, or neurosurgical consultation should be considered.

6.6   Neurologic

6.6.1   Intellectual Capacity

Although cognitive impairment is common, many adults with cerebral palsy have a normal intellectual capacity. The exact prevalence of intellectual disability among adults with CP is difficult to assess. In a report published by the U.S. Centers for Disease Control and Prevention, more than 40% of children with CP had an intellectual disability, defined by an IQ <70 [16]. In addition to an intellectual disability, learning deficits and language impairments may be present. There are no reports of associated dementia or other neurocognitive impairment or changes with aging.

6.6.2 Seizures

Seizure disorders are relatively common in persons with CP [41]. Overall, approximately 35–41% of persons with CP have co-occurring epilepsy [16, 95]. The prevalence of seizures, however, varies depending on the neurologic subtype of CP. In a sample from the Quebec Cerebral Palsy Registry, seizure disorders ranged from 6% in spastic diplegia to 31% in those with spastic quadriplegia [96]. The frequency of seizures increased from 6% in those with GMFCS I to 44% in those with GMFCS V [96]. The high prevalence of seizures disorders is particularly important given its association with increased mortality, increased inpatient admissions, and decreased functional status [97, 98]. Side effects from some anti-epileptic medications may contribute to osteopenia and should be recognized.

6.6.3 Speech and Hearing

Speech and hearing impairments also vary based on the type and severity of CP. Although some speech impairments may be present, most adults with spastic hemiplegia or diplegia are able to communicate verbally. However, up to 45% of those with spastic quadriplegia are nonverbal [96]. Nonverbal status increases from 1% in those with GMFCS I to 82% in those with GMFCS V [96]. Hearing impairment is less common but occurs in up to 14% of those with spastic quadriplegia and 21% of those with a GMFCS V [96]. The changes with hearing seen in a general aging population should also be considered in adults with CP, with evaluation as needed.

6.6.4 Visual Impairment

Cortical blindness and visual impairment are less common in CP and is mostly limited to those with spastic quadriplegia (21%) and those with GMFCS V (33%) [96]. Presence of a vision impairment has an independent effect on the probability of survival. As in the general aging population, vision changes may be seen and ophthalmologic evaluation should be considered.

6.6.5   Spasticity and Motor Control

Spasticity is the most common motor abnormality seen in CP. Management is required throughout the lifespan, and monitoring for change is important. Often increases in hypertonia or decrease in motor control are the early signs of additional or progressing health conditions. The upper motor neuron syndrome (UMNS) consists of negative symptoms (motor control) and positive symptoms (hypertonia) (see Table 6.2). Clinicians usually report the hyperactive symptoms, but more often it is the difficulties with motor control that are more problematic for function. Additionally, spasticity may actually assist with function (e.g., extensor posturing in lower limbs used for transferring), so not all spasticity is negative. If changes are noted, further assessment by a knowledgeable clinician is in order. Determining the reason for changes (e.g., infection, fracture, pressure ulcer, venous thromboembolism) as well as making modifications to management requires expert knowledge and skill. Side effects of oral medications often limit dosing. Targets for botulinum toxin injections should be directed by goals and biomechanics. Intrathecal baclofen is beneficial, and may increase survival [99]. Pain management should also be addressed.

6.6.6   Spinal Stenosis and Myelopathy

Spinal stenosis must be considered whenever significant functional change is noted, particularly for change in or loss of walking skills, increased leg spasticity, change in bladder habits, neck pain, vague sensory changes, and (late) changes in arm and hand function [100, 101]. Most studies report on adults with athetoid or dyskinetic CP [102]; however, more recent reports show these problems are present in spastic forms of cerebral palsy as well. There may be a predisposition to cervical stenosis in those with a congenitally narrow canal, especially at C4-C5 [100]. Diagnosis is made through history, clinical examination, and imaging studies. Surgical decompression may help to prevent further, often catastrophic, loss of function, but does not assure return of lost function, particularly in cases of longstanding compression with spinal cord atrophy. Recurrence at levels above or below surgical correction may be noted [103]. Postoperative management planning should accommodate changes in functional capabilities and care needs. The presence of dystonic movements will affect postoperative spine stabilization. Botulinum toxin injections can assist with neck stabilization, with or without halo vest immobilization, in the face of involuntary neck movements [104]. Caution must be taken to identify implant failures in the postoperative period for those with significant involuntary neck movements. When no surgical intervention is undertaken, a frank discussion of possible increasing loss of function, including respiratory compromise, and the future need for ventilator and other assistance should be undertaken.

6.6.7 Peripheral Neuropathy

Peripheral neuropathies may also occur in adults with CP. Compression of the median and ulnar nerves is the most common peripheral neuropathies. Compression may be related to transfer techniques, use of crutches or wheelchairs, or existing contractures. Carpal tunnel syndrome, or compression of the median nerve, has been reported and attributed to prolonged flexion of the wrist due to spasticity in some patients [105]. Electrodiagnostic testing is often necessary to define the etiology of the symptoms.

6.7 Cardiovascular

6.7.1 Hypertension

In a large population based study, adults with CP were found to have a higher age-adjusted prevalence of hypertension than the general population [46]. Other smaller studies have demonstrated elevated rates of hypertension as well [41]. The reason for elevated blood pressure in CP is unclear. It is also important to acknowledge that measurement inaccuracies related to spasticity are possible in CP. Hypertension in adults with CP should be treated like the general population, with extra care given to prevent orthostatic hypotension that may contribute to falls.

6.7.2 Metabolic Syndrome

Higher rates of obesity and metabolic syndrome have also been observed in persons with CP [40, 42, 43, 47]. Overall, the increased rates of obesity, hypertension, and metabolic syndrome all point to the silent threat that cardiovascular disease poses to adults with CP [42, 43, 47].

6.7.3 Vascular Disease

Overt vascular disease is also prominent in adults with CP. The age-adjusted prevalence of stroke in adults with CP has been reported as double that of those adults without CP (4.6% vs. 2.3%). In addition, mortality records reveal that death due to heart disease is higher among adults with CP [27]. Further details about cardiovascular and cerebrovascular disease are lacking. Given the increased risk of hypertension, stroke, and cardiac mortality, careful attention should be given to risk reduction through adequate control of blood pressure and assessing the need for statin or aspirin therapy. When assessing risk, it is important to recognize that traditional risk assessment tools, such as the ASCVD risk estimator, do not account for the increased risk apparent in cerebral palsy.

6.8 Obesity

Many studies report an increased prevalence of obesity in children with CP, however the documentation for adults is less clear. Additionally, because of muscle wasting and sarcopenia, Body Mass Index (BMI) may not accurately reflect the obesity status [34]. Using the U.S. Medical Expenditure Panel Survey (self-report), it appears that adults with CP are less likely to be in the normal range for BMI and more likely to be in the obese (not overweight) range [46]. The relationship of obesity to mobility status is not clear [106]. People with physical disabilities have higher utilization of and costs for health care than those without disability, and the presence of obesity significantly increases the burden [107]. Thus assessment of percent body fat should be a routine element of a clinical examination. Since adults with CP may have normal weight but increased body fat (the actual definition of obesity), use of waist circumference may better define cardiovascular or diabetic risk. Waist circumference may be more accurate than actual weight, particularly if modified scales are not available. Consideration of nutrition education or referral and discussion of physical activity is warranted.

6.9 Pulmonary

Respiratory illnesses are a leading cause of hospitalization and a significant contributor to excess mortality in adults with CP [27, 40, 46, 108]. Adults with CP should receive yearly influenza vaccine, and those with asthma or other risk factors shoulder receive PPSV23 (pneumococcal polysaccharide vaccine).

6.9.1 Asthma

Individuals with CP have been reported to have a higher rate of asthma than the general population [41, 46]. The reasons for the increased prevalence of airway reactivity is unclear, but aspiration may contribute in some individuals.

6.9.2 Aspiration

Adults with CP are at increased risk for aspiration. Aspiration risk correlates with the integrity of oral motor function the severity of CP. Advancing scoliosis may further increase the risks of aspiration. In addition to impaired swallowing, regurgitation of gastric contents may also result in aspiration. Recognizing impaired swallowing and aspiration is critical. Signs of aspiration with eating include choking, coughing, hoarse voice, vomiting, or heartburn. Potential aspiration should be evaluated with a clinical swallowing evaluation accompanied by video fluoroscopy. Gastric emptying studies may also be helpful to assess for delayed gastric emptying.

Speech or occupational therapists should be directly involved to assess swallowing integrity. Dieticians can help establish an appropriate diet consistent with recommendations of the speech therapist. Potential diets range from regular diets, to dysphagia diets, to pureed diets. When necessary, aspiration precautions should be established, slowing feeds, raising the head of the bed 30–45°, avoiding foods 2–3 h before bed [109].

6.10 Gastroenterology

Gastrointestinal symptoms are common in both children and adults with cerebral palsy.

6.10.1 Constipation

Adults with CP frequently experience constipation. In young adults, constipation is a common reason for inpatient admission [98]. Multiple factors likely contribute to constipation in adults. Abnormal gastrointestinal motility and immobilization both contribute to prolonged colonic transit time [110]. Adequate fiber intake and appropriate bowel regimens are the mainstay of treatment for constipation. Often other medications cause a decrease in bowel motility, such as spasmolytics and pain medications. Understanding the target of bowel medications assists with management: bulk forming medications assure uniform consistency; stool softeners change stool consistency, but may not promote bowel motility; laxatives increase motility through mucosal stimulation; suppositories and enemas stimulate distally. Commonly used medications are stool softeners, mild stimulant laxatives, and polyethylene glycol. Adults with chronic constipation should also be monitored for impaction. Impaction of stool can lead to dilation of the bowel and encopresis, a leakage of loose stool around hard impacted stool. An abdominal X-ray can help identify concerning stool patterns and dilatation of the proximal colon.

6.10.2 Gastric Reflux

In addition to constipation, neurogenic influences from CP can affect gastric motility, resulting in gastroesophageal reflux [110]. Gastroesophageal reflux disease (GERD) most commonly presents with a burning sensation after eating, regurgitation of food, or chronic cough. However, symptoms of GERD may present as behavioral changes in those not able to express the typical symptoms. GERD can result in erosive and non-erosive esophagitis and chronic reflux can, in turn, cause intestinal metaplasia. Upper endoscopy should be considered if the diagnosis is not clear or if the individual fails to respond to 4–8 weeks of acid suppressive therapy.

Initial treatment of GERD includes lifestyle and dietary modifications, including elevation of the head of the bed. Protein pump inhibitors are the mainstay of pharmacologic treatment for GERD. Gastroparesis may also contribute to refractory reflux. If objective evidence of delayed gastric emptying is confirmed, prokinetic medications, such as metoclopramide, may be useful to improve quality of life. However, prokinetic agents have not been shown to influence endoscopic response of GERD [111].

6.11   Genitourinary

6.11.1 Neurogenic Bladder

Neurogenic bladder is a common finding in persons with CP, with the prevalence ranging from 16% to 30% [112, 113]. A systematic review reports that more than 50% of people with CP experience one or more lower urinary tract symptoms [114]. Symptoms from neurogenic bladder peak in a bimodal distributions between 6 and 10 years and then again after the age of 30 years. Problems with bladder storage (incontinence) are more common than voiding symptoms (retention). People with CP with retention and pelvic floor overactivity are more prone to progress to upper urinary tract dysfunction through adult life [114]. It is possible that upper motor neuron bladders eventually become overstretched and progress to significant retention and poor detrusor function with advancing age [112]. Both the small irritable bladder and large hypotonic bladder can result in incontinence (overflow) and predispose individuals to urinary infection. Risk for significant urinary issues are those with spastic quadriplegia, CP subgroup GMFCS III or higher, and severe cognitive impairment [114]. Urodynamic studies can direct management. Most patients with neurogenic bladder can be treated with conservative therapies, including oxybutynin, biofeedback, relaxed toileting, and management of hypertonicity of the pelvic floor [112]. Changes in urinary function should be evaluated since these conditions are sometimes an early symptom of cervical myelopathy.

6.11.2 Urinary Tract Infections

Urinary tract infection (UTI) are a common reason for inpatient admission in individuals with CP [98]. Adults with more severe CP are at great risk and have a higher incidence of UTIs [115]. Urinary retention due to a neurogenic bladder predisposes individuals to develop a UTI, but only infrequently leads to upper urinary tract infections [112]. Depending on the cognitive function and sensory awareness, UTI may present with different symptoms ranging from the classic symptoms of dysuria and frequency to incontinence, behavioral changes, and restlessness. In addition to true infections, older institutionalized adults with CP may experience asymptomatic bacteriuria, which does not require treatment.

6.11.3 Incontinence

Urinary incontinence is more common in adults with CP than in the general population [41, 45]. Continence in individuals with CP is related to central nervous system functioning, bladder physiology, cognition, sensory awareness, and behavior. Identifying and addressing urinary incontinence is critical. Addressing continence is an important component of basic human dignity as well a key component to preventing skin break down. Urinary incontinence can be evaluated through urodynamic studies. If present, neurogenic and infectious causes of incontinence should be treated. When necessary, careful toileting routines and behavioral plans should be established; at times, anticholinergics can be considered, although there should be monitoring for side effects. Achieving continence and avoiding upper tract and renal dysfunction is important.

6.12   Behavioral and Mental Health

6.12.1 Depression and Anxiety

Depression and anxiety occur at higher rates in adults with cerebral palsy compared to the general population [36, 41]. Depression is also associated with increased pain, a common finding in adults with CP [68, 82, 116, 117]. Depending on the degree of symptoms and the individual's preferences, counseling and pharmacotherapy are options for treatment. Selective serotonin reuptake inhibitors (SSRIs) and serotonin norepinephrine reuptake inhibitors (SNRIs) are considered first-line pharmacotherapy. SNRIs, such as venlafaxine and duloxetine, may also have some benefit in treatment of chronic neuropathic pain, myofascial pain and musculoskeletal pain [118]. Treatment offers the potential to improve quality of life, health, physical functioning in adults with CP. Persons receiving treatment should receive routine follow-up to monitor progress.

6.12.2 Autism

Autism spectrum disorders (ASD) appear to occur at a higher prevalence in individuals with CP, with a documented prevalence of nearly 7% [95]. In children, co-occurring ASD was more common with non-spastic CP [95]. The reason for the co-occurrence of autism with cerebral palsy is not known, but may point to common neurologic risk factors and early neurologic insults.

6.12.3 Psychosis

Psychotic feature have also been reported in some individuals, although true psychosis is often difficult to assess in individuals with CP. The risk of psychotic features is related to the underlying cause, intellectual capacity, and co-occurring conditions.

6.13 Sexual Health

Sexual health in adults with CP is an important aspect to their overall health and well-being. Health care professionals' attitudes often limit services and education. Although challenging to discuss, adults with CP frequently want to address sexual health with their physicians. Sexual maturation in individuals with CP frequently differs from the general population and is related to nutritional status and degree of impairment [119]. Adolescent and adults with CP frequently report sexual interest but experience more difficulties with developing intimate and sexual relationships [120–122]. Both men and women report fewer sexual encounters than do age peers in the general population. The level of motor function is associated with sexual relationships [122]. Given the importance of sexual health, clinicians should provide a safe space to discuss sexual health with adults with CP. Office visit planning is required for those with significant motor impairments to assure a complete examination. Clinicians should anticipate concerns about body image and questions about sexual interactions.

6.13.1 Women

Contraception should be addressed in women who are sexually active. Women with CP are typically able to conceive and carry pregnancies to term without the expectation of major complications related to their CP. Family planning should also be addressed. Contraception may also be considered in women with menorrhagia or dysmenorrhea. Routine health maintenance activities, including pelvic examinations, Pap smears, and breast examinations, are frequently missed in individuals with cerebral palsy. Routine health maintenance exams offer a valuable opportunity to address preventive care as well as any concerns about sexual health.

6.13.2 Men

Men with CP also should receive information on sexual functioning, including information on contraception and protection from disease. There have been no reported problems with fertility. In addition to concerns about body image, men with CP have a higher incidence of cryptorchidism compared with the general population [123]. This may be due to spasticity of the cremasteric muscle.

6.14   Dental

Adults with cerebral palsy are at increased risk for many dental problems [124]. Oral health is increasingly recognized as a key component to overall health and well-being. Adults with CP are at increased risk for developing dental caries, dental erosions, and periodontal disease [124]. Bruxism, or grinding of the teeth, is also common in CP [124]. Adequate home dental hygiene should be encouraged. Routine dental exams are also essential. Occasionally, sedation is necessary prior to dental exams and procedures (see Chap. 11).

6.15   Promoting Health and Wellness

The steady improvements in medical care and social support systems have resulted in adults with CP being generally healthier, participating in community activities and employment, and living longer. The medical paradigm must now shift from that of illness and disease to one of health and wellness. Better definitions of health risks and outcomes related to common health conditions are now available for the general public, which in turn has directed public health initiatives focused on health promotion and prevention strategies. Routine immunizations and screening for common health risks and conditions along with interventions to arrest progression of the additional comorbidity process or reduce the consequences are the mainstay of a prevention program. Health promotion programs target improved health by enabling increased control over health and health determinants. These programs often are presented as opportunities for learning to improve health literacy and to develop life skills for improved health. These same strategies of preventive medicine and health maintenance should be included in health care systems for adults with CP. While some activities may require modifications to support learning, facilitate access, and address possible financial concerns, many require no change other than having the health care professional implement them. Referral to other specialty professionals may also be needed.

6.16   Immunizations and Screening

Health care maintenance and preventive health strategies should follow a typical preventive medicine schedule for adults. Table 6.4 identifies recommendations from the U.S. Preventive Services Task Force, with modifications for adults with CP. Adults with CP should receive immunizations based upon the standard immunization schedule for adults, with consideration for any comorbidities that may be

Table 6.4 Health care maintenance and preventive screening[a,b]

Health condition	Recommendation for general population	Modification needed
Hypertension	• Age ≥18 without risk factors: Screen every 3–5 years (Grade A)[c] • Age ≥18 with risk factors (African American, high normal BP, overweight): Screen annually • Age ≥40: Screen annually (Grade A) • Obtain measurements outside of the clinical setting for diagnostic confirmation	• Consider annual screening for all adults with CP. • Use appropriate sphygmomanometer for limb length and circumference • Watch for spasticity trigger
Immunizations	• Age and chronic condition dependent.	• No recommendations based on CP. • Other comorbidities may warrant immunizations.
Cardiovascular Lipid	• Men: Screen men aged 20–35 if at increased risk for coronary heart disease. Screen all men aged 35 and older for lipid disorders • Women: Screen women ≥20 years if at increased risk for coronary heart disease. Screen all women ≥45 years.	• None
Abdominal aortic aneurysm	• Perform a one-time screening for abdominal aortic aneurysm (AAA) with ultrasonography in men ages 65–75 years who have ever smoked (Grade B)[d]	• Accessible procedure environment
Cancer Men and Women: Colorectal	• Screen for colorectal cancer using fecal occult blood (annual), sigmoidoscopy (q3–5yr), or colonoscopy (q10yr), beginning at age 50 years and continuing until age 75 years (Grade A)	• Level-appropriate education for all tests and procedures • Accessible examination and procedure environment • May need sedation to complete procedure—must consider risks/benefits • May need 1:1 assist
Men and Women: Lung	• Screen patients annually who have a 30 pack-year smoking history and currently smoke or have quit within the past 15 years (Grade B)	
Women: Breast	• Screen women aged 50–74 years with mammography every 2 years (Grade B) • The American Cancer Society recommends offering annual screening at age 40–44 years and recommends starting annual screening at age 45	
Women: Cervical	• Screen women age 21–65 years with cytology (Pap smear) every 3 years (Grade A) • Screen women age 30–65 years who want to lengthen the screening interval with a combination of cytology and HPV testing every 5 year (Grade A)	
Men: Prostate	• PSA not recommended to screen for prostate cancer	

(continued)

Table 6.4 (continued)

Health condition	Recommendation for general population	Modification needed
Metabolic/ Endocrine Obesity	• Screening for all using BMI, counseling and behavior interventions offered if >30 kg/m²	• BMI does not reflect body fat, which is the measure of interest • Height/weight measurement may not be accurate in disability • Consider waist circumference measurement since this represents central adiposity and more accurately reflect high cardiovascular risks • Monitor for metabolic syndrome
Diabetes mellitus Type 2	• Screen for abnormal blood glucose in adults aged 40–70 years who are overweight or obese (Grade B)	• None
Mental health Depression	• Screen adults for depression when supports are in place to assure accurate diagnosis, effective treatment, and follow-up (Grade B)	• May require modification to screening tools • May need modifications to diagnose and treat
Cognitive impairment deterioration	• Current evidence is insufficient to assess role of screening	• Recommend evaluations in IDD since symptoms may present at younger than expected ages
Violence	• Current evidence is insufficient to assess role of screening	• Suspected high incidence of violence and abuse in disability • Offer opportunity to discuss
Tobacco use	• Recommend regular screening and offer cessation interventions	• None
Alcohol misuse	• Recommend regular screening and offer behavioral counseling to reduce misuse.	• Young adults and adults may use alcohol to control spasticity or dyskinesias, not often recognized without questioning.
Exercise	• Current evidence is insufficient to assess role of screening	• Exercise is an important activity for those with motor impairments • Exercise has been shown to be effective for improved performance, pain control, weight management • Refer to accessible programs or health professionals who can develop individual or identify existing individual or group programs
Fall Prevention	• Exercise interventions to prevent falls in community-dwelling adults 65 years or older who are at increased risk for falls. (B recommendation)	• Refer to accessible programs or health professionals who can develop customized programs

Table 6.4 (continued)

Health condition	Recommendation for general population	Modification needed
Aging Vision	• Presbyopia, cataract, macular degeneration, and glaucoma increases with advancing age • Current evidence is insufficient to assess role of screening	• Accessible examination
Hearing	• Hearing frequently decreases with advancing age >50 years • Current evidence is insufficient to assess role of screening	• Accessible examination

[a]Recommended Immunization Schedule for Adults Aged 19 Years or Older, United States, 2018, Centers for Disease Control and Prevention (https://www.cdc.gov/vaccines/schedules/hcp/adult.html) and United States Preventive Services Task Force (USPSTF) (https://www.uspreventiveservicestaskforce.org/)
[b]Modified from Turk, Gorter, & Logan. Aging with Pediatric Onset Disability and Diseases. In: Pediatric Rehabilitation: Principles and Practice, 5th edition (eds. Alexander MA & Matthews DJ). Demos Medical: 2016, Table 21.9 Health Preventive Screening Services, pp: 593–594
[c]Grade A = The USPSTF recommends the service. There is high certainty that the net benefit is substantial
[d]Grade B = The USPSTF recommends the service. There is high certainty that the net benefit is moderate or there is moderate certainty that the net benefit is moderate to substantial

present. Screening for common health conditions seen in an adult population should also be undertaken, especially since hypertension, obesity, depression/anxiety, and some cancers are commonly reported in adults with CP. Health behaviors differ for adolescents and adults compared to those age peers without CP. While there is usually less smoking and alcohol misuse, there is also less physical activity, less healthy food choices, and less socialization and friendship development [41, 125, 126].

6.17   Active Health Promotion Behaviors

Health promotion activities and programs for adults with CP frequently emphasize physical activity, nutrition, emotional health, recreation and leisure, and dental care (Table 6.5). Programs may focus on a single topic or involve a broader approach to increase health literacy. Both approaches support development of life skills for improved health. Positive health behaviors require social, health, and community resources. Primary care providers should be prepared to discuss an active approach to promoting health, or make referral to specialty care to assist.

Exercise and physical activity are areas of particular interest, since people with disability typically have much lower participation compared to those persons without disability and even modest increase in activity can decrease health care costs [128]. Additionally, adults with CP have been shown to have high risks associated with obesity, the metabolic syndrome, and limited exercise [28]. Exercise is a well-known and supported health-promoting behavior. There are many

Table 6.5 Typical targets for active healthy behaviors in adults with cerebral palsy[a]

Health activity target	Relevance to adults with cerebral palsy
General prevention	• Recognize risks for less healthy behaviors, and barriers and facilitators to behavior changes and participation • Specifically monitor for abuse and violence • Provide typical age-appropriate information about smoking, drinking, substance abuse, sexual contacts • Monitor for disability-specific health conditions • Encourage patient empowerment for interactions with health care professionals
Physical activity	• Promote exercise and activity as an expectation • Provide background education for adult with CP and family/support • Recognize exercise is not contra-indicated in the presence of spasticity or dyskinesia • Consider engaging rehabilitation professionals to initiate, monitor, and problem solve adaptations
Nutrition and obesity	• Recognize obesity can cause limitations, and can be the result of poor dietary habits and limited activity • Provide background education for adult with CP and family/support • Consider referral to nutritionist or other professional to engage patient and family
Emotional health	• Assess for sense of anxiety/depression, need for stress management, ability to adapt, and participation in social activities • Consider recreation and leisure activities to promote social support and ability to develop social skills • Consider medications and counseling as needed
Recreation and Leisure	• Assess social activities outside the home—promote importance for socialization, sense of self, support • Consider referral to community programs or rehabilitation professionals
Dental	• Discuss preventive dental care; daily maintenance care is needed • Suggest behavior strategies if there are problems engaging in dental appointments and refer for this service as needed

[a]Modified from Turk [127], Chapter 717: Health and Wellness for Children with Disabilities, Table 4: Targeting healthy behaviors for children with disabilities

barriers to people with disability engaging in exercise. Most common are the attitudes of health care professionals' not considering this approach and hesitancy among people with disability. However, the benefits of general self-initiated exercise are well established in persons with disability [129–135]. The benefits of a regular exercise program include improved fitness, weight reduction, improved mood, and improved sleep. It is also known that adults with CP must be judicious in participating in exercise programs, given the issues of fatigue and pain. Care must be taken in prescribing exercise, keeping in mind the need for modifications and access related to severity, environment, and self-efficacy. Recent evidence-based recommendations for exercise and physical activity prescription for people with CP define specific parameters for aerobic and resistance exercise and general physical activity related to dosing (frequency, intensity, time) and type [135]. Reports have also explored the use of video and other active gaming activities, which may offer other opportunities for increasing energy expenditure and physical activity [136, 137]. Although research has identified the importance of exercise and activity and the ability for people with CP to engage successfully in those activities, access to both individual and group programs remains limited. Programs may be locally available, and health care providers should be aware of those opportunities. Referral to professionals with expertise in exercise and physical activity and knowledge about modifications or local program opportunities should be considered. In order to achieve long-term participation in physical activity and exercise, such activities, whether at home, in a health club, or as part of an individual recreation program, and with or without modifications, should be initiated earlier than in adulthood. And, just as in the nondisabled population, people with CP may initially engage in activities, but adherence without continued contact or support may be limited [138, 139].

6.18 Conclusion

Most adults with CP are generally healthy, and the clear majority survive into adulthood. Health care can remain complex, involve a variety of clinical resources and medical technologies, and require specialty services. Severity, as defined by motor function scales, and the number of severe impairments related to the associated conditions affect survival. More severe motor impairment (i.e., higher GMFCS) is related to higher health care utilization. Epilepsy is a leading cause of death and hospitalization in adults with CP.

Many of the same associated conditions seen in children with CP are seen in adults. Adults may also develop other health conditions, such as secondary conditions that may manifest during young adulthood, or other conditions commonly seen in the general population with advancing age. The most common health conditions seen in adults with CP relate to their motor function, and include musculoskeletal conditions, pain, and fatigue. These conditions, with aging, are often considered to manifest earlier in adults with CP than in the general population. In particular, issues related to sedentary behavior, sarcopenia, and obesity should be recognized early. Hypertension is relatively common. Pulmonary illnesses are a leading cause of hospitalization and a significant contributor to excess mortality in CP. Lower gastrointestinal problems, especially constipation, persist into adulthood, as does incontinence. Both need to be monitored to prevent possible increasing medical concerns. Depression and anxiety are also common concerns, need to be recognized, and can be responsive to treatment. Sexual health should not be ignored.

It is time to reconsider the model of illness and disease for people with CP and adopt a health and wellness model. Environmental, communication, attitudinal, and systems barriers must be overcome in order for health care providers and adults with CP to work together for the best possible outcomes. Use of prevention and health promotion strategies should consist of implementing typical screening schedules, increasing health literacy, and encouraging or referring to other professionals for active health promotion.

References

1. Rosenbaum P, Paneth N, Leviton A, Goldstein M, Bax M, Damiano D, Dan B, Jacobsson B. A report: the definition and classification of cerebral palsy. Dev Med Child Neurol. 2007;49(Suppl 109):8–14. https://doi.org/10.1111/j.1469-8749.2007.tb12610.x.
2. Smithers-Sheedy H, Badawi N, Blair E, Cans C, Himmelmann K, Krägeloh-Mann I, McIntyre S, Slee J, Uldall P, Watson L, Wilson M. What constitutes cerebral palsy in the twenty-first century? Dev Med Child Neurol. 2014;56:323–8. https://doi.org/10.1111/dmcn.12262.
3. Cans C, De-la- Cruz J, Mermet M-A. Epidemiology of cerebral palsy. Paediatr Child Health Canada. 2008;18:393–8.
4. Palisano R, Rosenbaum P, Walter S, Russell D, Wood E, Galuppi B. Development and reliability of a system to classify gross motor function in children with cerebral palsy. Dev Med Child Neurol. 1997;39:214–23.
5. Palisano RJ, Rosenbaum P, Bartlett D, Livingston MH. Content validity of the expanded and revised gross motor function classification system. Dev Med Child Neurol. 2008;50:744–50.
6. Eliasson A-C, Krumlinde-Sundholm L, Rösblad B, Beckung E, Arner M, Öhrvall A-M, Rosesnbaum P. The manual ability classification system (MACS) for children with cerebral palsy: scale development and evidence of validity and reliability. Dev Med Child Neurol. 2006;48:549–54.
7. McCormick A, Brien M, Plourde J, Wood E, Rosenbaum P, McLean J. Stability of gross motor functional classification system in adults with cerebral palsy. Dev Med Child Neurol. 2007;49:265–9.
8. Öhrvall A-M, Krumlinde-Sundholm L, Eliasson A-C. The stability of the manual ability classification system over time. Dev Med Child Neurol. 2014;56:185–9. https://doi.org/10.1111/dmcn.12348.
9. Jeevananthan D, Dyszuk E, Bartlett D. The manual ability classification system: a scoping review. Pediatr Phys Ther. 2015;27:236–41. https://doi.org/10.1097/PEP.0000000000000151.
10. Compagnone E, Maniglio J, Camposa S, Vespino T, Losito I, DeRinaldis M, Gennaro L, Trabacca A. Functional classification for cerebral palsy: correlations between the gross motor function classification system (GMFCS), the manual ability classification system (MACS) and the communication function classification system (CFCS). Res Dev Disabil. 2014;35:2651–7. https://doi.org/10.1016/j.ridd.2014.07.005.
11. Odding E, Roebroeck ME, Stam HJ. The epidemiology of cerebral palsy: incidence, impairments and risk factors. Disabil Rehabil. 2006;28:183–11. https://doi.org/10.1080/09638280500158422.
12. Arneson CL, Durkin MS, Benedict RE, Kirby RS, Yeargin-Allsopp M, Van Naarden Braun K, Doernberg NS. Prevalence of cerebral palsy: autism and developmental disabilities monitoring network, three sites, United States, 2004. Disabil Health J. 2009;2:45–8.
13. Maenner MJ, Blumberg S, Kogan MD, Christensen D, Yeargin-Allsopp M, Schieve LA. Prevalence of cerebral palsy and intellectual disability among children identified in two U.S. National Surveys, 2011-2013. Ann Epidemiol. 2016;26:222–6. https://doi.org/10.1016/j.annepidem.2016.01.001.
14. Paneth N, Hong T, Korzeniewski S. The descriptive epidemiology of cerebral palsy. Clin Perinatol. 2006;33:251–67.
15. Winter S, Autry A, Boyle C, Yeargin-Allsopp M. Trends in the prevalence of cerebral palsy in a population-based study. Pediatrics. 2002;110:1220–5.
16. Bhasin TK, Brocksen S, Avchen RN, Van Naarden Braun K. Prevalence of four developmental disabilities among children aged 8 years – Metropolitan Atlanta Developmental Disabilities Surveillance Program, 1996 and 2000. MMWR Surveill Summ. 2006a;55:1–9.
17. Oskoui M, Coutinho F, Dykeman J, Jetté N, Pringsheim T. An update on the prevalence of cerebral palsy: a systematic review and meta-analysis. Dev Med Child Neurol. 2013;55:509–19.
18. Van Naarden Braun K, Doernberg N, Schieve L. Birth prevalence of cerebral palsy: a population-based study. Pediatrics. 2016;137(1):e20152872.

19. Brooks JC, Strauss DJ, Shavelle RM, Tran LM, Rosenbloom L, Wu YW. Recent trends in cerebral palsy survival. Part I: Period and cohort effects. Dev Med Child Neurol. 2014a;56:1059–64. https://doi.org/10.1111/dmcn.12520.
20. Brooks JC, Strauss DJ, Shavelle RM, Tran LM, Rosenbloom L, Wu YW. Recent trends in cerebral palsy survival. Part II: Individual survival prognosis. Dev Med Child Neurol. 2014b;56:1065–71. https://doi.org/10.1111/dmcn.12519.
21. Westbom L, Bergstrand L, Wagner P, Nordmark E. Survival at 19 years of age in a total population of children and young people with cerebral palsy. Dev Med Child Neurol. 2011;53:808–14. https://doi.org/10.1111/j.1469-8749.2011.04027.x.
22. Strauss D, Shavelle R. Life expectancy of adults with cerebral palsy. Dev Med Child Neurol. 1998;40:369–75.
23. Strauss D, Ojdana K, Shavelle R, Rosenbloom L. Decline in function and life expectancy of older persons with cerebral palsy. NeuroRehabilitation. 2004;19:69–78.
24. Day SM, Wu YW, Strauss DJ, Shavelle RM, Reynolds RJ. Causes of death in remote symptomatic epilepsy. Neurology. 2005;65:216–22. https://doi.org/10.1212/01.wnl.0000169018.44950.68.
25. Brooks JC, Shavelle RM, Strauss DJ. Survival in children with severe cerebral palsy: a further international comparison. Dev Med Child Neurol. 2012;54(4):383–4. https://doi.org/10.1111/j.1469-8749.2012.04236.x.
26. Hemming K, Hutton JL, Pharoah PO. Long-term survival for a cohort of adults with cerebral palsy. Dev Med Child Neurol. 2006;48:90–5.
27. Strauss D, Cable W, Shavelle R. Causes of excess mortality in cerebral palsy. Dev Med Child Neurol. 1999;41:580–5.
28. Peterson MD, Gordon PM, Hurvitz EA, Burant CF. Secondary muscle pathology and metabolic dysregulation in adults with cerebral palsy. Am J Physiol Endocrinol Metab. 2012;303:E1085–93. https://doi.org/10.1152/ajpendo.00338.2012.
29. Berens JC, Peacock C. Implementation of an academic adult primary care clinic for adolescents and young adults with complex, chronic childhood conditions. J Pediatr Rehabil Med. 2015;8:3–12. https://doi.org/10.3233/PRM-150313.
30. Nieuwenhuijsen C, Van Der Slot WMA, Dallmeijer AJ, Janssens PJ, Stam HJ, Roebroeck ME, Van Den Berg-Emons HJG, Transition Research Group South West Netherlands. Physical fitness, everyday physical activity, and fatigue in ambulatory adults with bilateral spastic cerebral palsy. Scand J Med Sci Sports. 2010;21(4):535–42. https://doi.org/10.1111/j.1600-0838.2009.01086.x.
31. Young NL, Gilbert TK, Mccormick A, Ayling-Campos A, Boydell K, Law M, Williams JI. Youth and young adults with cerebral palsy: their use of physician and hospital services. Arch Phys Med Rehabil. 2007;88:696–702. https://doi.org/10.1016/j.apmr.2007.03.005.
32. Pons C, Brochard S, Gallien P, Nicolas B, Duruflé A, Roquet M, Garlantezec R. Medication, rehabilitation and health care consumption in adults with cerebral palsy: a population based study. Clin Rehabil. 2016;31:957–65. https://doi.org/10.1177/0269215516663286.
33. Morgan P, McGinley J. Gait function and decline in adults with cerebral palsy: a systematic review. Disabil Rehabil. 2013;36:1–9. https://doi.org/10.3109/09638288.2013.775359.
34. Peterson MD, Gordon PM, Hurvitz EA. Chronic disease risk among adults with cerebral palsy: the role of premature sarcopoenia, obesity and sedentary behaviour. Obes Rev. 2013;14:171–82. https://doi.org/10.1111/j.1467-789x.2012.01052.x.
35. Roebroeck ME, Jahnsen R, Carona C. Adult outcomes and lifespan issues for people with childhood-onset physical disability. Dev Med Child Neurol. 2009;51:670–8.
36. Van der Slot WM, Nieuwenhuijsen C, Van Den Berg-Emons RJ. Chronic pain, fatigue, and depressive symptoms in adults with spastic bilateral cerebral palsy. Dev Med Child Neurol. 2012;54:836–42. https://doi.org/10.1111/j.1469-8749.2012.04371.x.
37. Young NL, Rochon TG, McCormick A, Law M, Wedge JH, Fehlings D. The Health and quality of life outcomes among youth and young adults with cerebral palsy. Arch Phys Med Rehabil. 2010;91:143–8. https://doi.org/10.1016/j.apmr.2009.08.152.
38. Murphy KP, Molnar GE, Lankasky K. Medical and functional status of adults with cerebral palsy. Dev Med Child Neurol. 1995;37:1075–84.

39. Ballin L, Balandin S. An exploration of loneliness: communication and the social networks of older people with cerebral palsy. J Intellect Dev Disabil. 2007;32:315–26. https://doi.org/10.1080/13668250701689256.
40. Cremer N, Hurvitz EA, Peterson MD. Multimorbidity in middle-aged adults with cerebral palsy. Am J Med. 2017;130:744.e9–744.e15. https://doi.org/10.1016/j.amjmed.2016.11.044.
41. Fortuna RJ, Holub A, Turk MA, Meccarello J, Davidson PW. Health conditions, functional status, and healthcare utilization in adults with cerebral palsy. Fam Pract. 2018; https://doi.org/10.1093/fampra/cmy027.
42. Ryan JM, Crowley VE, Hensey O, Broderick JM, McGahey A, Gormley J. Habitual physical activity and cardiometabolic risk factors in adults with cerebral palsy. Res Dev Disabil. 2014a;35:1995–2002.
43. Ryan JM, Crowley VE, Hensey O, McGahey A, Gormley J. Waist circumference provides an indication of numerous cardiometabolic risk factors in adults with cerebral palsy. Arch Phys Med Rehabil. 2014b;95:1540–6.
44. Turk MA. Health, mortality, and wellness issues in adults with cerebral palsy. Dev Med Child Neurol. 2009;51(Suppl 4):24–9.
45. Turk MA, Geremski CA, Rosenbaum PF, Weber RJ. The health status of women with cerebral palsy. Arch Phys Med Rehabil. 1997;78(12 Suppl 5):S10–7.
46. Peterson MD, Ryan JM, Hurvitz EA, Mahmoudi E. Chronic conditions in adults with cerebral palsy. JAMA. 2015;314:2303–5. https://doi.org/10.1001/jama.2015.11025.
47. van der Slot WM, Roebroeck ME, Nieuwenhuijsen C, et al. Cardiovascular disease risk in adults with spastic bilateral cerebral palsy. J Rehabil Med. 2013;45(9):866–72.
48. Turk MA, Gorter JW, Logan LR. Aging with pediatric onset disability and diseases. In: Alexander MA, Matthews DJ, editors. Pediatric rehabilitation: principles and practice. 5th ed. New York, NY: Demos Medical; 2016.
49. Anderson LL, Humphries K, McDermott S, Marks B, Sisirakm J, Larson S. The state of the science of health and wellness for adults with intellectual and developmental disabilities. Intellect Dev Disabil. 2013;51:385–98.
50. Bauer SE, Schumacher JR, Hall A. Disability and physical and communication-related barriers to health care related services among Florida residents: a brief report. Disabil Health. 2016;9:552–6.
51. Krahn GL, Hammond L, Turner A. A cascade of disparities: health and health care access for people with intellectual disability. Ment Retard Dev Disabil Res Rev. 2006;12:70–82.
52. Iezzoni LI. Make no assumptions: communication between persons with disabilities and clinicians. Assist Technol. 2006a;18:212–9.
53. Iezzoni LI. Going beyond disease to address disability. N Engl J Med. 2006b;355:976–9.
54. Ostapczuk M, Musch J. Estimating the prevalence of negative attitudes towards people with disability: a comparison of direct questioning, projective questioning and randomised response. Disabil Rehabil. 2011;33:399–411.
55. US Bone and Joint Initiative. The burden of musculoskeletal diseases in the United States. 3rd ed. Rosemont, IL: U.S Bone and Joint Initiative; 2016. Accessed from: http://www.boneandjointburden.org/.
56. Mathewson MA, Lieber RL. Pathophysiology of muscle contractures in cerebral palsy. Phys Med Rehabil Clin N Am. 2015;26:57–67. https://doi.org/10.1016/j.pmr.2014.09.005.
57. Prabhu RK, Swaminathan N, Harvey LA. Passive movements for the treatment and prevention of contractures. Cochrane Database Syst Rev. 2013;12:CD009331.
58. Katalinic OM, Harvey LA, Herbert RD, Moseley AM, Lannin NA, Schurr K. Stretch for the treatment and prevention of contractures. Cochrane Database Syst Rev. 2010;9:CD007455.
59. Carter DR, Tse B. The pathogenesis of osteoarthritis in cerebral palsy. Dev Med Child Neurol. 2009;51(Suppl 4):79–83.
60. Sulko J, Radlo W. Resekcja głowy kości udowej w zastarzałym zwichnięciu stawu biodrowego u dzieci z mózgowym porażeniem dziecięcym. [Femoral head resection in dislocated hip in cerebral palsy children]. Chir Narzadow Ruchu Ortop Pol. 2006;71:29–32.
61. Zaffuto-Sforza CD. Aging with cerebral palsy. Phys Med Rehabil Clin N Am. 2005;16:235–49.

62. Boldingh EJ, Bouwhuis CB, van der Heijden-Maessen HC, Bos CF, Lankhorst GJ. Palliative hip surgery in severe cerebral palsy: a systematic review. J Pediatr Orthop. 2014;23:86–92.
63. Leet AI, Chhor K, Launay F, Kier-York J, Sponseller PD. Femoral head resection for painful hip subluxation in cerebral palsy: is valgus osteotomy in conjunction with femoral head resection preferable to proximal femoral head resection and traction. J Pediatr Orthop. 2005;25:70–3.
64. Schorle CM, Manolikakis G. Surgical treatment of secondary hip dislocation in cerebral palsy. Der Orthop. 2004;33:1129–37.
65. King G, Hunt LP, Wilkinson JM, Blom AW. Good outcome of total hip replacement in patients with cerebral palsy. Acta Orthop. 2016;87:93–9. https://doi.org/10.3109/17453674.2015.1137439.
66. Stout JL, Gage JR, Schwartz MH, Novacheck TF. Distal femoral extension osteotomy and patellar tendon advancement to treat persistent crouch gait in cerebral palsy. J Bone Joint Surg Am. 2008;90:2470–84.
67. Houdek MT, Watts CD, Wyles CC, Trousdale RT, Milbrandt TJ, Taunton MJ. Total knee arthroplasty in patients with cerebral palsy: a matched cohort study to patients with osteoarthritis. J Am Acad Orthop Surg. 2017;25:381–8.
68. Jahnsen R, Villien L, Aamodt G. Musculoskeletal pain in adults with cerebral palsy compared with the general population. J Rehabil Med. 2004;36:78–84.
69. Hägglund G, Pettersson K, Czuba T, Persson-Bunke M, Rodby-Bousquet E. Incidence of scoliosis in cerebral palsy. Acta Orthop. 2018;14:1–5. https://doi.org/10.1080/17453674.2018.1450091.
70. Gu Y, Shelton JE, Ketchum JM. Natural history of scoliosis in nonambulatory spastic tetraplegic cerebral palsy. Am J Phys Med Rehabil. 2011;3:27–32.
71. Porter D, Michael S, Kirkwood C. Patterns of postural deformity in non-ambulant people with cerebral palsy: what is the relationship between the direction of scoliosis, direction of pelvic obliquity, direction of windswept hip deformity and side of hip dislocation. Clin Rehabil. 2007;21:1087–96.
72. Cloake T, Gardner A. The management of scoliosis in children with cerebral palsy: a review. J Spine Surg. 2016;2:299–309.
73. Mercado E, Alman B, Wright JG. Does spinal fusion influence quality of life in neuromuscular scoliosis? Spine. 2007;32(19 Suppl):S120–5.
74. Mergler S, Evenhuis HM, Boot AM. Epidemiology of low bone mineral density and fractures in children with severe cerebral palsy: a systematic review. Dev Med Child Neurol. 2009;51:773–8.
75. Sheridan KJ. Osteoporosis in adults with cerebral palsy. Dev Med Child Neurol. 2009;51(Suppl 4):38–51.
76. Smeltzer SC, Zimmerman VL. Usefulness of the SCORE index as a predictor of osteoporosis in women with disabilities. Orthop Nurs. 2005;24:33–9.
77. Harcke HT, Taylor A, Bachrach S, Miller F, Henderson RC. Lateral femoral scan: an alternative method for assessing bone mineral density in children with cerebral palsy. Pediatr Radiol. 1998;28:241–6.
78. Kim W, Lee SJ, Yoon Y, Shin Y, Cho S, Rhee Y. Adults with spastic cerebral palsy have lower bone mass than those with dyskinetic cerebral palsy. Bone. 2015;71:89–93. https://doi.org/10.1016/j.bone.2014.10.003.
79. Sees JP, Sitoula P, Dabney K, et al. Pamidronate treatment to prevent reoccurring fractures in children with cerebral palsy. J Pediatr Orthop. 2016;36:193–7.
80. Fehlings D, Switzer L, Agarwal P, Wong C, Sochett E, Stevenson R, Gaebler D. Informing evidence- based clinical practice guidelines for children with cerebral palsy at risk of osteoporosis: a systematic review. Dev Med Child Neurol. 2012;54:106–16.
81. Jahnsen R, Villien L, Stanghelle JK, Holm I. Fatigue in adults with cerebral palsy in Norway compared with the general population. Dev Med Child Neurol. 2003;45:296–303.
82. Klingbeil H, Baer HR, Wilson PE. Aging with a disability. Arch Phys Med Rehabil. 2004;5(7 Suppl 3):S68–73.

83. Liptak GS. Health and well-being of adults with cerebral palsy. Curr Opin Neurol. 2008;21:136–42.
84. Turk MA, Scandale J, Rosenbaum PF, Weber RJ. The health of women with cerebral palsy. Phys Med Rehabil Clin N Am. 2001;12:153–68.
85. Brunton LK, Bartlett DJ. Description of exercise participation of adolescents with cerebral palsy across a 4-year period. Pediatr Phys Ther. 2010;22:180–7. https://doi.org/10.1097/pep.0b013e3181db8aaa.
86. Vogtle LK. Pain in adults with cerebral palsy: impact and solutions. Dev Med Child Neurol. 2009;51:113–21. https://doi.org/10.1111/j.1469-8749.2009.03423.x.
87. Penner M, Xie WY, Binepal N, Switzer L, Fehlings D. Characteristics of pain in children and youth with cerebral palsy. Pediatrics. 2013;132:e407–13.
88. Hirsh AT, Kratz AL, Engel JM, Jensen MP. Survey results of pain treatments in adults with cerebral palsy. Am J Phys Med Rehabil. 2011;90:207–16.
89. Hong Y, Geraci M, Turk MA, Love BL, McDermott SW. Opioid prescription patterns for adults with longstanding disability and inflammatory conditions compared to other users, using a nationally representative sample. Arch Phys Med Rehabil. 2018; https://doi.org/10.1016/j.apmr.2018.06.034. S0003-9993(18)30929-8.
90. Engel JM, Kartin D, Jensen MP. Pain treatment in persons with cerebral palsy: frequency and helpfulness. Am J Phys Med Rehabil. 2002;81:291–6.
91. Engel JM, Jensen MP, Schwartz L. Outcome of biofeedback-assisted relaxation for pain in adults with cerebral palsy: preliminary findings. Appl Psychophysiol Biofeedback. 2004;29:135–40.
92. Malone LA, Vogtle LK. Pain and fatigue consistency in adults with cerebral palsy. Disabil Rehabil. 2009;32:385–91. https://doi.org/10.3109/09638280903171550.
93. Gringras P. Sleep disorders in cerebral palsy. Dev Med Child Neurol. 2016;59:349–50. https://doi.org/10.1111/dmcn.13335.
94. Lélis AL, Cardoso MV, Hall WA. Sleep disorders in children with cerebral palsy: an integrative review. Sleep Med Rev. 2016;30:63–71. https://doi.org/10.1016/j.smrv.2015.11.008.
95. Christensen D, Van Naarden Braun K, Doernberg NS. Prevalence of cerebral palsy, co-occurring autism spectrum disorders, and motor functioning - Autism and Developmental Disabilities Monitoring Network, USA. Dev Med Child Neurol. 2008;2014(56):59–65.
96. Shevell MI, Dagenais L, Hall N, Consortium R. Comorbidities in cerebral palsy and their relationship to neurologic subtype and GMFCS level. Neurology. 2009;72:2090–6.
97. Claassen J, Lokin J, Fitzsimmons B-F, Mendelsohn F, Mayer S. Predictors of functional disability and mortality after status epilepticus. Neurology. 2002;58:139–42.
98. Young NL, McCormick AM, Gilbert T, Ayling-Campos A, Burke T, Fehlings D, Wedge J. Reasons for hospital admissions among youth and young adults with cerebral palsy. Arch Phys Med Rehabil. 2011;92:46–50. https://doi.org/10.1016/j.apmr.2010.10.002.
99. Krach LE, Kriel RL, Day SM, Strauss DJ. Survival of individuals with cerebral palsy receiving continuous intrathecal baclofen treatment: a matched-cohort study. Dev Med Child Neurol. 2009;52(7):672–6. https://doi.org/10.1111/j.1469-8749.2009.03473.x.
100. Harada T, Ebara S, Anwar MM. The cervical spine in athetoid cerebral palsy. A radiological study of 180 patients. J Bone Joint Surg Br. 1996;78:613–9.
101. Nagashima T, Kurimura M, Nishimura M. Late deterioration of functional abilities in adult cerebral palsy. Rinsho Shinkeigaku. 1993;33:939–44.
102. Rosenfeld M, Friedman JH. Cervical stenosis and dystonic cerebral palsy. Mov Disord. 1999;14:194–5.
103. Azuma S, Seichi A, Ohnishi I. Long-term results of operative treatment for cervical spondylotic myelopathy in patients with athetoid cerebral palsy: an over 10-year follow-up study. Spine. 2002;27:943–8.
104. Furuya T, Koda M, Sakuma T, Iijima Y, Saito J, Kitamura M, Yamazaki M. Spinal instrumented fusion in combination with botulinum toxin treatment for cervical myelopathy in patients with athetoid cerebral palsy. Med Res Archiv. 2016;4:2375–1924. Accessed from: http://www.journals.ke-i.org/index.php/mra/article/view/853.

105. Alvarez N, Larkin C, Roxborough J. Carpal tunnel syndrome in athetoid-dystonic cerebral palsy. Arch Neurol. 1982;39(5):311–2.
106. McPhee P, Gorter J, Cotie L, Timmons B, Bentley T, Macdonald M. Descriptive data on cardiovascular and metabolic risk factors in ambulatory and non-ambulatory adults with cerebal palsy. Data Brief. 2015;5:967–70. https://doi.org/10.1016/j.dib.2015.10.045.
107. Peterson MD, Mahmoudi E. Healthcare utilization associated with obesity and physical disabilities. Phys Med Rehabil. 2014;6(8, Suppl 2):S131. https://doi.org/10.1016/j.pmrj.2014.08.179.
108. Blackmore AM, Bear N, Blair E. Factors associated with respiratory illness in children and young adults with cerebral palsy. J Pediatr. 2016;168:151–157.e151.
109. Gustafsson PM, Tibbling L. Gastro-oesophageal reflux and oesophageal dysfunction in children and adolescents with brain damage. Acta Paediatr (Oslo, Norway: 1992). 1994;83:1081–5.
110. Del Giudice E. Cerebral palsy and gut functions. J Pediatr Gastroenterol Nutr. 1997;25(Suppl 1):S22–3.
111. Ren LH, Chen WX, Qian LJ, Li S, Gu M, Shi RH. Addition of prokinetics to PPI therapy in gastroesophageal reflux disease: a meta-analysis. World J Gastroenterol. 2014;20:2412–9.
112. Murphy KP, Boutin SA, Ide KR. Cerebral palsy, neurogenic bladder, and outcomes of lifetime care. Dev Med Child Neurol. 2012;54:945–50.
113. Wang MH, Harvey J, Baskin L. Management of neurogenic bladder in patients with cerebral palsy. J Pediatr Rehabil Med. 2008;1:123–5.
114. Samijn B, Laecke EV, Renson C, Hoebeke P, Plasschaert F, Walle JV, Broeck CV. Lower urinary tract symptoms and urodynamic findings in children and adults with cerebral palsy: a systematic review. NeurourolUrodyn. 2016;36:541–9. https://doi.org/10.1002/nau.22982.
115. Henderson CM, Rosasco M, Robinson LM. Functional impairment severity is associated with health status among older persons with intellectual disability and cerebral palsy. J Intellect Disabil Res. 2009;53:887–97.
116. Engel JM, Jensen MP, Schwartz L. Coping with chronic pain associated with cerebral palsy. Occup Ther Int. 2006;13:224–33.
117. Murphy KP. The adult with cerebral palsy. Orthop Clin North Am. 2010;41:595–605.
118. Aiyer R, Barkin RL, Bhatia A. Treatment of neuropathic pain with venlafaxine: a systematic review. Pain Med (Malden, Mass). 2017;18:1999–2012.
119. Worley G, Houlihan CM, Herman-Giddens ME, et al. Secondary sexual characteristics in children with cerebral palsy and moderate to severe motor impairment: a cross-sectional survey. Pediatrics. 2002;110(5):897–902.
120. Wiegerink D, Roebroeck M, Bender J, Stam H, Cohen-Kettenis P. Sexuality of young adults with cerebral palsy: experienced limitations and needs. Sex Disabil. 2011;29:119–28.
121. Wiegerink DJ, Roebroeck ME, Donkervoort M, Cohen-Kettenis PT, Stam HJ. Social, intimate and sexual relationships of adolescents with cerebral palsy compared with able-bodied age-mates. J Rehabil Med. 2008;40:112–8.
122. Wiegerink DJ, Stam HJ, Gorter JW, Cohen-Kettenis PT, Roebroeck ME. Development of romantic relationships and sexual activity in young adults with cerebral palsy: a longitudinal study. Arch Phys Med Rehabil. 2010;91:1423–8.
123. Smith JA, Hutson JM, Beasley SW, Reddihough DS. The relationship between cerebral palsy and cryptorchidism. J Pediatr Surg. 1989;24:1303–5.
124. Jan BM, Jan MM. Dental health of children with cerebral palsy. Neurosciences (Riyadh, Saudi Arabia). 2016;21:314–8.
125. Steele C, Kalnins I, Jutai J, Stevens E, Bortolussi J, Biggar D. Lifestyle health behaviours of 11–16-year- old youth with physical disabilities. Health Educ Res. 1996;11:173–86.
126. Stevens SE, Steele CA, Jutai JW, Kalnins IV, Bortolussi JA. Adolescents with physical disabilities: some psychosocial aspects of health. J Adolesc Health. 1996;19:157–64.

127. Turk MA. Health and wellness for children with disabilities. In: Kliegman R, Stanton B, St. Geme JW, Schor NF, editors. Textbook of pediatrics. 20th ed. Philadelphia, PA: Elsevier; 2015.
128. Xu X, Ozturk OD, Turk MA, McDermott SW. Physical activity and disability: an analysis on how activity might lower medical expenditures. J Phys Act Health. 2018;27:1–8. https://doi.org/10.1123/jpah.2017-0331.
129. Durstine JL, Painter P, Franklin BA, Morgan D, Pitetti KH, Roberts SO. Physical activity for the chronically ill and disabled. Sports Med. 2000;30:207–19.
130. Fragala-Pinkham MA, Haley SM, Goodgold S. Evaluation of a community-based group fitness program for children with disabilities. Pediatr Phys Ther. 2006;18:159–67.
131. Kilmer DD. Response to resistive strengthening exercise training in humans with neuromuscular disease. Am J Phys Med Rehabil. 2002;81:S121–6.
132. Petajan JH, White AT. Recommendations for physical activity in patients with multiple sclerosis. Sports Med. 1999;27:179–91.
133. Rimmer JH, Rowland JL. Health promotion for people with disabilities: Implications for empowering the person and promoting disability-friendly environments. Am J Lifestyle Med. 2008;2(5):409–20.
134. Robinson-Whelen S, Hughes RB, Taylor HB. Improving the health and health behaviors of women aging with physical disabilities: a peer-led health promotion program. Womens Health Issues. 2006;16:334–45.
135. Verschuren O, Peterson MD, Balemans AC, Hurvitz EA. Exercise and physical activity recommendations for people with cerebral palsy. Dev Med Child Neurol. 2016;58:798–808. https://doi.org/10.1111/dmcn.13053.
136. Deutsch JE, Guarrera-Bowlby P, Myslinski MJ, Kafri M. Is there evidence that active videogames increase energy expenditure and exercise intensity for people poststroke and with cerebral palsy? Games Health J. 2015;4:31–7. https://doi.org/10.1089/g4h.2014.0082.
137. Knights S, Graham N, Switzer L, Hernandez H, Ye Z, Findlay B, Fehlings D. An innovative cycling exergame to promote cardiovascular fitness in youth with cerebral palsy: a brief report. Dev Neurorehabil. 2014;19(2):135–40. https://doi.org/10.3109/17518423.2014.923056.
138. Clanchy KM, Tweedy SM, Trost SG. Evaluation of a physical activity intervention for adults with brain impairment. Neurorehabil Neural Repair. 2016;30(9):854–65. https://doi.org/10.1177/1545968316632059.
139. Rimmer JH, Wang E, Pellegrini CA, Lullo C, Gerber BS. Telehealth weight management intervention for adults with physical disabilities. Am J Phys Med Rehabil. 2013;92(12):1084–94. https://doi.org/10.1097/phm.0b013e31829e780e.

Regression in Adolescents and Adults with Down Syndrome

7

Brian Chicoine and George Capone

7.1 Introduction

There is a growing number of clinical case reports of adolescents and adults with Down syndrome who have shown unexpected and severe regression in cognitive and adaptive functioning, motor function, communication skills, and behavior [12, 32, 38, 45, 50]. As reported by their families, this regression is reported to occur following a period of stable functional skill acquisition in young adolescents or adults.

While there have been several articles published about regression in adolescents and adults with Down syndrome, there remains a great deal that is still unknown. In this chapter, we will refer to this phenomenon as "adult regression syndrome." We will provide information from published studies and reports, describe why autism and Alzheimer's disease are excluded from consideration (as they are separate entities), report on a working definition of adult regression syndrome, and describe clinical features, evaluation, treatment, and prognosis. Emphasis will be given to some of the most challenging patients who manifest catatonia, auto-immunity, sleep apnea, and severe mental health symptoms.

B. Chicoine (✉)
Advocate Medical Group, Adult Down Syndrome Center, Park Ridge, IL, USA

Faculty, Family Medicine Residency, Advocate Lutheran General Hospital, Park Ridge, IL, USA
e-mail: brian.chicoine@advocatehealth.com

G. Capone
Pediatrics, Johns Hopkins School of Medicine, Baltimore, MD, USA

Down Syndrome Clinic & Research Center, Kennedy Krieger Institute, Baltimore, MD, USA
e-mail: capone@kennedykrieger.org

© Springer Nature Switzerland AG 2019   121
V. P. Prasher, M. P. Janicki (eds.), *Physical Health of Adults with Intellectual and Developmental Disabilities*, https://doi.org/10.1007/978-3-319-90083-4_7

7.2   Background

Reports of changes in young individuals with Down syndrome go back as far as the 1940s, when Rollin [42] described the development of catatonic psychoses in 28 of 73 (38%) individuals with Down syndrome living in a residential facility. More recently, Prasher [38] was the first, to report regression occurring over 1–2 years followed by a plateau in functioning in young adults with Down syndrome. He noted that there was a "gradual but severe deterioration in function after a period of normal development" and described these observations in his letter titled Young Adults with a Disintegrative Syndrome (YADS) (p. 101). Similarly, Devenny and Matthews [12] described individuals with a relatively rapid onset of decline in adaptive functioning with a loss of previously acquired cognition, socialization, and activities of daily living, and a concomitant increase in maladaptive behaviors following a period of stable adult function.

Akahoshi et al. [1] described acute regression in 13 adolescents or young adults with Down syndrome (mean age: 21.2 years) who developed acute neuropsychiatric disorders, including withdrawal, depression, obsessive-compulsive behaviors, and occasional delusions or hallucinations. Worley et al. [50] described a new onset of autistic-like regression they labeled "Down syndrome disintegrative disorder". The individuals had symptoms that included psychomotor slowing, withdrawal, mutism, apathy, emotional instability, anorexia, insomnia, obsessive-compulsive behaviors, and occasionally delusions or hallucinations. Some individuals were also diagnosed with major depressive, obsessive-compulsive, delusional, or adjustment disorders according to clinical criteria.

Ghaziuddin et al. [17] described four individuals with Down syndrome and regression along with motor disturbances such as slowing or increased motor activity and were diagnosed with catatonia. They were treated with benzodiazepines and electroconvulsive therapy with recovery to their baseline. Mircher et al. [32] described 30 individuals with Down syndrome, aged 11–30 years old with history of regression. The mean age at regression was 18 years in girls and 21 years in boys and occurred unrelated to baseline cognitive level. Patients presented with psychiatric symptoms (catatonia, depression, delusions, stereotypies, etc.), partial or total loss of independence in activities of daily living (dressing, toileting, meals, and continence), language impairment (silence, whispered voice, etc.), and loss of academic skills.

This decline in adolescents and adults with Down syndrome has been given various names. For this chapter, we use the term, 'adult regression syndrome'.

7.3   Disease Exclusions

It is now known that children with Down syndrome experience a higher incidence of autism [6, 9, 16, 22, 41] and adults with Down syndrome have a higher incidence of Alzheimer's disease [29, 51] compared to the general population. Both co-morbidities are associated with a characteristic age of onset and timeline that is distinguishable from the adult regression syndrome. Careful history-taking and diagnostic assessment for autism and Alzheimer's disease are needed to determine the age of onset, preexisting level of function, and pattern of change over time. Medical assessment to rule-out, and/or treat other contributing conditions or illnesses is also necessary [19, 22, 39, 43].

7.4 Autistic Regression

Although, as in Worley et al.'s study [50], autism or autistic-like has been used to describe these individuals, they are "too old" for the onset of childhood autism. Although ICD-10 criteria include onset by age 3 years of age, the onset of childhood autism has a later onset in children with Down syndrome. Castillo et al. [9] studied the symptom onset among children with autism and Down syndrome, comparing it to the onset in children with autism without Down syndrome. They found that 12 of 24 (50%) of the children with autism in their Down syndrome cohort had a history of loss of previously acquired language and socio-communicative skills. The mean age at language loss in children with autism with Down syndrome was 61.8 months (SD 22.9) compared to 19.7 months (SD 5.8) for those with autism without Down syndrome (p .01). The mean age at other skill loss was 46.2 months (SD 19.1) and 19.5 months (SD 5.6), respectively (p .006). Although the onset of symptoms for children with autism and Down syndrome was later than for those with autism and without Down syndrome, this decline occurred at a much younger age than the decline in those being diagnosed with adult regression syndrome. Even when considering late-onset autism or 'childhood disintegrative disorder', as referred to by Worley et al. [50], those criteria include onset by 10 years of age which is still much younger than most of those being described with adult regression syndrome [1, 32].

7.5 Alzheimer's Regression

Alzheimer's-type dementia in individuals with Down syndrome typically occurs after 45 years of age. Tyrrell et al. [46] reported a mean age of onset of 54.7 years and Lai and Williams [27] reported a mean age of onset of 54.2 years. The onset of adult regression syndrome in teens and early twenties is much too early to represent onset of Alzheimer's-type dementia marked by of progressive impairment in cognitive, adaptive and motor function often accompanied by seizures [18, 51].

However, some of the symptoms of regression syndrome, that will be described more fully later in the chapter, are also seen in Alzheimer's disease. Most people with Down syndrome who present with Alzheimer's disease also experience psychological or behavioral changes [10, 33], motor function changes, such as Parkinson-like symptoms [20, 47], and changes in speech. Wisniewski et al. [49] found that Alzheimer's disease-like pathological changes (e.g., neuronal loss, neurofibrillary tangles, or plaques) were present after 35 years of age in most individuals and that basal ganglia calcification was common in such individuals. Akahoshi et al. [1] found that people with Down syndrome and regression showed evidence of atrophy or hypoplasia on brain imaging. Such changes were even found in a patient as young as 10 years of age and likely reflect hypoplastic changes. However, clinically Alzheimer's disease is unlikely to present in patients with Down syndrome younger than 35–40 years [33].

In addition, there are other differences between Alzheimer's disease and regression syndrome. Regression syndrome often can plateau (sometimes for many years) after a rapid onset of symptoms. Due to these differences and the very young age that some of these individuals present we have proposed excluding Alzheimer's disease as causal. Akahoshi et al. [1] similarly concluded that these disorders (regression) present features and a clinical course that is different from those presented in typical Alzheimer's disease with Down syndrome. Therefore, we will define this as a separate entity from Alzheimer's disease. Given the evidence, we have excluded Alzheimer's disease and autism as a cause of the type of adult regression syndrome being described here.

7.6   Defining Adult Regression Syndrome: What Diagnosis to Include?

While these individuals don't fit either the autism or Alzheimer's disease diagnoses, they can similarly present with significant regression in skills, language, and other symptoms. The term adult regression syndrome has been suggested for the diagnosis for these individuals in the middle-age range who have developed this form of decline. These individuals are commonly in their teens or twenties (although older and younger individuals have been described) and their decline occurs mostly in association with other neuropsychiatric symptoms/conditions (e.g. depression, psychosis, obsessive compulsive disorder, or catatonia) and rarely in isolation from other psychiatric symptoms [38]. The changes often occur over weeks to months and affect individuals at all cognitive levels, many without prior mental health concerns [1].

A thorough evaluation may lead to a known diagnosis (e.g., depression, sleep apnea) and the appropriate treatment can be successfully provided. A subset of individuals has been described that may have a less clear or unknown etiology, are often more challenging to treat, and sometimes don't recover fully or only recover in a limited manner.

With a limited understanding of this syndrome now, there is ongoing discussion as to the definition of adult regression syndrome. One area of discussion is whether any individual who is regressing (who doesn't have Alzheimer's disease or autism) has adult regression syndrome. For example, do we include those who have regression of their skills, who are found to have a known comorbidity diagnosis (e.g. depression, sleep apnea), who are successfully treated, and whose skills return? Or should only those for whom the diagnosis is less clear, have severe regression, and/ or have limited recovery be included? There is a question about whether these individuals with severe regression in some way form a unique diagnostic group, or whether they are on a continuum of the expression of maladaptive behaviors or psychopathology [12].

There is debate as to the answer to these questions—but for this chapter, we will include all those individuals who are regressing for a variety of reasons (excluding those with Alzheimer's disease or autism) who present with a certain pattern of symptoms (*see Clinical Features below*). We will explore the differential diagnosis and give emphasis to those whom the diagnosis is less clear, tend to be more severely affected, and tend to provide a greater treatment challenge. The emphasis on the more severely affected group will be more evident in the next section describing clinical features. Many conditions in the differential often don't present with the breadth of symptoms described (although they can). Therefore, those with regression, but without the breadth of symptoms, while excluded from the diagnosis of adult regression syndrome, could be described as having some regression as part of the symptomatology of their co-morbid condition.

Presently, with this model of understanding, adult regression syndrome is a description of symptoms with a wide possible differential; a recognition that the brain/cognitive function of individuals with Down syndrome can be "fragile" and susceptible to further decline for a variety of reasons; and an acknowledgement that further study is needed to improve our understanding of diagnosis and treatment of individuals with Down syndrome who present with a significant and early decline in skills. In the sections that follow, we will present a case and then discuss different aspects of adult regression syndrome, including clinical presentation, differential diagnoses, and evaluation.

7.7 Clinical Presentation

Lucy was a 30-year-old woman with Down syndrome who presented for her first annual evaluation at a Down syndrome clinic. Lucy did not speak during the assessment, was reported to have no verbal skills, had repetitive motions through much of the assessment, and had little or no eye contact or interaction with the clinician. At first glance, the patient appeared to have autism, but the history was not classic for that diagnosis. Lucy had been a typically developing girl with Down syndrome with mild cognitive impairment, good verbal skills, and good self-care skills who attended school and a variety of activities prior to age 17. According to her mother, Lucy developed an upper respiratory infection at age 17, was treated with an antibiotic, and suddenly regressed. Over the following years, she had an extensive work-up including blood tests, imaging, and sleep study. She had been given a variety of diagnoses, including depression, anxiety, late-onset autism, early Alzheimer's disease, and psychoses. She had been treated with several psychotropic medications and supplements with little or no improvement. However, she also did not display further cognitive decline. She had neither improved nor deteriorated over the 13-year period.

7.8 Clinical Features of Adult Regression Syndrome

To improve the understanding of adult regression syndrome and to begin working towards a standardization of diagnostic, and evaluation procedures members of the Down Syndrome Medical Interest Group-USA (DSMIG-USA) Working Group [https://www.dsmig-usa.org/], [13] have operationalized a definition to provide a framework for case finding and further study. The discussions by this group have led to an operational definition outlined in Table 7.1.

Based on the consensus of experienced clinicians, all five core features are very commonly part of the presentation: cognitive-executive dysfunction, social withdrawal, loss of acquired skills, loss of functional use of language, and duration >3 months. Some or all the other variable features are often present. Figure 7.1 depicts the broad effect adult regression syndrome has on individuals.

The symptoms often emerge over an extended period. The core findings of regression/loss of skills may not be apparent initially or may be less significant than other symptoms, particularly behavioral or psychological, and, therefore, are not immediately recognized. For example, diagnosis and treatment of depression may or may not lead to amelioration of mood disturbance, whereas symptoms of skill loss may only become apparent over time.

Table 7.1 Core and Variable features

Core features
Cognitive—executive dysfunction
Social withdrawal
Loss of acquired skills
Loss of functional use of language
Duration >3 months
Exclusions
Not autism—affects children 3–7 years
Not Alzheimer-type dementia—affects adults >45 years
Variable features
Maladaptive behavior
Psychiatric symptoms
Failure to acquire new skills
Inattention-disorganization
Motor slowing
Vegetative symptoms—appetite/weight loss, incontinence, sleep pattern disturbance
Demographics
Typically between 15 and 30 years
Male = Female

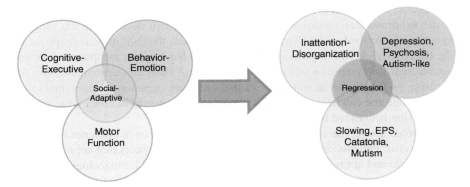

Fig. 7.1 A depiction of the core domains consistently affected in adult regression syndrome and their transition into clinically appreciable symptoms

7.9 Evaluation

John, a 23-year-old man with Down syndrome presented at a Down syndrome clinic with increasing cognitive impairment (from his baseline of a stable, mild intellectual disability) over several months. His family reported social withdrawal and reduced verbal communication, motor slowing interspersed with times of increased motor activity and emotional agitation, reduced ability to perform his self-care, times of increased sleep for weeks followed by weeks of difficulty sleeping, and inability to perform at his place of employment. His medications included levothyroxine which had been prescribed 8 months prior to his initial clinic appointment for a new diagnosis of hypothyroidism. Subsequent thyroid blood testing had been normal 5 months prior to the initial appointment. At the time of the appointment, his lab results revealed a very low thyroid stimulating hormone (TSH) level and high free thyroxine (fT4). Dose adjustment and eventual discontinuation of his levothyroxine did not result in a return to normal of those lab values (his TSH remained low and his f T4 remained high). With further assessment, it became clear that John's thyroid was fluctuating back and forth from a hyperthyroid state to a hypothyroid state. Ultimately, radioactive ablation and chronic levothyroxine treatment stabilized his thyroid function and his presenting symptoms improved over several months.

In John's case, fluctuating thyroid function likely contributed to the psychological, motor, and cognitive symptoms. As described by Popova et al. [37], a presentation of fluctuating thyroid function can occur in people with Down syndrome and, in John's case, seemed to cause significant morbidity that ultimately resolved with the appropriate diagnosis and treatment of his fluctuating thyroid function.

The assessment of a person with Down syndrome who is regressing requires an extensive search for underlying health problems. While the differential is substantial, there are conditions that are more common in people with Down syndrome and commonly present with some degree of regression. Sleep apnea, celiac disease, depression, adjustment to life changes, and other conditions common in people with Down syndrome can contribute to regression. Some will develop the full range of symptoms described above (Sect. 7.7) and, thus meet the definition as proposed by the DSMIG-USA Working Group, and some will have milder symptoms. It is also not unusual for symptoms to fluctuate over time. A thorough assessment, initially focusing on conditions as noted above that are more common in individuals with Down syndrome can help direct the diagnosis and treatment in either case. Further information is outlined below in Sect. 7.10.

As noted above, the complete picture of adult regression is often not evident on the first visit. Patients or families may focus on certain aspects that are particularly problematic and not recognize or report other symptoms. Pharmacologic treatment may improve some psychiatric symptoms making other symptoms (e.g. psychomotor slowing) more evident. In some cases, there may be an intensification of all symptoms over time until they stabilize. Recurrent assessment for symptom emergence and amelioration will often make the clinical picture clearer.

Table 7.2 describes one approach to individuals who are experiencing regression. This outline can guide the assessment. As noted above, for many reasons, all the symptoms may not be part of the initial presentation and review of the evaluation at subsequent appointments may clarify the diagnosis over time. Furthermore, as the patient is assessed and treated over time, the initial impressions can change based on current symptoms and the response to specific treatment.

Table 7.2 Evaluation of individuals with adult regression syndrome

History of present illness and examination
• Duration, age onset, duration of symptoms (weeks-months-years)
– Prior episodes
– Developmental-Behavioral-Psychiatric history
• Specific adaptive skill loss, based on previously established skills
– Cognitive-executive skills
– Social skills
– Speech/language skills
– Acquisition of new skills, learning
– Loss of control of bodily functions
– Episodes/spells
– Incontinence
– Autonomic dysfunction
• Psychiatric symptoms
– Mood, irritability
– Inattention, distractibility, disorganization
– Obsessive compulsive behavior, perseveration
– Agitation, aggression
– Apathy, mutism, abulia
– Stereotypy, mannerisms
• Maladaptive behaviors
– Self-injury, scratching, poking, skin-picking

Table 7.2 (continued)

History of present illness and examination
• Motor symptoms
– Catatonia-muscular rigidity/immobility/slowing
– Extrapyramidal symptoms
– Tics
• Vegetative symptoms
– Sleep disturbance
– Appetite/weight loss
• Focused systems review
– Level of function prior to onset
– Snoring, pauses in breathing, daytime drowsiness
– History of surgery and/or general anesthesia and relationship in time to the onset of symptoms
– Personal or family stressors
– Trauma, victimization
– Life changes (school, family changes, deaths)
– Recent infections
– Menstrual changes, dysmenorrhea
– Puberty
– Vision or hearing changes
– Change in gait, weakness
– Headaches
• Medication Review
– Changes, additions, subtractions relative to temporal onset of symptoms
• Examinations
– Observation-Mental Status-Physical-Neurologic examination
– DSM 5 or DM-ID criteria checklists
– DSMIG-USA operational criteria checklist
• Neuropsychology assessment
– Adaptive
– Cognitive-executive
– Maladaptive behavior
– Psychiatric symptoms
– Motor-movement (catatonia)

7.10 Differential Diagnoses

Sandy, a 33-year-old woman with Down syndrome was brought to a Down syndrome clinic for an evaluation for a reduced ability to manage her activities of daily living. Her family and her support staff were very concerned that she was developing Alzheimer's disease because of the changes over the last 6 months. Sandy was not participating in activities, was speaking less, and was withdrawn from contact with others. She was not sleeping well and would often decline to sleep in her bedroom preferring to sleep on the couch in the family room which tended to be brighter from outside lighting. She had a decreased appetite and seemed "nervous," according to family and support staff. During an exam approximately 18 months before, no cataracts had been visible on her eye exam. However, at this evaluation, dense cataracts were noted. Sandy was diagnosed with cataracts and depression, possibly related to her emotional response to the rapid loss of vision. Cataracts are common in adults with Down syndrome [25]. The evaluation did not reveal any other causes. Treatment included both referral to an ophthalmologist for cataract surgery and an anti-depressant. Over the next several months, Sandy returned to her previous level of function.

As has been mentioned above, the brain function of people with Down syndrome is susceptible to a variety of known medical conditions that can lead to further cognitive, behavioral, motor, and communication impairment. Therefore, a wide differential diagnosis may potentially need to be explored to properly diagnose and treat these individuals.

Table 7.3 describes a wide differential. As noted above, there are conditions that are more common in people with Down syndrome and, if consistent with the symptoms, should be part of the initial evaluation. In most cases, multiple co-morbid conditions are the rule rather than the exception. Additionally, people with Down syndrome often have limited verbal skills and limited ability to report physical symptoms. This can lead to a higher likelihood of a primary physical problem developing into secondary mental health symptoms. Therefore, when assessing an individual with Down syndrome with regression, multiple medical and psychosocial etiologies need to be considered.

Table 7.4 lists a number of tests that can be performed to evaluate those potential etiologies. In addition, Jacobs et al. [21] have described a tiered method that can guide the assessment of a person with Down syndrome and regression. This tier approach does focus on the more likely diagnoses in the lower tiers and the more obscure as one works down the tiers. Clinical assessment, the conditions diagnosed, and the response to treatment can guide the practitioner to decide which tests in Table 7.4 are indicated and/or how far to go through the tiers. Table 7.4 contains much of what Jacobs et al. [21] would consider tiers 1 and 2. The work-up for most would not require going further through tiers 3–5 as the diagnostic yield as one progresses through the tiers diminishes accordingly.

One additional note in assessment is that regression may be associated with changes on MRI/CT. Akahoshi et al. [1] reportedly found atrophy or hypoplasia in the basal ganglia but there was no data on controls with Down syndrome who did not have regression.

One of the yet unanswered questions is: in the most challenging cases with a negative medical work-up (tiers 1–2) are we dealing with a known pathophysiology, or is there some other neurobiological predisposition due to trisomy 21 that increases the likelihood of regression? In our clinical experience, it appears that some individuals are experiencing an unexplained and/or yet untreatable condition.

Table 7.3 Differential diagnoses

1) Medical conditions
a) Medication side effects
b) Sleep apnea
c) Seizures
d) Vitamin B12 deficiency
e) Cervical myelopathy
i) Subluxation, spinal stenosis
f) Chronic pain
g) Dental
h) Sinus
i) Cervical spine
j) Menstrual
k) Gastrointestinal, severe constipation
l) Cardiovascular disease
i) Uncorrected congenital heart disease with pulmonary hypertension, congestive heart failure
ii) Eisenmenger's syndrome
iii) Stroke: thrombotic or hemorrhagic
m) Infectious disease
i) Urinary tract infection
ii) Pneumonia
iii) Sepsis
iv) Viral/bacterial meningitis/encephalitis
v) Lyme's disease
n) Toxic-metabolic
i) Numerous etiologies
2) Neuropsychiatric disorders
a) Catatonia
b) Mood disorder
c) Obsessive compulsive disorder
d) Psychotic disorder
e) Complex tic disorder
f) Post-traumatic stress disorder
g) Parkinsonism, dystonia
h) Adjustment to life events—transitions and relationships
i) Loss of family, friends, pets
ii) School graduation, work setting changes, physical relocation
iii) Response to hospitalization or medical condition
3) Sensory
a) Visual impairment
i) Glaucoma
ii) Retinal detachment
iii) Cataracts
iv) Keratoconus

(continued)

Table 7.3 (continued)

b) Hearing impairment
i)   Hypoacusis or Hyperacusis
ii) Tinnitus
iii) Vertigo
4) Endocrine disorders
a) Hypo or hyperthyroidism
b) Adrenal insufficiency
c) Diabetes mellitus
d) Puberty-associated
e) Menopause-associated
5) Autoimmune disorders (additional evidence required)
a) Hashimoto's encephalopathy
b) Pediatric autoimmune neuropsychiatric disorders associated with streptococcal infections (PANDAS)
c) Central nervous system manifestation of Celiac disease
d) Central nervous system manifestation of systemic lupus erythematosus (SLE)
e) Autoimmune encephalopathy
f) Limbic encephalitis

Table 7.4 Tests to consider when assessing a person for adult regression syndrome

• Metabolic panel and CBC for electrolyte abnormalities, anemia, diabetes, and liver disease
• TSH and free T4
• Thyroid antibodies
• Folate, Vitamin B12, 25-OH Vitamin D
• Anti-tissue transglutaminase IgA and IgG and Total IgA
• Polysomnogram
• Hearing test
• Vision assessment for vision impairment, cataracts, and keratoconus
• Abdominal x-ray for constipation
• Depression screen
• Psychological assessment
• Brain MRI
• Lyme antibodies
• Anti-streptolysin antibodies
• Anti-nuclear antibodies, erythrocyte sedimentation rate, and C-reactive protein
• Rapid plasma reagin and human immunodeficiency virus load for syphilis or human immunodeficiency virus

While there are unanswered questions, it seems to be clear that agreement on the definition, thorough assessments based on the wide differential, and the compilation of cases, including treatment, will increase the likelihood of improved understanding. To that end, a review and development of a list of differential diagnoses and a recommended assessment protocol has been discussed and data are being compiled [31].

7.11 Treatment

Treatment for commonly diagnosed conditions will not be extensively reviewed here. Thyroid replacement for hypothyroidism, Continuous positive airway pressure for sleep apnea, anti-depressants for depression, and others may all be part of treating different individuals with Down syndrome and regression syndrome. Some of the most challenging symptoms are behavioral or psychological. Akahoshi et al. [1] described diagnosing a variety of psychiatric diagnoses including anxiety, depression, and psychosis with variable response to treatment—from non-responsive to fully responsive. A combination of medications may be necessary.

Worley et al. [50] found that no medication or combination of medications was consistently effective, but risperidone, fluoxetine, sertraline, trazodone, donepezil, and rivastigmine each helped at least one patient to some degree. They concluded that no medication can be recommended for all and that the improvement in core symptoms experienced by eight of 11 cases was mostly spontaneous and not due to an intervention.

Mircher et al. [32] described that causes of regression are unknown and treatment is most of the time symptomatic. Most patients received several types of drugs simultaneously or consecutively. Benzodiazepines (but not at high doses as recommended for catatonia), selective serotonin reuptake inhibitors (SSRI) (paroxetine, fluoxetine, escitalopram, sertraline), and antipsychotic drugs (haloperidol, propericiazine, amisulpiride for the older cases, and more recently, risperidone and aripiprazole) were the more frequently used. Antiepileptic drugs used as mood stabilizers were used less frequently. One woman needed six electroconvulsive treatment (ECT) sessions and recovered completely. The evaluation of treatment efficacy was impossible in this study, but aripiprazole, risperidone, and paroxetine were reported as the most frequently effective to treat social withdrawal and psychotic symptoms. Jacobs et al. [21] described an individual who returned to 85% of baseline with the use of clozapine.

Providers, who are members of DSMIG-USA, often prescribe treatment that focuses on target symptoms such as psychiatric, behavior, attention, motor, sleep, and other medical symptoms with a focus on those that are most impairing and most likely to respond. Treatment often includes an approach that includes pharmacology, ecological adaptations, and treatment of medical conditions. Occupational therapy, physical therapy, speech therapy and behavioral therapy may all be part of the treatment regimen. Prioritization of the multimodal treatments is based on clinician experience, family preferences, and patient tolerability. Caretaker support is generally part of the treatment regimen and may include assisting with adaptation to a new reality and the future.

One additional key factor for many of these individuals is a withdrawal from activities and/or a limitation in leaving home. Many of these individuals will need a gradual, "safe" re-entry into activities. Successful participation in activities that are unlikely to provoke significant anxiety or fear is required to prevent abrupt reversal of improvement. This gradual re-entry without fear and anxiety is therapeutic as well.

As indicated earlier in this chapter, we included patients who have a variety of etiologies and often respond well to treatment for those conditions. These might include symptoms that improve after the diagnosis of sleep apnea and treatment with continuous positive airway pressure, diagnosis of depression and treatment with an anti-depressant, diagnosis of celiac disease with B12 deficiency, and treatment with gluten-free diet and B12 supplementation, or the diagnosis of recurrent seizures and the treatment with appropriate seizure medication. However, as indicated there is a subset of individuals for whom the diagnosis and treatment have been more challenging at times. Although, some providers would only include these individuals in the diagnosis of adult regression syndrome, we are more inclusive in this chapter but do want to give special attention to these individuals. Of note are some of the conditions that have been found in some of the most challenging patients to treat.

7.11.1 Catatonia

Jane, a 23-year-old woman, developed a rash after taking a hike in the woods. When the rash did not respond to oral antihistamine medication and topical steroids and the pruritus worsened, she was given a short course of oral prednisone. However, within a few days of starting the prednisone, Jane's mood and behavior changed dramatically. She declined to participate in activities, including self-care, and was agitated and withdrawn. Over the next few months, despite treatment with various anti-depressant and anti-psychotic medications, she continued to decline. She stopped eating and was hospitalized. Ultimately, a percutaneous endoscopic gastrostomy (PEG) tube was placed to provide adequate hydration and nutrition. In addition, she developed muscular rigidity and would lie motionless for hours. She underwent a series of electroconvulsive therapy (ECT) treatments and had a dramatic recovery. She was weaned off her medications. Approximately 1 year later, she had a milder recurrence and was successfully treated with medications alone.

Ghaziuddin et al. [17] described catatonia in a small series of people with Down syndrome. Catatonia is a condition that traditionally was associated with psychoses, but it is now recognized that it can be associated with a variety of psychiatric or medical conditions [11]. It has also been proposed that it be a separate diagnosis not associated with other psychiatric or medical conditions [14, 15, 35, 44]. Loss of motor skills or, conversely, constant hyperactive motor activity are symptoms. Catatonic patients will sometimes hold rigid poses for hours and will ignore any external stimuli. They may also show stereotyped, repetitive movements. The Bush-Francis Questionnaire [24] is a diagnostic tool recommended for diagnosing catatonia.

Treatment can include high-dose lorazepam and ECT treatments [17]. Miles [31], a co-author on the paper with Ghaziuddin et al. [17], described successful use of N-methyl-D-aspartate receptor (NMDA) antagonists, dextromethorphan-quinidine (Nuedexta), memantine (Namenda), and amantadine. She reported best success with dextromethorphan-quinidine. In the non-Down syndrome population,

Daniels [11] reported successful treatment with NMDA antagonists in individuals whose catatonia was resistive to lorazepam. A dysregulation of dopamine, gamma-Aminobutyric acid (GABA) and glutamate is proposed as being involved in catatonia. Lorazepam enhances GABA activity and the NMDA antagonists reduce the effect of glutamate.

Ghaziuddin et al. [17] reported that all four of their cases were treated with a benzodiazepine combined with ECT and recovered their baseline functioning. They noted that the need for prolonged maintenance ECT for people with Down syndrome and catatonia raises questions about the possibility of difference in pathophysiological mechanisms, which may underlie catatonia in individuals with Down syndrome and other intellectual disability versus those with typical development. The authors concluded that they suspect catatonia is a common cause of unexplained deterioration in adolescents and young adults with Down syndrome. Lorazepam and ECT were successful treatments in their series. However, a recent meta-analysis of the use of ECT in people without Down syndrome, who were diagnosed with catatonia, reported that in seven studies the adverse effects included mental confusion, memory loss, headache, or adverse effects associated with anesthesia [28]. The study further concluded that the "literature consistently describes improvement in catatonic symptoms after ECT"; "however, the published studies fail to demonstrate efficacy and effectiveness" (p. 1). Further study is warranted to understand the role of ECT in people with Down syndrome and catatonia.

7.11.2 Auto-immunity

It is known that the immune system of people with Down syndrome functions differently than those without Down syndrome [26, 36]. A higher rate of infections associated with impaired immunity and a higher rate of auto-immune conditions are found in people with Down syndrome. Is it possible that the immune system is involved in the changes associated with regression syndrome?

As noted above, Worley et al. [50] proposed an auto-immune etiology for the regression they found in a series of patients. Ten of 11 (91%) children and adolescents presenting with regression had elevated ("positive") thyroperoxidase antibody titers compared to only five of 21 (23%) age-matched control subjects with Down syndrome (p < .001). All cases with "Down syndrome disintegrative disorder" in their series had thyroid autoimmunity on at least one test. However, the only two cases who received steroids had no response to them. Interestingly, Armangue et al. [3] reported that Hashimoto's encephalitis is one of several autoimmune disorders that has been associated with development of catatonia.

In our experience, a common clinical description is that the onset of symptoms was preceded by an infection. In the case of Lucy in the Sect. 7.7, she had a respiratory infection prior to the onset of her symptoms. This has led some to question whether an infection may trigger the immune system causing regression syndrome. Viral infections are proposed to trigger the immune system in the development of Type 1 diabetes [23, 40] and celiac disease [5] both of which are more common in people with Down syndrome [2, 4, 30]. However, presently there are only limited data suggesting a role of auto-immunity in regression. Further study is needed to clarify this potential link.

7.11.3 Sleep Apnea

Sleep disturbances are extremely common in adolescents and adults with Down syndrome who experience new onset or exacerbation in mental health status [8]. Capone et al. [8] noted that 28 individuals meeting criteria for major depressive episode and nine controls without psychopathology were referred for overnight polysomnography. Functional decline was reported in 19 (68%) of cases with depression, but none of the controls. Twenty-four (86%) of the individuals with depression had obstructive sleep apnea compared with only four (44%) of controls. Moderate-severe obstructive sleep apnea was present in 15 (54%) of those with depression compared to only one (11%) of controls. Intermittent sleep-associated hypoxia and Rapid Eye Movement (REM) sleep deficits were also more frequent in those with depression.

In practice, many of the individuals presenting with mental health disturbances are not able to tolerate the overnight polysomnogram procedure required for definitive diagnosis and treatment. In such cases a home audio-video recording or in-home sleep study (screener) may prove informative enough to warrant an otolaryngology or sleep medicine referral for airway management. Many individuals also appear to benefit from pharmacologic treatment to improve insomnia and fragmented sleep if caution is exercised not to make obstructive apnea symptoms worse (Capone, 2018, personal observation).

7.11.4 Severe Depression

Severe depression is another possible cause of regression. Devenny and Matthews [12] reported that all but one of the individuals they studied with regression "showed at least one behavior that was within the domain of 'depression'." Capone et al. [7] suggested that psychosocial stressors, such as a growing awareness of being different and bereavement, may exacerbate symptoms of depression in adolescents. Some of these individuals appear to have regression in relation to a life event (or events). However, the nature of these events and their potential for triggering neuropsychiatric change is not at all clear and there are no data on life events in individuals without regression. In individual cases we have assessed and treated, reconstructing a timeline of how or when a medical illness, life-event or stress-related factor might have triggered an alteration in mental function is likely to be problematic when approached retrospectively, not least because of selective, recall bias. Mircher et al. [32] reported that all the patients experienced severe emotional stress prior to regression and hypothesized that this severe emotional stress may be considered the trigger. Prasher [38] proposed that 1) "disruption in routines and the loss of support that follows transitioning from child-based to adult-based community services" or 2) "a disruption in self-identity that may accompany maturation and the realization of limited social and career options" may contribute to regression. No doubt there exists neurobiological vulnerabilities that contribute to the severity and complexity of depression in individuals with trisomy 21 [7, 34, 48].

While mood disturbances such as depression are often part of the adult regression syndrome and many patients are treated with anti-depressants, the causal relationship between depression and regression, sleep disturbance and stressful life events is unclear presently.

7.12 Prognosis

The recovery of individuals with regression is highly dependent on both the cause and the certainty of the diagnosis. For those with more challenging regression, recovery may take many months or years and adaptive skills may take an even longer time to recover or relearn. About half of all individuals do not appear to regain skills up to their previous baseline. In Mircher et al.'s [32] series, the recovery was reported as: worsening in 10%, stabilization without recovery in 37%, partial recovery in 43%, and complete recovery in 10%. As noted above, Ghaziuddin et al. [17] reported that all four of their catatonia cases treated with a benzodiazepine combined with ECT recovered their baseline functioning.

7.13 Conclusion

Adult regression syndrome is a proposed name for the decline seen in adolescents and young adults with Down syndrome. Individuals with Down syndrome can regress due to many co-morbid conditions. For those that have more challenging clinical courses, four possible etiologies were reviewed: catatonia, auto-immune disease, sleep apnea, and severe depression. It is not clear that any one of these can explain all of the most challenging cases or that there aren't additional diagnoses for some of those most severely affected. Clearly, further study is needed to define and optimize treatment for these individuals.

References

1. Akahoshi K, Matsuda H, Funahashi M, Hanaoka T, Suzuki Y. Acute neuropsychiatric disorders in adolescents and young adults with Down syndrome: Japanese case reports. Neuropsychiatr Dis Treat. 2012;8:339–45. https://doi.org/10.2147/NDT.S32767.
2. Anwar AJ, Walker JD, Frier BM. Type 1 diabetes mellitus and Down's syndrome: prevalence, management, and diabetic complications. Diabet Med. 1998;15:160–3. https://doi.org/10.1002/(SICI)1096-9136(199802)15:2<160::AID-DIA537>3.0.CO;2-J.
3. Armangue T, Petit-Pedrol M, Dalmau J. Autoimmune encephalitis in children. J Child Neurol. 2012;27:1460–90. https://doi.org/10.1177/0883073812448838.

4. Bergholdt R, Eising S, Nerup J, Pociot F. Increased prevalence of Down's syndrome in individuals with type 1 diabetes in Denmark: a nationwide population-based study. Diabetologia. 2006;49:1179–82. https://doi.org/10.1007/s00125-006-0231-6.
5. Bouziat R, Hinterleitner R, Brown JJ, Stencel-Baerenwald JE, Ikizler M, Mayassi T, Jabri B. Reovirus infection triggers inflammatory responses to dietary antigens and development of celiac disease. Science. 2017;356:44–50. https://doi.org/10.1126/science.aah5298.
6. Capone GT, Grados MA, Kaufmann WE, Bernard-Ripoll S, Jewell A. Down syndrome and comorbid autism-spectrum disorder: characterization using the aberrant behavior checklist. Am J Med Genet. 2005;134:373–80. https://doi.org/10.1002/ajmg.a.30622.
7. Capone GT, Goyal P, Ares W, Lannigan E. Neurobehavioral disorders in children, adolescents, and young adults with Down syndrome. Am J Med Genet C Semin Med Genet. 2006;142:158–72.
8. Capone G, Aidikoff J, Taylor K, Rykiel N. Adolescents and young adults with Down syndrome presenting to a medical clinic with depression: co-morbid obstructive sleep apnea. Am J Med Genet A. 2013;161:2188–96.
9. Castillo H, Patterson B, Hickey F, Kinsman A, Howard JM, Mitchell T, Molloy CA. Difference in age at regression in children with autism with and without Down syndrome. J Dev Behav Pediatr. 2008;29:89–93. https://doi.org/10.1097/DBP.0b013e318165c78d.
10. Castro P, Zaman S, Holland A. Alzheimer's disease in people with Down's syndrome: the prospects for and the challenges of developing preventative treatments. J Neurol. 2017;264:804–13. https://doi.org/10.1007/s00415-016-8308-8.
11. Daniels J. Catatonia: clinical aspects and neurobiological correlates. J Neuropsychiatry Clin Neurosci. 2009;21:371–80. https://doi.org/10.1176/appi.neuropsych.21.4.371.
12. Devenny DA, Matthews A. Regression: atypical loss of attained functioning in children and adolescents with Down syndrome. In: Hodapp RM, editor. International review of research in developmental disabilities, vol. 41. Oxford: Academic Press; 2011. p. 233–64.
13. Down Syndrome Medical Interest Group-USA Work Group on Regression. July 2017. https://www.dsmig-usa.org.
14. Fink M, Shorter E, Taylor MA. Catatonia is not schizophrenia: Kraepelin's error and the need to recognize catatonia as an independent syndrome in medical nomenclature. Schizophr Bull. 2010;36:314–20. https://doi.org/10.1093/schbul/sbp059.
15. Francis A, Fink M, Appiani F, Bertelsen A, Bolwig TG, Braunig P, Caroff SN, Carroll BT, Cavanna AE, Cohen D, Cottencin O, Cuesta MJ, Daniels J, Dhossche D, Fricchione GL, Gazdag G, Ghaziuddin N, Healy D, Klein D, Kruger S, Lee JW, Mann SC, Mazurek M, McCall WV, McDaniel WW, Northoff G, Peralta V, Petrides G, Rosebush P, Rummans TA, Shorter E, Suzuki K, Thomas P, Vaiva G, Wachtel L. Catatonia in the diagnostic and statistical manual of mental disorders, fifth edition. J ECT. 2010;26:246–7. https://doi.org/10.1097/YCT.0b013e3181fe28bd.
16. Ghaziuddin M, Tsai LY, Ghaziuddin N. Autism in Down's syndrome: presentation and diagnosis. J Intellect Disabil Res. 1992;36:449–56.
17. Ghaziuddin N, Nassiri A, Miles JH. Catatonia in Down syndrome: a treatable cause of regression. Neuropsychiatr Dis Treat. 2015;11:941–9. https://doi.org/10.2147/NDT.S77307.
18. Head E, Powell D, Gold BT, Schmitt FA. Alzheimer's disease in Down syndrome. Eur J Neurogen Dis. 2012;1:353–64.
19. Hepburn S, Philofsky A, Fidler DJ, Rogers S. Autism symptoms in toddlers with Down syndrome: a descriptive study. J Appl Res Intellect Disabil. 2008;21:48–57. https://doi.org/10.1111/j.1468-3148.2007.00368.x.
20. Hestnes A, Daniel SE, Lees AJ, Brun A. Down's syndrome and Parkinson's disease. J Neurol Neurosurg Psychiatry. 1997;62:289.
21. Jacobs J, Schwartz A, McDougle CJ, Skotko BG. Rapid clinical deterioration in an individual with Down syndrome. Am J Med Genet A. 2016;170:1899–902. https://doi.org/10.1002/ajmg.a.37674.
22. Kent L, Evans J, Paul M, Sharp M. Comorbidity of autistic spectrum disorders in children with Down syndrome. Dev Med Child Neurol. 1999;41:153–8.

23. Kinik ST, Ozcay F, Varan B. Type I diabetes mellitus, Hashimoto's thyroiditis and celiac disease in an adolescent with Down syndrome. Pediatr Int. 2006;48:433–5. https://doi.org/10.1111/j.1442-200X.2006.02238.x.
24. Kirkhart R, Ahuja N, Lee JW, Ramirez J, Talbert R, Faiz K, Ungvari GS, Thomas C, Carroll BT. The detection and measurement of catatonia. Psychiatry (Edgmont). 2007;4:52–6.
25. Krinsky-McHale SJ, Jenkins EC, Zigman WB, Silverman W. Ophthalmic disorders in adults with Down syndrome. Curr Gerontol Geriatr Res. 2012;2012:974253. https://doi.org/10.1155/2012/974253.
26. Kumar V, Rajadhyaksha M, Wortsman J. Celiac disease-associated autoimmune endocrinopathies. Clin Diagn Lab Immunol. 2001;8:678–85. https://doi.org/10.1128/CDLI.8.4.678-685.2001.
27. Lai F, Williams RS. A prospective study of Alzheimer disease in Down syndrome. Arch Neurol. 1989;46(8):849–53.
28. Leroy A, Naudet F, Vaiva G, Francis A, Thomas P, Amad A. Is electroconvulsive therapy an evidence-based treatment for catatonia? A systematic review and meta-analysis. Eur Arch Psychiatry Clin Neurosci. 2017; https://doi.org/10.1007/s00406-017-0819-5.
29. Mann DM. The pathological association between Down syndrome and Alzheimer disease. Mech Ageing Dev. 1988;43:99–136.
30. Mårild K, Stephansson O, Grahnquist L, Cnattingius S, Söderman G, Ludvigsson JF. Down syndrome is associated with elevated risk of celiac disease: a nationwide case-control study. J Pediatr. 2013;163:237–42. https://doi.org/10.1016/j.jpeds.2012.12.087.
31. Miles J. Catatonia as a cause of regression in Down syndrome. Presentation at the annual symposium of the Down Syndrome Medical Interest Group-USA, Sacramento, CA. 2017.
32. Mircher C, Cieuta-Walti C, Marey I, Rebillat AS, Cretu L, Milenko E, Conte M, Sturtz F, Rethore MO, Ravel A. Acute regression in young people with Down syndrome. Brain Sci. 2017;7:E57. https://doi.org/10.3390/brainsci7060057.
33. Moran JA, Rafii MS, Keller SM, Singh BK, Janicki MP, American Academy of Developmental Medicine and Dentistry, Rehabilitation Research and Training Center on Aging with Developmental Disabilities at University of Illinois at Chicago, American Association on Intellectual and Developmental Disabilities. The National Task Group on Intellectual Disabilities and Dementia Practices consensus recommendations for the evaluation and management of dementia in adults with intellectual disabilities. Mayo Clin Proc. 2013;88:831–40. https://doi.org/10.1016/j.mayocp.2013.04.024.
34. Myers BA, Pueschel SM. Major depression in a small group of adults with Down syndrome. Res Dev Disabil. 1995;16:285–99.
35. Padhy SK, Parakh P, Sridhar M. The catatonia conundrum: controversies and contradictions. Asian J Psychiatr. 2014;7:6–9. https://doi.org/10.1016/j.ajp.2013.07.006.
36. Pellegrini FP, Marinoni M, Frangione V, Tedeschi A, Gandini V, Ciglia F, Mortara L, Accolla RS, Nespoli L. Down syndrome, autoimmunity and T regulatory cells. Clin Exp Immunol. 2012;169:238–43. https://doi.org/10.1111/j.1365-2249.2012.04610.x.
37. Popova G, Paterson WF, Brown A, Donaldson MD. Hashimoto's thyroiditis in Down's syndrome: clinical presentation and evolution. Horm Res. 2008;70:278–84. https://doi.org/10.1159/000157874.
38. Prasher V. Disintegrative syndrome in young adults [Letter to the editor]. Irish J Psychol Med. 2002;19:101.
39. Prasher VP, Sachdeva N, Tarrant N. Diagnosing dementia in adults with Down's syndrome. Neurodegen Dis Manag. 2015;5:249–56. https://doi.org/10.2217/nmt.15.8.
40. Principi N, Benoli MG, Bianchini S, Esposito S. J Clin Virol. 2017;96:26–31. https://doi.org/10.1016/j.jcv.2017.09.003.
41. Rasmussen P, Borjesson O, Wentz E, Gillberg C. Autistic disorders in Down syndrome: background factors and clinical correlates. Dev Med Child Neurol. 2001;43:750–4.
42. Rollin H. Personality in mongolism with special reference to the incidence of catatonic psychosis. Am J Ment Defic. 1946;51:219–37.

43. Sabbagh M, Edgin J. Clinical assessment of cognitive decline in adults with Down syndrome. Curr Alzheimer Res. 2016;13:30–4.
44. Shorter E. Making childhood catatonia visible, separate from competing diagnoses (Comment). Acta Psychiatr Scand. 2012;125:3–10. https://doi.org/10.1111/j.1600-0447.2011.01788.x.
45. Stein DS, Munir KM, Karweck AJ, Davidson EJ, Stein MT. Developmental regression, depression, and psychosocial stress in an adolescent with Down syndrome. J Dev Behav Pediatr. 2013;34:216–8. https://doi.org/10.1097/DBP.0b013e31828b2b42.
46. Tyrrell J, Cosgrave M, McCarron M, McPherson J, Calvert J, Kelly A, McLaughlin M, Gill M, Lawlor BA. Dementia in people with Down's syndrome. Int J Geriatr Psychiatry. 2001;16:1168–74.
47. Vieregge P, Ziemens G, Piosinski A, Freudenberg M, Kömpf D. Parkinsonian features in advanced Down's syndrome. J Neural Transm Suppl. 1991;33:119–24.
48. Warren AC, Holroyd S, Folstein FM. Major depression in Down's syndrome. Br J Psychiatry. 1989;155:202–5.
49. Wisniewski KE, French JH, Rosen JF, Kozlowski PB, Tenner M, Wisniewski HM. Basal ganglia calcification (BGC) in Down's syndrome (DS) – Another manifestation of premature aging. Ann N Y Acad Sci. 1982;396:179–89.
50. Worley G, Crissman BG, Cadogan E, Milleson C, Adkins DW, Kishnani PS. Down syndrome disintegrative disorder: new-onset autistic regression, dementia, and insomnia in older children and adolescents with Down syndrome. J Child Neurol. 2015;30:1147–52. https://doi.org/10.1177/0883073814554654.
51. Zigman WB, Lott IT. Alzheimer's disease in Down syndrome: neurobiology and risk. Ment Retard Dev Disabil Res Rev. 2007;13:237–46. https://doi.org/10.1002/mrdd.20163.

Visual Impairment

8

Susan C. Danberg

8.1   Introduction

The terms *vision* and *sight* are often confused and misused in defining how a person sees. Sight refers to the clarity of an image, whereas vision refers to how the brain attends to and interprets visual information and in turn uses that information to make meaningful action and motor reaction in response to what is seen. Vision problems are not directly related to the clarity of an image (indeed, persons with 6/6 or 20/20 vision can still have a problem with vision), however, adults who do not obtain good clear sight by being denied available remedies can be at a disadvantage when performing day-to-day tasks. Visual input begins in the eye where photoreceptors and bipolar cells transfer the energy of light to retinal ganglion cells, which transmit the messages to the brain. The eye develops from the fore part of the brain, and the biochemistry of the retina is similar to that of the brain. Conscious seeing is a cerebral function and therefore it is not surprising that people with cerebral dysfunction often have visual impairment.

Across the developed world, adults with intellectual disability can expect an increasing life-span. All older people will find that their vision changes with age and the majority will need eyeglasses (or spectacles). This is considered a normal phenomenon provided that visual acuity with eyeglasses is normal. Older adults are also at risk of visual impairment due to cataracts, age-related macular dystrophy, glaucoma, and other less common disorders. In glaucoma the optic nerve suffers, and high pressure in the eyes is an important risk factor. Patients with glaucoma often do not observe loss of their peripheral vision because the central vision remains intact for a long time.

Adults with intellectual disability have additional risks. Adults with Down syndrome often present with cataracts and keratoconus, and they have an increased risk of developing diabetes, which may induce retinal pathology over time. Individuals

S. C. Danberg (✉)
Private Practice, Special Olympics Global Health Program, Glastonbury, CT, USA

© Springer Nature Switzerland AG 2019
V. P. Prasher, M. P. Janicki (eds.), *Physical Health of Adults with Intellectual and Developmental Disabilities*, https://doi.org/10.1007/978-3-319-90083-4_8

with Down syndrome also tend to develop early onset dementia (typically related to Alzheimer's disease) with compared to the neurotypical population. A number of visual problems have been reported stemming from Alzheimer's disease. Individuals with chromosomal aberrations often have malformations of the eyes; other syndromes are associated with disorders of the cornea, lens, or retina. Adults with intellectual disability who have moderate, severe or profound visual impairment usually do not complain of poor vision since they do not know how well others can see, and a considerable number may have limited communication skills, hence, regular monitoring of vision is important.

This chapter reviews the principal issues of visual impairment in people with intellectual disability. The majority of research has been undertaken on people with moderate, severe or profound intellectual disability and this chapter reflects this. Further, not all the abnormalities associated with visual impairment are discussed; however, the most of the prevalent topics are covered.

8.2   Definitions of Visual Impairment

Visual acuity is defined as the smallest letter recognized at a distance of 6 m (20 feet). Generally, adults with normal vision can just recognize alphabet letters at 6 m away (20 feet); thus, their visual acuity is 6/6, or 1.0, or 20/20. If adults can recognize only larger letters at a distance of 6 m, they are deemed to have a visual impairment which is expressed as 6/9; 6/12; 6/18; 6/24; 6/36, or 6/60 (in accord to the distance at which normal individuals can recognize the same letters). These fractions are often converted to decimals. The letters are constructed so that the distance between the strokes is equal to the width of the strokes. The letters used are termed optotypes or Snellen letters. Picture charts are constructed in most countries in such a way that they are comparable to optotypes. Assessments with single letters or single pictures give better visual acuity measures than assessment with optotypes in a line.

The Lea Symbol Acuity chart developed by Finnish pediatric ophthalmologist Lea Hyvärinen, provides an accurate and sufficient assessment in 95.9% of the 149 preschool-age children tested [1, 2]. Lea Acuity is used for both distance and near testing. The distance Lea chart is measured at a distance of 3 m (10 feet). It comes in single symbol, crowded, and un-crowded formats. The crowded (Massachusetts Visual Acuity Test format) has the highest sensitivity for detecting amblyopia. The Lea symbol charts consist of four characters: house, apple, square, and circle. Below threshold acuity each symbol will appear to be a circle. The test is very reliable and the names of the characters can be given by children as young as 2 years old. The Lea symbol test has been successfully used by Special Olympics Lions Clubs International Opening Eyes Visual screenings for over 20 years, where the test is administered monocularly and the athlete is asked to either name or point to the match on a test card (Fig. 8.1).

While the optotype test shows that the person can recognize the letters or pictures, the Teller Acuity Test (Fig. 8.2) [3], the Cardiff Acuity Test [4] and Lea Paddles are less demanding (Fig. 8.3). In these tests, the examiner observes if the person fixates on the gratings or the pictures or possibly points at them, meaning

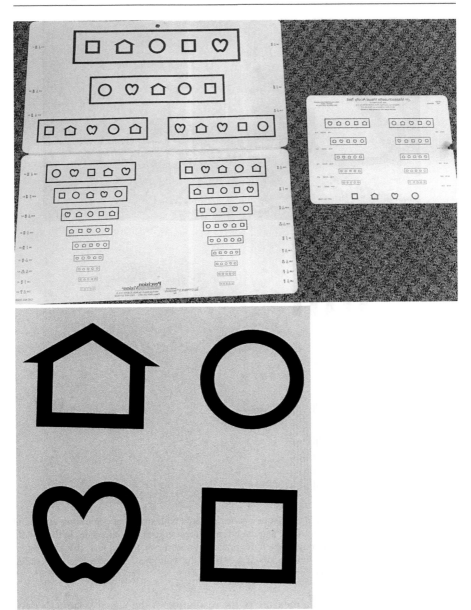

Fig. 8.1 Lea Acuity Chart (Massachusetts Visual Acuity Test format) with accompanying symbols chart for matching

that he or she can resolve one stripe from the next. These tests are often classified as "preferential looking" tests, because everybody prefers to look at objects that can be seen rather than at blank surfaces (Fig. 8.2b). Assessments of vision with the Teller Acuity Test cards, Cardiff Acuity Test cards, or the Lea Paddles are near tests; hence, the results are not comparable with optotype assessment at a distance.

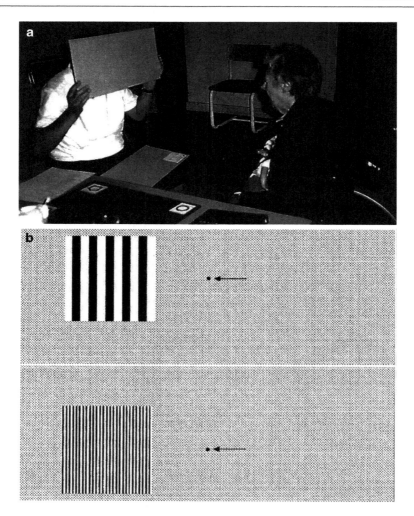

Fig. 8.2 (a) Teller Acuity Cards consist of a series of cards with stripes of decreasing width and separation. The stripes are on one side, and there is a uniform grey at the other side. In the middle there is a peephole (arrow) through which the practitioner observes the subject. (b) Assessment with Teller Acuity Card. The clinician sits 55 cm from the examinee, and observes the fixation pattern through the central hole

Moreover, grating acuity is a measure of the resolution of the visual system, but not of recognition of shapes.

The results of grating acuities have been compared with the results of optotype acuities in children; several studies have shown a reasonable agreement, but Mayer et al. [5] showed that grating visual acuity tests overestimate visual acuity as compared to recognition tests, the greater the degree of vision loss being tested. The Lea Grating and Cardiff Acuity Cards are comparing different aspects of vision. The Lea Paddles utilize gratings, which at best tell us the resolution acuity and do not truly

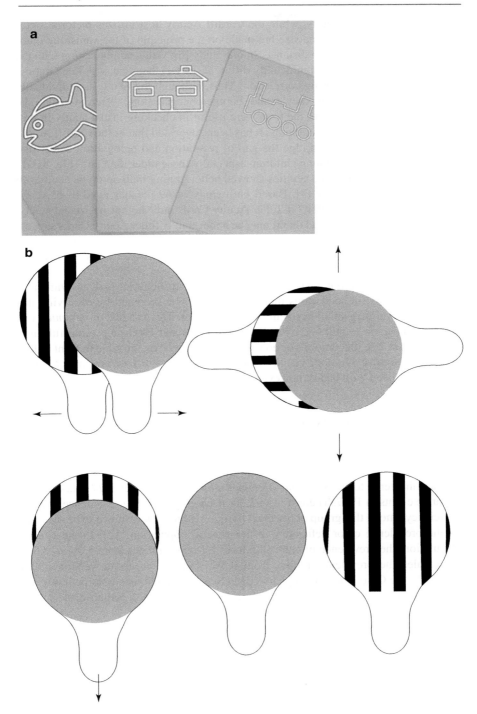

Fig. 8.3 (**a**) Cardiff cards. (**b**) Lea paddle

represent recognition acuity, while the Cardiff Acuity Test utilizes pictorial opto-types, which are of the same size but made on the principle of the vanishing opto-types beyond the resolution distance. In one study [6], visual acuity testing with the Cardiff Acuity Cards was significantly different (better) than that with Lea Grating, but the two showed a strong correlation. Thus, although the two tests individually would give reliable results, they cannot be interchanged along different visits. The study also showed that both the tests were useful in checking visual acuity in pre-verbal children older than 6 months. It has been suggested that as the Cardiff Acuity Cards is pictorial, it may bridge the gap of resolution and recognition acuity and generate more interest among children, especially those older than one (Fig. 8.3a).

Similarly, poor optotype acuities showed better grating than optotype acuities in children born prematurely [7]. Based on a study of 69 persons aged 8–40 years, Kushner et al. [8] found that "if Teller Acuity Cards indicate normal visual acuity, there is still a high likelihood that it may be abnormal; if Teller Acuity Cards suggest abnormal vision, there is a high likelihood that it is abnormal", and vice versa: "If Snellen visual acuity was normal in one or both eyes, it was always normal with Teller cards."

Even preferential looking tests are sometimes too difficult for patients with intel-lectual disability, in such cases their eyesight may be screened by observing if a person can find very small beads in front of him/her. This is a test of *minimum vis-ibility*. If a person cannot find a bead of 1 mm (100s and 1000s; e.g., colorful sugar beads used as cake decorations or nonpareil sugar beads) on the table in front of him when the contrast is good, vision is presumably below 0.1 (<6/60 or <20/200). Assessing vision with beads, however, is very imprecise [9].

8.2.1   Color Vision Testing

Studies have shown that the color vision is highly testable among adults with intel-lectual disability [10]. The Color Vision Testing Made Easy (CVTME; [11]) test was administered to 1078 Special Olympics athletes (age range: 8–77 years) at four separate events in 1997. There was a 93.2% testability rate. The prevalence of color deficiency among this group of Special Olympics athletes was shown to be the same as the prevalence color deficiency in the general population [12]. In the general population, the prevalence of color blindness for males ranges from 5.0% to 8.0%; in females the prevalence ranges from 0.5% to 1.0%. A newer version of the CVTME, the ColorCheck Complete Vision Screener, combines both pediatric and adult color plates and uses the Lea symbols for better ease with pediatric and special needs populations (Fig. 8.4) [13].

Visual impairment is defined by constriction of the visual fields and the degree of visual impairment in the best eye with best correction (i.e., best spectacles). In other words, it is a definition referring to vision at a distance, but unfortunately, many people with intellectual disability can only be tested at near range, usually with the Teller, Lea Paddles or the Cardiff technique.

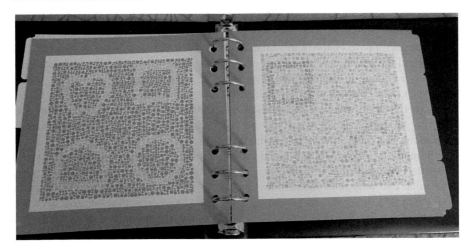

Fig. 8.4 CVTME

Fig. 8.5 Nearsighted person. Even with his strong minus glasses he has a very short viewing distance to the pictures

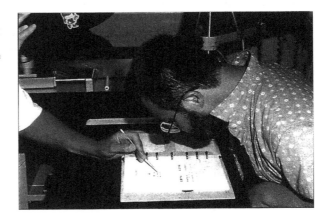

For adults with intellectual disability, vision at near range is usually more important than distance vision because occupational activities usually involve near work. There is no accepted definition of poor vision at near; near-sighted people have good acuity for near (Fig. 8.5) and poor vision for distance without glasses, and older farsighted adults have poor vision both at near range and distance without their spectacles. Poor near vision after the age of 45 years is called presbyopia and is a condition that everyone will experience. Many activities beyond reading may require the use of corrective lenses for presbyopia (such as eating, shaving, preparing food, and using assistance technology—such as word boards, tablets, mobile phones, etc.). Caregivers should be mindful that the adult is wearing the correct prescription for that activity. Bifocals may be prescribed, but should be used with caution for those patients who have balance or ambulation issues. In such cases use of separate prescription glasses for near and/or distance correction maybe more appropriate.

There is more to vision than visual acuity and visual fields. Some disorders of the retina and the optic nerve can affect color vision, dark adaptation (i.e., adjusting the eyes to a change in illumination), seeing in reduced illumination (such as during twilight), and contrast sensitivity. Understanding the message transmitted by the eyes to the brain involves recognition, perception of movement, orientation, discerning the difference between picture and background and more complex gnostic functions. Vision requires sensory integration in the brain.

If an adult has one good eye and the other one has poor vision, there is a visual disorder, but no visual impairment; such adults often do not realize that they see with one eye only, and monocular low vision is common in persons with squint (strabismus). Strabismus is present in 25–50% of people with moderate, severe or profound intellectual disability [14, 15]. Depth Perception Testing is method to assess binocular vision, especially if the patient is not compliant enough to do a cover test or Hirschberg estimation of the angle of turn. For example, the Special Olympics organization uses the Randot E or the Smile test (PASS) and Polaroid glasses are used to present a stereoscopic image. The examination is a forced choice test where the athlete must decide which plate has the picture of the either the "E" (Randot E) or the Smiley face (PASS). The patient must get 5/6 correct answers to pass the test. Stereo acuity is based on test distance used: 504 s of arc at 50 cm or 630 s of arc at 40 cm (Figs. 8.6 and 8.7).

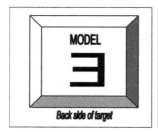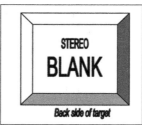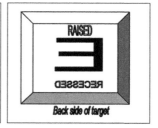

Fig. 8.6 RANDOT E

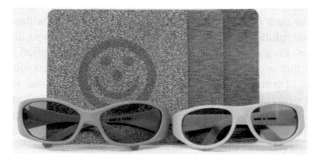

Fig. 8.7 Smile Test (PASS)

Lay people generally have difficulty recognizing visual impairment in adults; the impairment does not always give rise to handicap in well-known environments and in environments that have been adapted to visually impaired people. This means good contrast borders around doors, good general illumination, and variable acoustic or scented information. People with intellectual disability who have visual impairment may be mistakenly assessed as clumsy or unwilling to take part in near work, some may reject participating in walks because they have problems seeing the flagstones, or they might have difficulty seeing in too bright or too dim light. Caregivers should be oriented to look for clues of vision difficulties or abnormalities and the report their observations to vision specialists.

8.3   Prevalence of Visual Impairment

8.3.1   General Population

The prevalence of low vision in the general population varies both with the social and geographical environment, the age groups analyzed, and the methods used, but studies generally show a much lower prevalence than that found in adults with intellectual disability. The prevalence of best-corrected visual acuity ≤0.3 was 3.8% and visual impairment ≤0.1 was observed in 1.5% of people of European heritage in the Baltimore, Maryland (USA) area [16]. In Finland, Hirvelä and Laatikainen [17] found that 10% of normal subjects over 70 years of age had low vision and approximately 2% were blind.

8.3.2   Individuals with Intellectual Disability

There are many studies on visual impairment in children with intellectual disability [18–20]. In 1979, Warburg et al. [21] found that about half of children in Denmark who were blind also had intellectual disability, and the rate of blindness (visual acuity ≤0.1) in the children with intellectual disability was 200-fold that of other children. In Sweden, 50% of children with visual impairment (visual acuity <0.3) had intellectual disability [22], and that early mortality (that is, during the first 19 years of life) was as much as 120 times higher in children with visual impairment and ID than age peers in the general population [23]. This may explain why the prevalence of visual impairment in adults with intellectual disability is lower than in children.

There are few surveys of visual function in adults with intellectual disability as compared with those performed during the last 30 years in children. The majority showed that 20–30% of adults with intellectual disability were moderately visually impaired, and 1–5% were severely visual impaired or blind [24–32]. In a Danish study of 837 persons with moderate, severe, or profound intellectual disability, Warburg [33] found that 50% had either low visual acuity, or low near vision, or both. Most studies have been concerned with a few hundred individuals, and the aetiology and degree of impairment of the study population varied from one investigation to the next. Other large surveys were performed by questionnaires or notification of the affected persons by staff or medical personnel without actual assessment of acuity [26, 28, 29]. The prevalence of visual impairment in these studies was 20–30%.

The largest of the series of studies of adults with intellectual disability comprised 45,500 individuals [26]. In this study, visual impairment was reported by the staff and increased from 17% in the 35–39 years-old to 34% in people aged 60–69 and 53% in 271 persons 80–89 years of age. Van Schrojenstein Lantman-de Valk et al. [29] found similar figures based on questionnaires to the staff of 1583 persons with intellectual disability. They found the prevalence of visual impairment increased from 11% at the age of 20–29 to 17% at age 30–39. Of those in the age group, 60–69, 22% were considered to be visual impaired by the staff.

Visual impairment was noted in the case reports or observed by the staff of a large hospital in 24% of 99 adults aged 65 and above [34]. The prevalence of visual impairment increased from 18% in the 65–69 year-olds to 37% in the over 75 year-olds, but no definition of visual impairment was given, and no mention was made as to whether the staff referred to binocular or monocular visual impairment.

8.4   Special Olympics Healthy Athletes Program's Vision Screening

The United Nations Convention on the Rights of Persons with Disabilities (UNCRPD) and the World Health Organization [35] World Report on Disability have helped to change public perception of people with disabilities as objects of charity to viewing them as equal members of society who should be supported to be as independent as possible. In this context, the Special Olympics International (SOI) organization provides year-round sports training and athletic competition to approximately five million children and adults with intellectual disability in more than 170 countries. Its purpose is promoting the UNCRPD principle of full and effective participation and inclusion in society via providing opportunities for athletes, which includes a focus on health. Participation in SOI's athletics programs begins at age 8 and there is no upper age limit. Besides personal development, SOI gives people with intellectual disability continuing opportunities to conditioning and physical fitness, gain confidence and develop skills, and develop and maintain friendships with other athletes. The SOI global health strategy calls for a concerted effort to achieve inclusive health for people with intellectual disability. In addition to sports, SOI maintain several health oriented programs, including Healthy Athletes (HA), Healthy Communities, Fitness programs, and Family Health Forums. SOI's underwrites health assessments and produces health data which aid in revealing health disparities for people with ID, including the unique challenges individuals and families encounter as they navigate the complexities of often fragmented healthcare systems. SOI created the HA program in 1997 to identify and address these health disparities faced by people with intellectual disability. The HA program provides SO athletes with free health screenings, education, and referrals for follow-up care absent the barriers that people with intellectual disability often encounter during a

Table 8.1 Healthy Athletes program aspects

SOI screening program	Function of program
Fit Feet	Podiatric screenings
FUN fitness	Physical therapy screenings
Health Promotion	Screening focused on health education with clinical exams in bone density, blood pressure, and BMI
Healthy Hearing	Hearing screening
MedFest	Sports physicals
Special Olympics-Lions Clubs International Opening Eyes	Vision and eye health assessments
Special Smiles	Oral health screenings
Strong Minds	Interactive learning activities focused on developing coping and stress management skills

visit to a doctor, dentist, or other healthcare professional in their home community. The HA also enables healthcare professionals to gain skills on how to treat people with intellectual disability in their own practices. Within this program, each participating discipline has a specific scientifically validated protocol that must be followed. The HA program includes eight disciplines in its health screenings (see Table 8.1).

Through this program, SOI enabling athletes to master skills that increase confidence and ability to succeed in life; documenting and addressing disparities in access to sport, schooling, and healthcare for people with intellectual disability; Increasing families' knowledge and expectations of what athletes can achieve; and changing attitudes to create inclusion in schools, communities, and society at large.

HA data are representative of people with intellectual disability who are Special Olympics athletes and are not separated by syndromes or medical diagnoses. It is not known how these data compare with all people with ID, and it is possible that SO athletes may be healthier than non-SO athletes; however, these data still provide valuable insight in the organic health status of one large group of adults with intellectual disability.

As of 2016, there were 4,931,754 Special Olympics athletes participating in the program, representing 172 countries. During 2016, 14,391 Special Olympics athletes from 46 countries ages 8–98 were assessed at the Special Olympics Lions Clubs International Opening Eyes™ (SOLCIOE) program. Visual assessments were done using the SOLCIOE™ protocols which included Distance and Near Lea Acuity, Cover Test, Stereo Acuity with (Randot E™) Color Vision Test Made Easy (CVTME™), as well as assessment of internal and external eye health, and tonometry.

It was found that 35% of SO athletes tested had entering visual acuity between 20/40–20/60 (6/12–6/18) and 0.6% had visual acuities of less than 20/200 (6/60). Data on eye diseases, included external eye health problems (such as lid anomalies, conjunctivitis, blepharitis), and internal eye health problems (such as cataracts, retinal anomalies, and coloboma). Some 16.1% (n = 26,133) of the athletes had some type of eye disease (internal or external). Among the internal diseases, 3.9% (n = 4795 have cataracts; 1.3% (n = 1629) are suspected to have glaucoma; and 1.1% (n = 1299) have an optic nerve anomaly. Other internal diseases observed include colobomas and retinal anomalies. Among the external diseases, 3.2% (n = 4211) had blepharitis; 2.35 (n = 3068) had conjunctivitis; 1.1% (n = 1407) had a lid anomaly, and 1.4% (n = 1865) had a corneal anomaly. Other external diseases included lid anomalies, pterygium, pinquecula, and ptosis.

It was also found that 38.3% (n = 62,361) of the athletes needed a new prescription for vision assistance.

8.4.1 Vision and Down Syndrome

Individuals with Down syndrome have a higher prevalence of visual impairment than do adults with other etiologies, and their risk begins earlier [36]. The rates often vary, depending upon the source of study subject populations. In one study, of 243 persons with Down syndrome, visual impairment was observed in 23% of individuals aged 20–29, in 32% of the 40–49 year-olds, and in 64% in the 60–69 year olds (Van Schrojenstein Lantman-de Valk et al. [29]). In another study, binocular vision was assessed in 96 persons with Down syndrome (visual impairment was defined as ≤0.3) and it was found that it increased from 3% in 30–39 year-olds to 13% in 50–59 year olds [37]. Studies have shown that although there is high prevalence of refractive errors in Down syndrome, these are not always present in early infancy. There is also a higher prevalence of myopia than hypermetropia, and higher rates of myopic refractive errors. Studies have shown that the prevalence of nystagmus, strabismus, and congenital cataracts is significantly higher in children with Down syndrome [38], and all of these are considered amblyogenic factors. If these conditions are not diagnosed and treated in early infancy and childhood, amblyopia will ensue and with aging impact the individual's ability to do certain tasks.

Early onset of Alzheimer's disease is of particular concern to the optometrist or ophthalmologist treating adults with Down syndrome. In addition to the difficulties in reporting visual changes, changes in behavior may be attributed to diagnostic over-shadowing rather than symptoms of visual changes associated with this condition [39–41]. Studies have shown that adults ages 40–49 years old and 50–59 may have prevalence rates of dementia as high as 55%. Above age 60 the rates can increase to 77%. There are a number of visual problems that can occur with Alzheimer's disease, including changes in visual acuity and color vision, problems with smooth pursuit and saccadic eye movements, problems with reading, visuo-spatial function, and in the naming and identification of objects [42]. In addition, many adults may have trouble with figure ground skills, such as finding a known object in a new environment. Caregivers must note these changes and be mindful that these changes can be attributed to early onset of Alzheimer's disease rather than Down syndrome.

8.5   Staff Estimation of Visual Impairment

Questionnaires and notifications give different information of visual impairment than individual clinical assessment. Lay caregivers generally underestimate normal vision and blindness and overestimate mild and moderate visual impairment as compared to assessment of vision by professional methods [33]. Kerr et al. [43] found that caregivers often underestimate the severity of visual impairment. In 506 subjects, nurses with ready access to the medical and nursing records reported 'perfect vision, requiring no intervention' in 49%, reduced vision in 47%, and blindness in 4%. At actual assessments, vision was judged completely normal in only four people (0.8%) and 4% required blind registration. Cataracts were present or had been removed in 140 subjects. Glaucoma was diagnosed in 4%. Tests found little or no residual vision in those whom caregivers had considered blind. Spectacles were considered appropriate, after discussion between the optometrist and the staff, in 106 individuals (21%).

8.6   Errors of Refraction

Errors of refraction are very common in adults with intellectual disability. The largest survey [15] demonstrated that 57% of adult residents in a large institution had ametropias comprising both spherical and astigmatic errors. Similar prevalence rates have been found by others [32, 44]. Refractive errors are treatable with glasses, contact lenses, or surgery. Many studies have shown that more than one half of prescribed spectacles are in use at the time of follow-up [14, 44–47].

Many caregivers have difficulty in understanding the difference between visual acuity and refractive errors. Refraction, as a rule of the thumb, is prefixed by a minus or plus sign. In the absence of amblyogenic factors, a person who wears the correct glasses should be correctable to normal visual acuity, even when the refractive error is high. The caregiver may find both the visual impairment and the power of the glasses in documentation from the optometrist or the ophthalmologist, for instance, visual impairment 1.0 –5.00 × −1.25(80°) which means that the subject has normal visual acuity (i.e., 1.0, 20/20) with myopia (−5.00) and astigmatism (−1.25) glasses in the 80° meridian.

8.6.1   Presbyopia

Correction both for near and distance is usually necessary in elderly persons, and bifocal spectacle lenses or progressive glasses are recommended [46]. Patients with this condition are usually fond of their glasses, but their elderly parents, on the other hand, claim that bifocals are much too difficult to use, and persuading the parents to permit an attempt to be made can be difficult. Unfortunately, the same attitude can be found in some professionals.

Some practitioners advise a gradual increase in time during which the glasses are worn whereas others consider that adaptation to the glasses requires some time whenever the glasses are in use; therefore they recommend that the spectacles should be worn all day from the very beginning. In practice, the caregivers individualize according to their understanding of each person.

8.6.2 Medical Causes of Visual Impairment

Older adults with intellectual disability have the same eye disorders as all others of the same age, but so far, the life expectancy of adults with moderate, severe or profound intellectual disability is lower than in the remainder of the population, hence most causes of visual impairment in aging adults have been present from a younger age. The majority of ocular causes of low vision, however, are uncorrected errors of refraction (i.e., lack of appropriate spectacles). Medical disorders with visual impairment are mainly optic nerve atrophy, unoperated cataract, keratoconus, high myopia, retinitis pigmentosa, glaucoma and rare syndromes [14, 32, 33, 48]. In fact, more than 345 rare syndromes, most of them genetic, present with both visual impairment and intellectual disability [49]. Many of these syndromes are reviewed in Chap. 4.

8.6.3 Optic Nerve Atrophy

Optic nerve atrophy is seen in a large number of cerebral disorders, both congenital and acquired. It has usually run its course in adults, and the resulting visual impairment will be permanent. Optic nerve atrophy can be mild and difficult to assess in patients with spastic cerebral paresis; however, hemianopia (loss of one half of the visual field) is common and its signs should be described to the care personnel. Optic nerve atrophy can be a sign of progression of the cerebral disorder, for example in hydrocephalus. People with optic nerve atrophy need better contrast than others, which means good illumination, contrasting borders around doors, tablecloths of one color only, contrasting plates and cutlery. Caregivers should approach adults in their seeing visual field, and adults should be positioned in the room and at tables so that activities are presented in their seeing field. Using an identification button, such as the Rummel Hemianopsia Button™, can alert caregivers as to which side the patient has useable vision (available from Bernell (citation, date)) (Fig. 8.8).

8.6.4 Cataracts

Cataracts (Fig. 8.9) are seen as a cloudy reflection behind the pupil. They are common in Down syndrome, both as congenital and acquired cataracts; moreover more than 150 syndromes present both cataracts and intellectual disability [49]. Cataracts may also be found in adults with psychoses who hit themselves in the face.

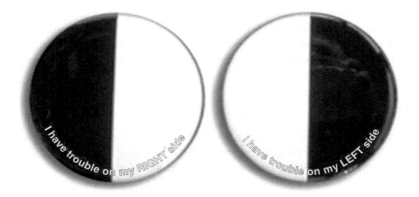

Fig. 8.8 Rummel Hemianopsia button

Fig. 8.9 Cataract of the
right eye. The pupil has
been dilated, there is a grey
reflex in the pupil instead
of the normal black

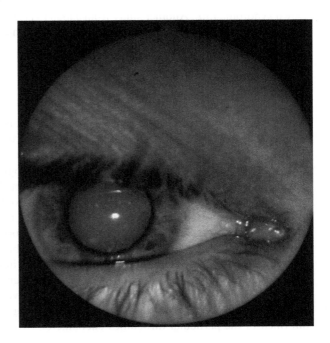

Unoperated cataracts are common findings in older adults with intellectual disability [14, 48]. Their vision becomes progressively blurred, and surgery with removal
of the cloudy lens and implantation of an intraocular plastic lens is the standard
procedure, irrespective of whether a cataract presents in people with Down syndrome or in others. A 24-h watch is recommended for the first 48 h after the operation to prevent the patients from rubbing their eyes (but the use of shields may draw
the attention of the patients to their eyes and cause them to try to remove the occlusion). Use of a restraint such as the L-Bow Arm Restraint™, which limits the elbow

flexion, can be used to prevent patients from touching their face or eyes. Some people with intellectual disability with poor vision may become agitated, aggressive, or bang their heads against a wall due to their vision problems, but after they have regained their eyesight their behavior usually becomes far more manageable.

8.6.5   Glaucoma

Glaucoma is a group of conditions that affect the health of the optic nerve. Open angle Glaucoma is the most common form of Glaucoma and is usually characterized by higher than normal intraocular pressure. Intraocular pressure is measured with a tonometer, which usually requires the use of a topical anesthetic. Tonometry is often a difficult test to perform on uncooperative patients, however some of the handheld tonometers such as iCare and Tonopen may be a better choice in this patient population. Glaucoma is estimated to be present in 1–7% of children with Down syndrome [50]. Another study from Japan [51] showed a significantly higher incidence of glaucoma 11.5% (P = 0.014) in adults with Down syndrome compared to those in the control group.

8.6.6   Retinitis Pigmentosa

Retinitis pigmentosa is the collective term for a number of progressive retinal disorders. These result in loss of peripheral vision (so called "tunnel vision"), and reduced or absent night vision; however, visual impairment may remain acceptable for many years while tunnel vision progresses. The ophthalmologist observes that the retina is thin and translucent, and the blood vessels are attenuated. Dark star shaped retinal pigmentations appear later together with pallor of the optic nerve. Physicians with little experience of retinitis pigmentosa will notice the optic nerve atrophy, but the initial attenuation of the retinal vessels is often overlooked. Retinitis pigmentosa has a higher prevalence in people with intellectual disability than that in the general population [52]; it is presumably even under diagnosed in these patients who are not subjected to regular eye examination. Although at present there is no medical treatment, the identification of retinitis pigmentosa improves the social adaptation of people with an intellectual disability when the caregivers and staff have been informed of the particular difficulties encountered by these persons. Persons with retinitis pigmentosa need a high-contrast environment similar to those with optic nerve atrophy. There are more than 1100 syndromes of intellectual disability, but only just over 80 where both retinitis pigmentosa and intellectual disability is pronounced [49]; hence, the identification of retinitis pigmentosa in a person improves the establishment of a correct syndromic diagnosis.

The commonest causes of retinitis pigmentosa in adults with intellectual disability are Leber congenital amaurosis, a heterogeneous group of retinitis pigmentosa-like phenotypes that has been studied intensively in children, but few have been followed to old age, and the prognosis as to longevity is unknown. Retinitis pigmentosa presenting in adults with intellectual disability also comprises of Cohen syndrome, muscle-eye-brain syndrome, retinitis pigmentosa-mental retardation, and other rare syndromes. The Bardet-Biedl syndrome is variably associated with intellectual disability [53, 54].

8.6.7 Malformations

Malformations of the eye often lead to visual impairment. Such conditions are extremely rare in the general population, and although they are more common in persons with intellectual disability, they remain rare. The commonest malformations are sector-shaped defects of the iris or the retina and choroid (Fig. 8.10) called colobomata, which in some patients are associated with microphthalmia. Other malformations may be observed in the interior of the eye (viz., the vitreous), or the retina, which may be detached or folded (falciform folds). Nystagmus is a rapid oscillation of the eyes, but the environment is perceived as stationary. Congenital or infantile nystagmus is present in several eye disorders, all characterized by low vision. Some patients will adapt an unusual head position if there is a null zone. A null zone is where the nystagmoid movement is at its lowest and the vision is at its most stable. Yoked prisms can be used to shift the patient's line of sight into the null zone. Careful examination by a behavioural optometrist or ophthalmologist should be done to check for null point position.

A number of previously undescribed or unknown syndromes have been observed in the latter years in adults with intellectual disability, the majority of them are

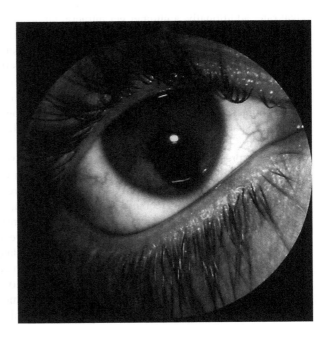

Fig. 8.10 Coloboma of the iris. Colobomas are common malformations. If they present in the iris only, there is no visual impairment, but if the retina and choroid are involved visual impairment is often present

genetic and thus of immense interest to the families in which they occur. Some of them give rise to serious visual impairment or blindness, while others are not associated with poor vision, but all of them are important handles in the search for a precise differential diagnosis. Microphthalmia and colobomata are particularly common in persons with chromosomal aberrations, and all individuals with intellectual disability and colobomata or microphthalmia should be subjected to a chromosomal examination [55].

8.7 Cerebral Visual Impairment

Cerebral visual impairment is a condition with poor use of vision caused by brain lesions or malformations of the brain; the eyes are normal or there is an eye disorder, which does not fully explain the reduced vision. The retinal photoreceptors, bipolar and ganglion cells are but relay stations for vision, and the areas which process sight are spread over most of the cortex of the brain, hence, cerebral lesions may give rise to a variety of visual defects.

Cerebral visual impairment was not regarded as a cause of visual impairment some 20 years ago, but in the industrialized world it is now the most prominent cause of visual impairment in people with intellectual disability next to uncorrected ametropia. The cause of this paradox is that people with intellectual disability were not subjected previously to regular eye examinations and those who appeared to have healthy eyes without using their vision were classified as severely intellectually impaired and not as visually impaired. Cerebral visual impairment is becoming more prevalent, mainly because extremely premature babies now have a higher survival rate; additionally, a number get intracranial haemorrhage during birth, which may lead to cerebral visual impairment and to intellectual disability.

The most striking feature in adults with cerebral visual impairment is the indifference to objects presented at a clinical examination, as if the meaning of the object or the understanding of the task of observing it was nonexistent. Some of these persons are well oriented in their usual environment and can respond to visual clues in their homes. Eyesight varies from day to day and from time to time. Adults with cerebral visual impairment may present visual field defects, and nystagmus is seen in a minority [56].

Minor expressions of cerebral visual impairment have not yet been described in adults with intellectual disability, but it is well known both in children who were born prematurely and in older adults who have suffered a stroke. Some of these individuals have problems recognizing people; others have poor orientation, so that they cannot find their way to neighbouring rooms, for instance the toilet, or the corridor with their overclothes. Examination of cooperative adults with cerebral visual impairment reveals mild to moderate visual loss not related to eye disease and that stereoscopic vision may be impaired. Some adults with cerebral visual impairment move about quite easily, while others have visual field loss and bump into the furniture. In some cases, the adult has difficulty in detecting moving objects (for instance, cars), while others have difficulty seeing stationary objects if they themselves are

Table 8.2 Clinical Questions relating to cerebral visual impairment

Does the person (P) recognize the parents, the staff, other persons?
Can the P recognize shape, do picture lottery?
Does the P name and or match colors?
Does the P get lost in the house? the street? The workshop?
Can the P climb the stairs? See the curbstone?
Can the P walk in the dusk?
Can the P recognize pets? houses? cars? etc., when moving in a car or on a bus?
Can the P recognize pets? houses? cars? when the P is not moving?
Can the P find small objects on a patterned table cloth?
Can the P copy simple geometric drawings (triangle, circle S)?
Does the P gaze at lights?
Is visual attention fleeting?

moving (for instance, sitting in a car). A very characteristic feature of these adults is that they have problems with crowding (i.e., difficulty recognizing features in a crowd such as letters in a word or intricate pictures) [56, 57]. Crowding also may result in expressed difficulties with finding objects placed among other things, and some adults even find eating together at a table with a number of other persons disturbing. Cerebral visual impairment is difficult to diagnose in individuals with intellectual disability and there is a risk that the affected persons are considered to be more intellectually impaired than they really are. The retina in cerebral visual impairment can resemble retinitis pigmentosa without abnormal pigmentations if there is mild pallor of the optic disc, and a correct diagnosis requires electroretinographic assessment.

Neuropsychological assessment is of considerable assistance in these cases in order to better understand the specific nature of the visual problems. Modern cerebral imaging and electrophysiological examination of the brain may classify the causes, so that intervention will become more precise, but only general educational strategies are available at present. When orientation is difficult, doggerels or jingles have been of help, the person reciting or singing the route as he or she goes on. It is easier for those affected to recognize other people when they speak, walk, carry recognizable jewellery or scent and caregivers should reintroduce themselves every day. Table 8.2 shows a series of questions that may be helpful in the diagnosis.

8.8   Ocular Disorders in Adults with Down Syndrome

Down syndrome is the commonest single cause of intellectual disability, comprising 15–20% of people with intellectual disability [58]. The first large study of the ocular features in Down syndrome was published by Skeller and Øster [59]. Brushfield spots are seen in most persons with Down syndrome, other common features are blepharitis, strabismus (squint), keratoconus, cataract, nystagmus, and high myopia.

Blepharitis is inflammation of the eyelids. It will be present in all cases unless active prevention is carried out. The inflammation presents with a sticky discharge, redness and swelling of the eyelids and the conjunctiva (the mucous membrane covering the eyeball). The eyelids may be glued together in the morning, and tears run down the cheeks. Often, they have had several series of antibiotic medicine, but without permanent result. The cause of the inflammation is a sheet of dry skin cells and mucous surrounding the eyelashes where they project from the eyelids and chronic ulceration is often present underneath this debris. The eyelashes become distorted after many recurrences, and some of them break while others turn in toward the eyeball and scratch the cornea. Most of the eyelashes are lost eventually, and the eyelids lose part of their protective property. Such eyelids without lashes are quite common in aging persons with Down syndrome.

Prevention is simple; the lashes must be cleaned every day. This can be done by scrubbing the eyelashes with moist cotton wool while simultaneously stretching the lid slit (the palpebral rim) with a finger on the lateral side of the eye. All traces of debris must be removed and unless the lid is stretched it is impossible to scrub sufficiently well. If an ulcer appears after scrubbing, it is not the fault of the helper, the ulcer has been present all the time. A small drop of a simple ointment without antibiotics is applied afterwards and surplus ointment removed. Left untreated blepharitis can lead to more serious conditions such as corneal ulcers.

The small white dots on the iris—Brushfield spots—cause no harm (Fig. 8.11). Keratoconus is a condition in adults with Down syndrome where the central part of the cornea becomes tapering, projecting, and thin (Fig. 8.12). This is a rare condition in the general population where it will be treated initially with contact lenses, later with corneal transplantation. The central part of the cornea in adults with keratoconus may swell and become opaque (acute keratoconus); this is very painful, but extremely rare in the general population, and when it does occur in adults with Down syndrome it gives rise to much anxiety in caregivers and physicians alike. However, simple treatment with drops and antibiotics over a period of 1–3 months will leave the cornea with a central scar, which can be removed by operation once the active phase is over. Steroid drops are not recommended.

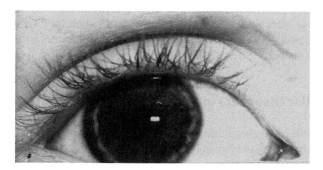

Fig. 8.11 Brushfield's spots are a concentric row of slightly elevated white nodules. They are also found in ordinary people, and have no untoward effect

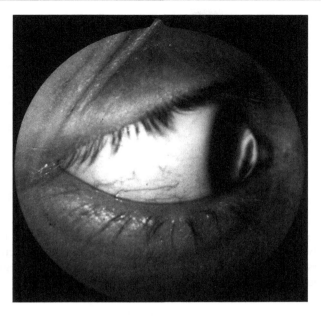

Fig. 8.12 Keratoconus. The patient looks to the left, the bright part in the corner of the eye is a protuberant clear part of the cornea—the keratoconus. Vision is severely impaired and spectacles do not improve vision. The treatment of choice is corneal transplantation

Congenital or juvenile cataract may have been removed in adults with Down syndrome at a time when intraocular lenses were not available, These adult thus need high plus lenses, usually bifocals, unless their eyes are myopic; without their strong lenses vision will be poor, but fortunately, implantation of intraocular lenses is now routine. There is a risk that new caregivers may not be informed about spectacles when the individual moves from one residence to another.

In adults with Down syndrome, age-related cataracts occur at an earlier age than in the general population. Age-related cataracts may be observed from the fourth decade; therefore it is advisable for persons with Down syndrome to be systematically examined from the age of 30 years by an ophthalmologist or optometrist, so that a cataract can be removed before vision becomes seriously impaired, and before the individual develops Alzheimer's disease. Vision is usually good postoperatively, but glasses may be necessary.

A high degree of myopia is also more common in persons with Down syndrome than in the general population. Sometimes the individuals refuse to wear spectacles, presumably because their world is a near world, and their ambulatory vision is sufficient without glasses. Myopia can be treated surgically with good functional results, but informed consent presents a difficult ethical question.

Accommodation is impaired earlier in adults with Down syndrome than in other adults and those who are not nearsighted will need glasses for near work [60, 61]. Further there is a higher prevalence of high ametropia [15, 32, 37, 44, 62]. Among persons needing glasses, compliance for using the glasses may be poor if they are

Fig. 8.13 Female adult Specs4us

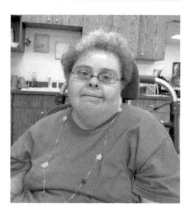

prescribed too late. It is recommended to use bifocal or progressive lenses so that the adults always wear the correct spectacles. If an adult with intellectual disability has two pairs of glasses, one for distance and one for near-work, caregivers may be confused and have difficulty in distinguishing between them.

Adults with Down syndrome have a flat nasal bridge, and spectacles have a tendency to slide down the nose. If this is remedied by shortening the sidebars (temples), it can result in wounds behind the ears and on the root of the nose. Then, of course, the patient will reject wearing them. Well-adapted spectacles should always be demanded. Two optical companies make frames suitable for this group, Specs4us™ and Miraflex™. Specs4us has a lower bridge and appropriately placed temples to accommodate the features of an individual with Down syndrome. Miraflex is made from soft plastic and come with an adjustable strap. They are made without any metal components and are hypoallergenic (Fig. 8.13).

Contact lenses must be prescribed with caution. Daily disposables are a good choice since they eliminate the need for cleaning and storing, as the lenses are discarded after each day of use. Contact lenses may slide up under the upper eyelid and give rise to irritation, when caregivers may believe that the lenses are in place. If the lenses are inserted by someone whose personal hygiene is poor, then the patient's cornea may become infected. A caregiver who has been trained to remove a contact lens must be available at all times; some caregivers find this a challenging responsibility.

Diabetes has a higher prevalence among individuals with Down syndrome than in the general population [63]. Diabetic retinopathy and glaucoma are sight-threatening complications of diabetes, particularly in individuals with poor dietary compliance. Regular monitoring of the eyes of diabetic patients is essential and cannot be ignored.

8.9   Cost of Treatment

Most eye surgery is carried out under topical anesthesia on an out-patient basis, but surgical interventions and preoperative examinations in individuals with intellectual disability require general anesthesia, post anesthetic observation, and postoperative surveillance. Often, each visit to the surgery requires a driver and escort by a caregiver known to the adult. Further, glasses are often broken or lost and must be renewed [44, 46, 47]. Because of these factors, the cost of surgery in people with intellectual disability is higher than for other people. However, the humanitarian benefit of regaining good vision is evident, aggression and fear are reduced when the adult can see what is happening, and help with basic daily living skills, such as walking, eating, dressing, and toileting, becomes easier for the caregivers.

8.10   Coping

If people have poor vision, they need predictability. Everything needs to be in its correct place. Doors must be fully either open or closed, for half-opened doors can cause serious accidents when the adult bumps into them. The preferred illumination is difficult to predict; some eye disorders are associated with reduced vision in poorly illuminated areas, other disorders give glare if the light is too strong. The solution is understanding the eye disorder and observation of the person in question. If the visual fields are restricted (for instance, below the horizontal) then the individual may tend to stumble over objects on the floor, such as low stools, toys, rolled-up carpets, and doorsteps. If the visual field is reduced to one side (hemianopia), the individual may bump into objects (furniture, persons, lamp posts) on the blind side. A dinner table laid with a multicolored cloth will make it difficult to find small objects, for instance the salt shaker, the (translucent) water bottle, or a piece of chocolate. Totally blind persons prefer to be told what they have on their plate and what to choose between. Visually impaired and blind persons use sound for orientation. Continuous background music or a non-stop TV noise is deleterious to their orientation. There are sports suitable for persons with visual impairment and blindness, for example, swimming, horseback riding, running between two ropes, and tandem bicycling. It is important to continue a good habit of physical exercise even if vision becomes impaired.

Caregivers should try to introduce themselves each time they come and go, and explain what is happening in the room, on the TV, and when they walk together with someone who is visually impaired in the street so that anxiety may be reduced. Special aids are often useful for people with mild intellectual disability. They can use the white cane or a notebook in the form of a small tape recorder; similarly, a tag with the Blind Logo of the country tells others to take care when they pass by. Compensation techniques may vary depending on the activity and the adult's level of responsiveness. In general, lighting levels need to be appropriate. In many institutional or home settings the lighting may not be adequate for the task. Natural or full spectrum lights give the best type of visibility, and a wide variety of lamps and bulbs are commercially available. Conversely excessive glare can be a problem for some individuals. Glare can come from reflected light from lightly colored or glossy painted surfaces. Reflected glare from windows may be a problem for adults especially if a window is near a television or computer screen. With new technology there are many computer aids that can be used for either viewing videos/movies, listening to music, and text-to-speech reading. There are also many speech adaptive equipment for adults with multiple sensory needs. An assessment by an occupational/low vision and/or speech therapist is best to assess each patient's needs.

8.11   Prevention

The prevention of visual impairment in intellectual disability is mainly concerned with cerebral visual impairment, prenatally acquired disorders, and genetic syndromes. The reduced mortality of very premature babies has initiated an epidemic of cerebral visual impairment and intellectual disability. The results are beginning to show up now, and professionals need to be prepared for diagnosis and treatment of these individuals; prevention of intracranial haemorrhage at birth (and later) will reduce the incidence. An International Association for the Scientific Study of Intellectual Disability (IASSID) sponsored international consensus statement recommends ophthalmological assessments when adults leave school, and when adults with Down syndrome are 30 years old and others at age 45, and then every 5 years thereafter [64].

The eye is part of numerous syndromes, and an ophthalmological examination is helpful in syndrome recognition. Many rare syndromes in people with intellectual disability are genetic, and genetic counselling requires a precise diagnosis. Modern molecular genetics has provided an opportunity for improving the delineation of disorders which were previously difficult to separate. Simultaneously, a large number of hitherto unknown—or undiagnosed—disorders have been described in people with intellectual disability. Identification of syndromes requires interdisciplinary cooperation. A considerable number of the "new disorders" or syndromes associated with intellectual disability have been recognized in children, but adults with intellectual disability have not been given the same opportunity of taking advantage of these new developments. The reason presumably is that adults with intellectual disability are treated only for acute diseases, for instance pneumonia, gastric ulcers, and epilepsy, and the identification of specific syndromes is not perceived as the obligation of the general physician.

A precise diagnosis is not only important in genetic counseling, but can also predict specific difficulties in later life. For example, in Williams disease, persons affected may expect visuospatial constructive disabilities [65], adults with Down syndrome may run the risk of developing a premature cataract or keratoconus, adults with Lowe disease may have kidney disorders, and individuals who are blind and who lose their hearing, such as some adults with Norrie disease, may evidence later hallucinations. Because many causes of visual impairment in people with intellectual disability are treatable, there is a need for firmly regulated referrals to ophthalmic or optometric care [66].

8.12   Conclusion

Among adult people with intellectual disability, almost 50% have some degree of visual impairment either at near or distance. Moderate visual impairment at distance is present in 20–30% of all, and severe visual impairment or blindness in 1–5%

dependent on the case mix and the methods used to assess vision. The most important causes of visual impairment are lack of appropriate spectacles for distance and near, cerebral visual impairment, optic nerve atrophy, cataract, and keratoconus. Conditions such age-related macular degeneration and glaucoma are common in older adults in the general population but the prevalence of such conditions in age peers with intellectual disability is still unknown. Diabetic retinopathy is a risk, particularly in persons with Down syndrome. Surgery in people with cataract, glaucoma, and keratoconus has a good prognosis in cooperative patients. Some adults with intellectual disability with high myopia may benefit from refractive surgery if conventional glasses cannot be worn. Individuals with optic nerve atrophy and retinitis pigmentosa need rooms with good illumination, good contrast and—most important—well informed staff. People with intellectual disability are living longer and longer and continued assessment of the individual's health status is needed. Prevention and correction of visual impairment in adults with intellectual disability helps them function better and be more physically and socially engaged. Therefore, adults with intellectual disability should have ophthalmic or optometric care at regular intervals.

Acknowledgment Work by the author was supported in part by the Ulla and Bernt Hjejle Memorial Foundation. With thanks to Mette Warburg who wrote the visual impairment chapter in *Physical Health of Adults with Intellectual Disabilities*.

References

1. Bertuzzi F, Orsoni JG, Porta MR, Paliaga GP, Miglior S. Sensitivity and specificity of a visual acuity screening protocol performed with the Lea symbols 15-line folding distance chart in preschool children. Acta Ophthalmol Scand. 2006;84:807–11.
2. Verweyen P. Measuring vision in children. Community Eye Health. 2004;17(50):27–9.
3. Mash C, Dobson V. Long-term reliability and predictive validity of the Teller acuity card procedure. Vision Res. 1998;38:619–26.
4. Woodhouse JM, Oduwaiye KA. The Cardiff test: a new visual acuity test for toddlers and children with intellectual impairment. A preliminary report. Optom Vis Sci. 1992;69:427–32.
5. Mayer DL, Fulton AB, Rodier D. Grating and recognition acuities of pediatric patients. Ophthalmology. 1984;91:947–53.
6. Mody KH, Kothari MT, Sil A, Doshi P, Walinjkar JA, Chatterjee D. Comparison of lea gratings with Cardiff acuity cards for vision testing of preverbal children. Indian J Ophthalmol. 2012;60:541–3. https://doi.org/10.4103/0301-4738.103791.
7. Dobson V, Quinn GE, Tung B, Palmer EA, Reynolds JD, for the cryotherapy for retinopathy of prematurity cooperative group. Comparison of recognition and grating acuities in very-low-birth-weight children with and without retinal residua of retinopathy of prematurity. Invest Ophthalmol Vis Sci. 1995;36:692–702.
8. Kushner BJ, Lucchese NJ, Morton GV. Grating visual acuity with Teller Cards compared with Snellen acuity in literate patients. Arch Ophthalmol. 1995;113:485–93.
9. Richman JE, Garcia RP. The bead test: a critical appraisal. Am J Optom Physiol Opt. 1983;60:199–203.
10. Block SS, Beckerman SA, Berman PE. Vision profile of the athletes of the 1995 Special Olympics World Summer Games. J Am Optom Assoc. 1997;68(11):699–708.
11. Color Vision Testing. CVTME research; 2017. Accessed from http://www.colorvisiontesting.com/color6.htm.
12. Erickson G, Block S. Testability of a color vision screening test in a population with mental retardation. J Am Optom Assoc. 1999;70:758–63.

13. GoodLite. ColorCheck complete vision screener; 2018. Accessed from https://www.good-lite. com/Details.cfm?ProdID=873.
14. Jacobson L. Ophthalmology in mentally retarded adults. A clinical survey. Acta Ophthalmol. 1988;66:457–62.
15. Woodruff ME, Cleary TE, Bader D. The prevalence of refractive and ocular anomalies among 1242 institutionalized mentally retarded persons. Am J Optom Physiol Opt. 1980;57:70–84.
16. Tielsch JM, Sommer A, Witt K, Katz J, Royall RM. The Baltimore Eye Survey Research Group: blindness and visual impairment in an American urban population. Arch Ophthalmol. 1990;108:286–90.
17. Hirvelä H, Laatikainen L. Visual acuity in a population aged 70 years or older; prevalence and causes of visual impairment. Acta Ophthalmol Scand. 1995;73:99–104.
18. Aitchison C, Easty DL, Jancar J. Eye abnormalities in the mentally handicapped. J Ment Defic Res. 1990;34:41–8.
19. Kwok SK, Ho PCP, Chan AKH, Gandhi SR, Lam DSC. Ocular defects in children and adolescents with severe mental deficiency. J Intellect Disabil Res. 1996;40:330–5.
20. Menacker SJ. Visual function in children with developmental disabilities. Pediatr Clin North Am. 1993;40:659–74.
21. Warburg M, Rattleff J, Kreiner-Moller J. Blindness among 7700 mentally retarded children in Denmark. In: Smith & Keen, editor. Visual handicap in children. London: Spastics International Medical Publications/Heinemann Medical Books; 1979. p. 56–67.
22. Blohmé J, Tornqvist K. Visual impairment in Swedish children. 1. Register and prevalence data. Acta Ophthalmol Scand. 1997;75:194–8.
23. Blohmé J, Tornqvist K. Visually impaired Swedish children. The 1980 cohort study—aspects on mortality. Acta Ophthalmol Scand. 2000;78:560–5.
24. Beange H, McElduff A, Baker W. Medical disorders of adults with mental retardation: a population study. Am J Ment Retard. 1995;99:595–604.
25. Haire AR, Vernon SA, Rubinstein MP. Levels of visual impairment in a day centre for people with a mental handicap. J R Soc Med. 1991;84:542–4.
26. Janicki MP, Dalton AJ. Sensory impairments among older adults with disability. J Intellect Dev Disabil. 1998;23:3–11.
27. Sacks JG, Goren MB, Burke MJ, White S. Ophthalmologic screening of adults with mental retardation. Am J Ment Retard. 1991;95:571–4.
28. Van Schrojenstein Lantman-de Valk HMJ, Haveman MJ, Maaskant MA, Kessels AGH, Urlings HFJ, Sturmans F. The need for assessment of sensory functioning in ageing people with mental handicap. J Intellect Disabil Res. 1994;38:289–98.
29. Van Schrojenstein Lantman-de Valk HMJ, van den Akker M, Maaskant MA, Haveman MJ, Urlings HFJ, Kessels AGH, Crebolder FJM. Prevalence and incidence of health problems in people with intellectual disability. J Intellect Disabil Res. 1997;41:42–51.
30. Warburg M. Visual impairment among people with developmental delay. J Intelllect Disabil Res. 1994;38:423–32.
31. Warburg M. Visual impairment in adult people with intellectual disability. A literature survey. J Intellect Disabil Res. 2001;45:424–38.
32. Woodhouse JM, Griffiths C, Gedling A. The prevalence of ocular defects and the provision of eye care in adults with learning disabilities living in the community. Ophthalmic Physiol Opt. 2000;20:79–89.
33. Warburg M. Visual impairment in adult people with moderate, severe, and profound intellectual disability. Acta Ophthalmol Scand. 2001;79:450–4.
34. Day KA. The elderly mentally handicapped in hospital: a clinical study. J Ment Defic Res. 1987;31:131–46.
35. World Health Organization. World report on disability 2011. Geneva: World Health Organization; 2011. ISBN-13: 978-92-4-156418-2
36. Cregg M, Woodhouse JM, Stewart RE, Pakeman VH, Bromham NR, Gunter HL, Trojanowska L, Parker M, Fraser WI. Development of refractive error and strabismus in children with Down syndrome. Invest Ophthalmol Vis Sci. 2003;44:1023–30. https://doi.org/10.1167/iovs.01-0131.

37. Van Buggenhout GJCM, Trommelen JCM, Schenmaker A, De Bal C, Verbeek JJMC, Smeets DFCM, Ropers HH, Devriendt K, Hamel BCJ, Fryns JP. Down syndrome in a population of elderly mentally retarded patients: genetic-diagnostic survey and implications for medical care. Am J Med Genet. 1999;85:376–84.
38. Arsen A, Ozgur O, Bozkurt OH, Guven A, Degerliyurt A, Munir K. Refractive errors and strabismus in children with down syndrome: a controlled study. J Pediatr Ophthalmol Strabismus. 2009;46(2):83–6.
39. Head E, Powell D, Gold BT, Schmitt FA. Alzheimer's disease in Down syndrome. Eur J Neurodegener Dis. 2012;1:353–64.
40. Janicki MP, Dalton AJ. Dementia, aging, and intellectual disabilities: a handbook. PA, USA: Taylor & Francis; 1999.
41. Urbano R. Health issues among persons with Down syndrome. International Review of Research in Mental Retardation. 39. Academic Press; 2010. ISBN: 0080922686, 9780080922683.
42. Armstrong RA. Alzheimer's disease and the eye. J Optom. 2009;2:103–11. https://doi.org/10.3921/joptom.2009.103.
43. Kerr AM, McCulloch D, Oliver K, McLean B, Coleman E, Law T, Beaton P, Wallace S, Newell E, Eccles T, Prescott RJ. Medical needs of people with intellectual disability require regular reassessment and the provision of client- and carer-held reports. J Intellect Disabil Res. 2003;47:134–45.
44. Haugen OH, Aasved H, Bertelsen T. Refractive state and correction of refractive errors among mentally retarded adults in a central institution. Acta Ophthalmol Scand. 1995;73:129–32.
45. Bader D, Woodruff ME. The effects of corrective lenses on various behaviors of mentally retarded persons. Am J Optom Physiol Opt. 1980;57:447–59.
46. Schwartz RE. An optometric clinic in a state institute for the severely retarded. J Am Optom Assoc. 1977;48:59–64.
47. Warburg M. Tracing and training of blind and partially sighted persons in institutions for the mentally retarded. Dan Med Bull. 1970;17:148.
48. McCulloch DL, Sludden PA, McKeown K, Kerr A. Vision care requirements among intellectually disabled adults: a residence-based study. J Intellect Disabil Res. 1996;40:140–50.
49. Winter RM, Baraitser M. Dysmorphology database, Oxford medical databases. Version 2. London: Oxford University Press; 1998.
50. Creavin AL, Brown RD. Ophthalmic assessment of children with Down syndrome: is England doing its bit? Strabismus. 2010;18:142–5.
51. Yokoyama T, Tamura H, Tsukamoto H. Prevalence of glaucoma in adults with Down's syndrome. Jpn J Ophthalmol. 2006;50:274. https://doi.org/10.1007/s10384-005-0305-x.
52. Haim M. Prevalence of retinitis pigmentosa and allied disorders in Denmark. II. Systemic involvement and age at onset. Acta Ophthalmol. 1992;70:417–26.
53. Green JS, Parfrey PS, Harnett JD, Farid ID, Cramer BC, Johnson G, McManamon PJ, O'Leary E, Pryse-Philips W. The cardinal manifestations of Bardet-Biedl syndrome, a form of Laurence-Moon-Bardet-Biedl syndrome. N Engl J Med. 1989;321:1002–9.
54. Riise R, Andréasson S, Borgström MK, Wright AF, Tommerup N, Rosenberg T, Tornqvist K. Intrafamilial variation of the phenotype in Bardet-Biedl syndrome. Br J Ophthalmol. 1997;81:378–85.
55. Warburg M, Friedrich U. Coloboma and microphthalmos in chromosomal aberrations. Chromosomal aberrations and neural crest cell developmental field. Ophthalmic Paediatr Genet. 1987;8:105–18.
56. Jacobson L, Ek U, Fernell E, Flodmark O, Broberger U. Visual impairment in preterm children with periventricular leukomalacia – visual, cognitive and neuropaediatric characteristics related to cerebral imaging. Dev Med Child Neurol. 1996;38:724–35.
57. Dutton G, Ballentyne J, Boyd G, Bradnam M, Day R, McCulloch D, Mackie R, Philips S, Saunders K. Cortical visual dysfunction in children: a clinical study. Eye. 1996;10:302–9.
58. Partington M, Mowat D, Einfeld S, Tonge B, Turner G. Genes on the X-chromosome are important in undiagnosed mental retardation. Am J Med Genet. 2000;92:57–61.
59. Skeller E, Øster J. Eye symptoms in mongolism. Acta Ophthalmol (Copenh). 1951;29:149–61.

60. Woodhouse JM, Meades JS, Leat SJ, Saunders KJ. Reduced accomodation in children with Down syndrome. Invest Ophthalmol Vis Sci. 1993;34:2382–7.
61. Woodhouse JM, Pakeman VH, Saunders KJ, Parker M, Fraser WI, Lobo S, Sastry P. Visual acuity and accommodation in infants and young children with Down's syndrome syndrome. J Intellect Disabil Res. 1996;40:49–55.
62. Hestnes A, Sand T, Fostad K. Ocular findings in Down's syndrome. J Ment Defic Res. 1991;35:194–203.
63. Anwar AJ, Walker JD, Frier BM. Type 1 diabetes mellitus and Down's syndrome: prevalence, management and diabetic complications. Diabet Med. 1998;15:160–3.
64. Evenhuis H, Nagtzaam LMD, editors. IASSID international consensus statement. Early identification of hearing and visual impairment in children and adults with an intellectual disability. IASSID, Special Interest Research Group on Health Issues; 1998.
65. Atkinson J, Anker S, Braddick O, Nokes L, Mason A, Braddick F. Visual and visuospatial development in young children with Williams syndrome. Dev Med Child Neurol. 2001;43:330–7.
66. Warburg M, Riise R. [Ophthalmological services to mentally retarded persons. A review and recommendations] in Danish. Ugeskr Laeger. 1994;156:6366–9.

Hearing Impairment

9

Sarah Bent, Siobhan Brennan, and Lynzee McShea

9.1   Introduction

Our ability to hear is a key component in our ability to communicate with others and to interact with the world around us. Those with impaired hearing from birth may rely on other senses, such as sight and touch, and other forms of communication, such as sign language, but for those whose hearing had changed during their life, or whose hearing was not known to be impaired, this is a significant disability. Universal newborn hearing screening has proven successful in identifying hearing impairment shortly after birth in countries such as the United Kingdom [1]; however, this has only been in place for just over a decade and is not globally available. In addition, hearing commonly deteriorates with age, with high impact on the individual, including risks of social isolation, mental health problems, and dementia. The World Health Organization reports that there are 360 million people with significant hearing impairment globally, approximately 5% of the world's population [2]. This varies in level and categorisation among countries. For example, in the United Kingdom, some 17% are affected by hearing impairment increasing to 40% of those adults age 50 years and older [3].

Hearing impairment affects still greater proportions of adults with intellectual disability and yet it is an overlooked and misunderstood condition in this group,

S. Bent (✉)
North Wales Audiology Service, Betsi Cadwaladr University Health Board, Wrexham Maelor Hospital, Wrexham, UK
e-mail: SARAH.BENT@wales.nhs.uk

S. Brennan
Manchester Centre for Audiology and Deafness (ManCAD), University of Manchester, Manchester, UK

L. McShea
Audiology Department, City Hospitals Sunderland Foundation Trust, Sunderland Royal Hospital, Sunderland, UK

© Springer Nature Switzerland AG 2019
V. P. Prasher, M. P. Janicki (eds.), *Physical Health of Adults with Intellectual and Developmental Disabilities*, https://doi.org/10.1007/978-3-319-90083-4_9

with low rates of hearing assessment [4, 5]. Often reliance is on self-report, with caregivers being unaware of signs and symptoms or hearing assessment being seen as of low value for individuals with multiple disabilities. The good news is that, for the majority of those adults with intellectual disability, hearing impairment can be either treated or rehabilitation provided with successful outcomes achievable [6, 7].

This chapter looks at firstly the demographics of hearing impairment for adults with intellectual disability and the evidence base underpinning this, with some detail on the common types of hearing impairment and the effects that this can have on daily life. We will explore the types of hearing assessment that are used and common adaptations or alternative test methods that are available for those adults with intellectual disability. And finally, by detailing the rehabilitation options and ways in which people with intellectual disability may be supported to maximise their communication and interaction, their appreciation of music and their environmental awareness, we hope to inspire readers and start to break down the myths about hearing impairment for this population.

Looking back at earlier work in this area, it is clear to see how much has developed in audiological practice and in our wider understanding of and support for adults with intellectual disability. With the UK National Institute for Health and Care Excellence (NICE) guidelines on hearing impairment [8] and with working groups looking at guidelines for hearing impairment in adults with intellectual disability across the world (e.g. British Society of Audiology, European Federation of Audiology Societies), the awareness and work towards common good practice standards are set to continue to improve.

9.2   Demographics of Hearing Impairment in Adults with Intellectual Disability

On average, about 40–45% of adults with intellectual disability have hearing impairment of a level that impacts communication [9–11]. As with the worldwide population, hearing impairment prevalence increases further with age, with reports of 59–68% for those adults with intellectual disability over 50 years old [5, 6, 9, 12, 13]. For adults with Down syndrome over 50 years old, this is even higher: 62–93% [5, 9, 12]. A review of the literature for older adults with learning disabilities found evidence of significant levels of undiagnosed hearing impairment, but little evidence relating to specific groups other than older adults with Down syndrome [14].

9.2.1   Quality of Evidence Available

Screening conducted at various Special Olympics events and with other 'high functioning' groups (where hearing assessments are completed for those attending) have provided some detailed evidence of hearing impairment. For these participants, the level of intellectual disability tends to be milder and additional co-morbidities less likely [15]. These data are comparable to those observed at a residential school for persons with intellectual disability [16].

Much of the evidence has relied on self-report or caregiver-report surveys [17] which tend to underestimate hearing impairment [18]. This is partly due to diagnostic overshadowing, as the signs and symptoms of hearing impairment are attributed to other health issues or the intellectual disability [19].

The literature that relies on existing healthcare services is limited by both the access of those services [20, 21] and the assessment methods used. Even where a question of hearing is included in the primary care annual health check (such as in the UK), this is not sufficiently sensitive to identify hearing loss [22], and in the UK only 70% of adults with intellectual disability are known to primary care services [23]. Whilst audiology services complete more in-depth assessment, only 30–45% of the general population who visit their general practitioner about hearing problems are referred onwards for assessment [24, 25]; there are additional barriers to access for those adults with intellectual disability due to attitudes and opinions of the referrer [22].

9.3 Main Types of Hearing Impairment and Common Causes

Hearing impairment may be described as conductive, sensorineural or mixed hearing impairment depending on the results of the hearing assessment, and these indicate the parts of the ear affected. Yeates [11] found that in adults with intellectual disability, 10% were found to have a conductive hearing impairment, 30% a sensorineural hearing impairment, 29% a mixed impairment and the remainder could not be diagnosed with the electro-physiological tests used. Of those adults with Down syndrome who had a diagnosed hearing impairment, some 64% had a mixed hearing loss.

9.3.1 Conductive Hearing Impairment and Ear Health

Conductive hearing impairment tends to be an acquired change due to abnormalities in the external ear (including the ear canal) or the middle ear (including the ear drum, ossicles, and middle ear space), reducing the level of the sound as it enters the ear. The most common causes are occluding wax blocking the ear canal, perforations of the ear drum, and otitis media with effusion (commonly known as 'glue ear').

The prevalence of occluding wax is high, particularly in adults with Down syndrome [26] due in part to the smaller anatomy of the external ear, increasing from 2% in the general population to 30% in adults with intellectual disability [27, 28]. In addition, Fransman [29] reported a link between lack of back teeth and wax impaction. Any occlusion of the outer ear may cause a mild reduction in hearing or an additional effect in addition to an underlying hearing impairment due to other cause.

The middle ear space behind the ear drum is normally filled with air, with the pressure equalized with the outside via the Eustachian tube that leads to the back of the throat. 'Glue ear' describes the presence of a sticky fluid in that space, usually resulting from an upper respiratory tract infection, typically draining away via the Eustachian tube within a few months. In adults with different facial anatomies, such as narrower Eustachian tubes in adult with Down syndrome [30], there may be increased risk of longstanding 'glue ear'. Whilst 'watchful waiting' is advised in the short term, prolonged untreated 'glue ear' may result in other damage, including perforated ear drums and inner ear damage.

Chronic ear infections may occur in anyone that had poor ear health, such as adults with poor hygiene generally, or may be due to regular trauma from picking, inserting objects in the ears, or banging the ears with hands. Otitis Externa is a chronic inflammation of the outer ear, and may also be present. Both may cause conductive hearing impairment through blockage of the outer ear, and also cause issues for hearing aid use.

9.3.2   Sensorineural Hearing Impairment and Presbyacusis

Sensorineural hearing impairment originates from the cochlea (the sensory organ) or from the auditory nerve. The most common cause is loss of inner hair cells in the cochlea with age (known as presbyacusis), but there may also be damage due to noise, ototoxicity from medication or other drugs, or be present from birth. This particularly affects hearing the higher frequencies found in speech (2–8 kHz), resulting in difficulties discriminating speech due to inability to hear clearly the more subtle consonants.

Mixed hearing impairment is a combination of the two above. This is common as adults with longstanding conductive hearing impairments age, and particularly in adults with Down syndrome due to premature aging [31].

9.3.3   Hyperacusis

In addition to (or instead of) hearing impairment, hearing difficulties may be experienced related to a heightened sensitivity to sound, known as hyperacusis. The prevalence in those adults with intellectual disability is not well documented; however, it is found in clinical practice primarily by those adults with sensory modulation disorders, such as with autism spectrum disorder.

9.4   Other Causes of Hearing Impairment

In addition to increased likelihood of acquired hearing loss throughout life, there are a range of pathologies and syndromes associated with intellectual disability that also affect the hearing system from birth [32, 33]. The etiology of hearing impairment in adults with intellectual disability was found in one study to be 48% with acquired hearing impairment, 21% congenital (17% inherited and 4% chromosomal) and in 30% with an unknown cause [34].

Inherited causes may be due to recessive genes (e.g. Pendreds, Ushers or Jervell-Lange-Nielson), dominant genes (pigment related—e.g., Waardenburgs, or congenital deformities—e.g. Treacher-Collins and Aperts) or x-linked genetic causes (e.g.

Hunters). The most common chromosomal abnormality is Down syndrome, but there are others related to hearing impairment (e.g. Patau's, Edward's and Cri-du-chat). Infections either peri- or post-natal are also associated with sensorineural hearing impairment, particularly rubella, cytomegalovirus, toxoplasmosis, meningitis, measles, and mumps. Other peri- and post-natal causes include prematurity, anoxia, and hyperbilirubinemia.

9.5 Effects of Hearing Impairment

For all persons with hearing impairment, the primary impact is on communication, but hearing also plays a significant role in our ability to appreciate the world around us, to enjoy music and other pleasurable experiences, and to interact independently with our surroundings. For adults with intellectual disability there also is a higher likelihood of requiring support with daily living or various health needs, which adds additional importance to communication; the essence of person-centered care in promoting choice and independence within a person's abilities relies on being able to communicate those wishes and foster those skills appropriately. Sensory stimulation, including enjoyment of music and awareness of surroundings, is recognized as valuable to good quality of life for adults with intellectual disability [35], with sensory deprivation having significant impact on all aspects of life [36].

The association between 'challenging behavior' and sensory impairment is well documented, particularly for adults with intellectual disability and hearing impairment who do not have access to effective amplification [37, 38]. Challenging behavior has long been linked to communication difficulties [39], but is now understood to be an expression of communication in itself [40] and indeed the signs of hearing impairment are often incorrectly labelled as challenging behaviors [41]. Conversely, using hearing aids has been shown to be effective in reducing challenging behavior [7].

This significant impact on a person's life creates a multiplicative effect of hearing impairment and intellectual disability, greater than of the individual effects added together [42]. Taking all this into account, the importance of hearing assessment in early life and then regular re-assessment throughout the lifespan for people with intellectual disability then starts to become clear.

9.6 Assessment Aspirations

When assessing hearing, the primary question that should be in the mind of the tester is "Why are we doing this?" and "What information is required?" Ideally the audiologist would like information about hearing ability across a range of frequencies for each ear individually. It may not be possible to obtain this information in a single test session and the audiologist, persons with intellectual disability and their caregivers should consider what the priorities are. The usual priority for audiology has been maximizing the person's ability to hear speech, but what if that is not the priority for the person him or herself? What if other sounds are of greater interest?

If information about each ear individually is not achieved, has information been gained about a person's functional hearing when the person is using both ears together? Is this sufficient for this individual?

The British Society of Audiology advises in "Adult Rehabilitation – Common Principles in Audiology Services" [43] that *"The International Classification of Functioning, Disability and Health (ICF) was officially endorsed by the World Health Organization in 2001 as the framework for disability and health sectors worldwide [44]. This biopsychosocial approach highlights individual health rather than disability, with the focus on impact rather than cause... This approach underpins the UK Action Plan on Hearing Loss [45] that emphasizes the responsibility for the health sector to provide care with individual level activity limitations (previously known as disability) and participation restrictions (previously known as handicap) as the focus of assessment, diagnosis and management of the hearing impairment (i.e., function)."*

9.7 Specific Hearing Tests

Audiology practitioners, as with many other healthcare disciplines, are becoming increasingly adept as optimizing care for adults with intellectual disability and this includes hearing assessment. Less than 1% of adults with intellectual disabilities referred for a hearing assessment require a general anesthetic to undertake the examination. This section will describe a variety of methods that are used to assess hearing and ear health, and are summarized in Table 9.1.

9.7.1 Otoscopy

Otoscopy refers to looking into a person's ears, which provides a practitioner with a view of the external ear, ear canal, and ear drum. The ear drum is usually opaque, and it is also often possible to gain some, albeit limited, information about the middle ear. Challenges to otoscopy include an obscured view of the ear drum from narrow ear canals or more often wax occluding the canal. While otoscopy should not be painful there are people who dislike or misinterpret physical contact and may not tolerate this procedure. As the aim of otoscopy is to identify issues such as ear infections or blockages in the external ear, omitting otoscopy from the test battery can have adverse implications on ear health.

9.7.2 Tympanometry

Tympanometry is a method of assessing the middle ear. It involves adjusting the pressure in the ear canal (and feels similar to ascending or descending in an airplane) and the movement of the ear drum in response to this pressure change is measured. This can not only inform the practitioner about the status of the ear drum, it can also provide information about the middle ear as there are certain pathologies

Table 9.1 Summary of some of more common components of a hearing assessment and their implications for the person and the tester

Test	Typical Duration	Contact with Person	Person Requirement	Part of the ear tested	Frequencies tested	Intensity tested
Otoscopy	< 1 minute	Tip into entrance of ear canal. External ear pulled gently	None	External ear, canal and ear drum	None	None
Tympanometry	< 1 minute	Tip into entrance of ear canal. External ear pulled gently	None	Ear canal, drum and middle ear	None	None
Acoustic Reflex	< 1 minute	Tip into entrance of ear canal. External ear pulled gently	None	Outer, middle and inner ear, early auditory brainstem	A range specific frequencies across the speech	Loud sound
otoacoustic Emissions (OAEs)	< 2 minutes	Tip into entrance of ear canal. External ear pulled gently	Minimal movement	Outer, middle and inner ear	Limited information about different frequencies	Quiet sound
Auditory Brainstem Response (BOA)	10 minutes - 1 hour	Electrodes on skin. Wearing earphones	Minimal movement	Outer, middle and inner ear, auditory brainstem	Low pitch and high pitch	Electro-physiolocical threshold
Auditory Steady State Responses (ASSR)	10 minutes - 1 hour	Electrodes on skin. Wearing earphones	Minimal movement	Outer, middle and inner ear, auditory brainstem and/or cortex depending on parameters used	A range specific frequencies across the speech spectrum	Electro-physiolocical threshold
Cortical Evoked Response Audiometry (CERA)	10 minutes - 1 hour	Electrodes on skin. Wearing earphones	Minimal movement	All of auditory pathway to auditory cortex	Low pitch and high pitch	Electrophysiolocical threshold
Behavioural Observation Audiometry (BOA)	10 minutes	None	Behavioural response to sound	All of auditory pathway	A range specific frequencies across the speech	Near threshold
Soundfield Performance Audiometry	10 minutes	Client holding an object to place in receptacle	Capacity to wait for and respond to sound	All of auditory pathway	A range specific frequencies across the speech	Threshold
Pure Tone Audiometry (PTA) or Play Audiometry	20 minutes	Client holding a button or object to place in receptacle. Wearing earphones	Capacity to wait for and respond to sound	All of auditory pathway	A range specific frequencies across the speech spectrum	Threshold
Speech Discrimination Testing	10 minutes	None	Sufficient receptive linguistic skill to differentiate words	All of auditory pathway	Frequencies across the speech spectrum	Near threshold

of the middle ear, such as 'glue ear' or ossification of the middle ear bones that will limit the ear drum's movement. The likelihood of an accurate tympanometry test is dependent on the ear canal being clear and the ability of the person to be relatively still for the duration of the measurement which is typically a few seconds. The audiologist should take into account the fact that some syndromes are associated with anatomical features that can affect the accuracy of tympanometry, such as Down syndrome, and different normative values should be used.

9.7.3 Audiometry

The most commonly used audiological measure is pure tone audiometry. This test is used to identify the quietest sound that a person can hear; usually described as the 'threshold'. This test typically involves the person wearing headphones and they are presented with decreasingly quiet sounds. The person is usually asked to press a button every time they hear a sound irrespective of how loud or soft the sound is. This test depends on the person's capacity to wait for a sound and act on it. If a person's intellectual disability are such that he or she can't do this sufficiently reliably for the tester to draw a conclusion on whether the person has heard the stimulus or not, the test should be modified or deemed inconclusive. There are a wide range of modifications that are available to the tester;

- More responses to sound occur when the sound is more interesting to the person. While the audiology practitioner would like the sound to be as 'frequency specific' as possible, using sounds that contain more frequencies tend to be more interesting (e.g., a warble tone or a narrow band sound).
- Pressing a button can be less accurate than when the person is asked to make a larger movement in response to sound. The button could be replaced by placing a peg in a basket, for example, commonly then known as 'play audiometry'.
- Responses can also be verified by asking the person to point to the ear where the sound is heard.
- For people who have a sensory modulation disorder and have a tactile defensiveness to the extent that headphones aren't tolerated, the sounds can be presented from a speaker, commonly known as 'soundfield performance audiometry'. Caution should be applied as each individual ear is not being tested, irrespective of where the speaker is in the room; the better ear will be being tested. A desensitization program can be used to help with the acceptance of headphones.

As an alternative to asking the person to respond to sound, behavioral observation audiometry (BOA) is where a sound is presented and any response (e.g., head turn, eye glance or stilling) is noted and could give an indication as to the level that is being heard. Extreme caution should be applied to the use of this test due to its highly subjective nature. Additionally, it is thought that responses to sounds using the test are not necessarily thresholds, but minimum response levels. The audiologist should work with the person's family or caregiver to identify and verify responses to sound as different to unrelated movements. Behavioral responses to sound in this group tend to vary considerably between people. Research continues to identify ways of improving this methodology for individuals with profound and multiple intellectual disabilities.

9.7.4   Speech Discrimination

If a hearing aid is required, the algorithms used to program it are based on these measured thresholds. However, understanding of speech is not only based on whether a sound is loud enough to hear, but also the ability of the ear to discriminate between the different elements to identify one sound from another. Speech discrimination is typically assessed by presenting words and the person repeats them back. The limitations to this type of testing include the clarity of the person's speech and their ability to articulate what they have heard. Another version includes presenting a range of pictures and asking the person to point to the picture of the word that they have heard. This requires the person being able to recognize the items being said. A choice of picture type or use of familiar objects can further promote engagement.

9.7.5 Auditory Electrophysiology

In the absence of accurate and/or reliable behavioral assessments there is a form of objective assessment known as auditory electrophysiological testing (AET). There are multiple tests of hearing under this banner and the practitioner should select one most suited to the age and level of alertness of the person. As far as the person is concerned this test involves three or four electrodes (depending on the method being used) being placed on the head and behind the ears. Sound will be delivered through either some form of earphones or a speaker. The test time is often around 20 minutes but this type of testing can vary in duration arguably more than any other audiological test, from 10 minutes to over an hour. Magazines or silent films can be provided to provide low impact distraction during the testing.

Different electrophysiological tests provide information about different parts of the auditory pathway. Cortical evoked response audiometry (CERA) informs the tester about the auditory pathway as far as the auditory cortex—which is the highest point in the auditory pathway that is typically tested in an audiology clinic. It is possible; however, that a neuropathology that may cause an intellectual disability may also affect the auditory cortex and so this test may have inaccuracies in this client group. Another disadvantage to this test is that the person needs to be alert throughout which can be difficult to ensure for the full duration of the test. Additionally, for an auditory electrophysiological test to provide accurate results it is necessary for movement from the person to be minimal. This can obviously be difficult to achieve in some circumstances. In this situation it is possible to assess hearing while the person is under general anesthetic by using the most commonly used auditory electrophysiological test known as the auditory brainstem response (ABR). It is common practice to align this test with other healthcare that needs to be provided under general anesthetic, so that the person has as few episodes of general anesthetic as possible. An electrophysiological method being used increasingly in the UK is the auditory steady state response (ASSR) which can test multiple frequencies and both ears simultaneously, making testing considerably quicker; however, the need for the person to be still and quiet remains the same.

9.7.6 Other Automated Tests

If duration of the test is particularly problematic, acoustic reflexes can be recorded. Acoustic reflexes are recorded by placing a small tip in the ear and a loud sound presented; no input from the person is required and this takes under a minute. This test does not provide information about threshold; however, it can be used to rule out a profound hearing impairment, along with supporting other diagnostic information.

Otoacoustics emissions (OAEs) are most commonly used for hearing screening. A small tip is placed in the ear and quiet sounds are presented. No behavioral response from the person is required; however, the person does need to remain relatively quiet and still for any responses to be recorded. This test takes typically less than 2 minutes per ear. OAEs are often used to rule out significant hearing losses; however, it is worth noting that it does not provide information about the auditory nerve.

9.8   After a Hearing Assessment

Thanks to increasing awareness of the need for hearing assessment and advances in assessment techniques, there is the potential for increasing numbers of people with intellectual disability to be diagnosed with hearing impairment. But a diagnosis isn't the end of the story, it some ways it is only the beginning. The rest of this chapter explores 'treatments' for hearing impairment, and considerations specific to people with intellectual disability.

9.8.1   Can Hearing Impairment Be Treated?

Generally speaking, conductive hearing impairments are usually treatable with medication or a surgical procedure. If the hearing impairment is present due to a physical obstruction such as wax, infection, or a foreign body, removal of the obstruction will restore hearing to previous levels. Conductive hearing impairment arising from conditions such as otitis media with effusion (fluid in the middle ear) or otosclerosis (abnormal bone growth) can be improved surgically.

Sensorineural hearing impairment (affecting the organ and nerve of hearing) is usually permanent and cannot be reversed. The most common 'treatment' for this type of hearing impairment is use of hearing aids. Though hearing aids cannot restore hearing, they have been proven to be an effective and beneficial option.

9.9   What Is (Re)Habilitation?

There is a subtle but important difference in terminology between the terms 'habilitation' and 'rehabilitation'. Rehabilitation is the term most frequently used, and describes a process, service or device that enables a person to *regain* an ability that has been lost (such as ability to hear sounds). Habilitation may involve the same interventions or treatments, but allows a person to *acquire* a skill or ability for the first time.

Audiologists therefore provide both habilitation and rehabilitation, depending on the age and circumstances of the individual. Rehabilitation is the term most frequently used with adults, as the majority of adults with hearing impairment are born with good hearing acuity, which diminishes over time. For those adults with intellectual disability, the lines between the two are arguably a little more blurry, as we may be less sure of their prior hearing abilities (for example, non-verbal adults with minimal response to external stimuli).

9.9.1 Options for Rehabilitation

Hearing impairment is categorized in terms of volume and frequencies. In simple terms, a hearing aid is an amplification device that makes the inaudible, audible. All hearing aids regardless of their size, shape, or appearance work in these basic terms. A microphone within the hearing aid detects external sounds, which are processed as a transformed output. Modern hearing aids use digital sound processing and are much more than just basic amplification devices. They are multichannel and can process different frequencies and intensities of sound to different degrees, dependent on the sound environment the wearer is in.

The most commonly used hearing aids are 'air conduction' types, where the device is worn on or in the ear. These devices detect ambient sounds via their microphones and transmit the processed sound along the whole hearing pathway (outer, middle, and inner ear). In contrast, bone conduction hearing aids bypass the outer and middle ear and transmit processed sound by vibrations across the skull, to be detected by the inner ear. Bone conduction hearing aids are considered when the outer and/or middle part of the ear is absent or compromised. They can be worn via a headband or attached directly to the skull (via a metal abutment). For those with profound hearing impairment, air or bone conduction hearing aids may provide limited benefit due to the extent of the inner ear damage and cochlear implants are increasingly used. These are electronic, medical devices that provide electrical (rather than acoustic) stimulation directly to the inner ear via an external and internal sound processor 'implanted' by a surgical operation.

Due to improved technology, cosmetic appearance and increased awareness of hearing issues, more people are seeking hearing aids than ever before. In one survey completed in the UK, 90% of adult respondents wearing hearing aids in the general population found hearing aids beneficial to their lifestyle [46]. However, this perceived benefit does not appear to have translated to adults with intellectual disability.

9.9.2 Rehabilitation for People with ID in the Literature

The health disparity faced by people with intellectual disability is well known and has been documented for a number of years [47]. Despite this, and the widespread availability of hearing aids, there is a shortage of literature addressing the issue of hearing rehabilitation for this group.

However, it is important to note that there is rarely a biological or physical reason why people with intellectual disability cannot be offered, and benefit from, hearing aids. There are misguided assumptions that this group will not tolerate hearing aids or benefit from them [48]. Attitudes, awareness and confidence are likely to play more of a role in uptake and use than any technical or medical factor. For example, all individuals fitted with hearing aids in a study by Coppens-Hofman et al. [49]

experienced demonstrable benefit from amplification, though this benefit was denied by 35% of caregivers.

This issue was investigated further by one of the authors in publications addressing the perceptions and practices of paid caregivers, general practitioners, and nurses [22, 50]. Findings suggested that caregiver and non-audiology healthcare practitioners generally lacked knowledge, skills, and confidence regarding hearing aids, which affected the use and maintenance of the devices issued to adults with intellectual disability. The UK's Hearing and Learning Disabilities (HaLD) Special Interest Group available at: http://www.hald.org.uk/ [accessed August 2018] is for professionals with this dual interest and shares at its meetings and in publications by members a wealth of stories from audiologists, regarding hearing aid benefit and the subsequent improvements in quality of life that follow (e.g. [7]). The future challenge remains to disseminate this anecdotal evidence widely, and in a format that will be integrated into program practice.

9.9.3 Rehabilitation Considerations Specific to People with Intellectual Disability

Over the last two decades, there have been significant technological advances in audiology; not only in the quality of hearing aid devices offered, but also in the techniques available for measurement and verification of their output. Devices can now be programmed to take into account individual hearing thresholds and ear canal properties. This makes the process of fitting a hearing aid more objective, thus increasing confidence that the device will be providing enhanced access to sound.

However, due to a shortage of research into rehabilitation for people with intellectual disability, hearing aids continue to be prescribed and issued to this group using evidence-based practice obtained from hearing aid wearers in the general population. Whilst this may prove to be valid, assumptions are made that results and findings are transferrable. In audiological terms, areas that require investigation and validation include:

• Prescription formulae selection
• Real ear to coupler difference (RECD) applications when verifying hearing aids
• Choice of real ear measurement protocol when verifying hearing aids
• Use of outcome measures and their relevance

As well as these more technical aspects, consideration should also be paid to individual ear size and position and other aspects pertaining to comfort and ease of use. Many individuals will wear glasses as well as hearing aids, which may cause practical concerns (i.e., how to fit both elements behind the ear). There are a range of solutions which should be explored and offered in order to remove this potential barrier to hearing aid use.

The literature has cautioned that the process of issuing hearing aids can become a ritualized encounter [51], where the client is only considered as a pair of ears to be treated and individual attitudes and opinions are not viewed to be necessary or relevant. Due to the heterogeneity of this group, and the lack of awareness and confidence in hearing aids from those who support them, a more personalized and holistic approach is essential for effective rehabilitation.

9.10 Support for Rehabilitation

Too often, rehabilitation is viewed simplistically with overemphasis on the hearing device itself and, as a consequence, rejection of the hearing aid often occurs following issue. In one study, less than half of users continued to wear hearing aids 8–16 years post fitting, but on the whole this was not because they did not receive benefit from them [52]. Audiologists have a duty of care to make their rehabilitation inclusive and collaborative, and to encourage motivation and engagement.

Despite this, many individuals do not receive follow up post intervention [38]. By not reviewing the progress of individuals, it is likely that this progress will be limited. Even in the general population, first time hearing aid users report feeling overwhelmed and leave the appointment with both informational and support needs neglected [53]. Paid caregivers have difficulties understanding the use and maintenance of hearing aids [41]. Even those who experience hearing aids as part of their work have poor practical skills. A survey by Pryce and Gooberman-Hill [54] revealed that 44% of staff working with older age hearing aid users, did not know how to fix broken devices.

The high prevalence of hearing impairment in people with intellectual disability justifies the need for training, as has been known for many years [48, 55]. Yet, the majority of caregivers have still had no formal training in hearing impairment [56]. In recent years, training has become more accessible and now exists in a variety of formats in audiology, including creation of individual support plans with clinicians [43], via online platforms [57], and face to face training in residential settings [58]. Importantly, training such as these do not focus solely on hearing aids, as not all individuals with hearing impairment will choose to wear them. Assistive listening devices such as personal amplifiers, vibrating alarm clocks, visual smoke detectors, and amplified telephones should also be considered. Training on communication tactics is also important as this helps to reinforce the idea that communication is a shared responsibility between the speaker and listener.

9.10.1 Support from a Multidisciplinary Team (MDT)

It is argued that assessment and management of hearing impairment should be multidisciplinary [41]. A multidisciplinary approach allows audiology, caregivers and primary care workers to come together to best support people with intellectual disability and hearing impairment. This inclusive approach is empowering and can lead to improved outcomes. Coppens-Hofman et al. [49] found that caregivers were more likely to rate hearing aids as beneficial for people they supported, if they had themselves been aware of concerns regarding the person's hearing prior to the hearing aids being issued.

An example of a multidisciplinary model used in Audiology (the 5As model) is described in McShea [59], and may be represented visually as shown in Fig. 9.1. Flexibility is built into this model as there is no minimum or maximum number of stakeholders, this can be determined according to the need and remit of the group. Initially, an assembly of stakeholders is necessary to consider the issue and determine membership. For hearing impairment and intellectual disability, several possible stakeholders can be identified (including community teams, social care, service commissioners, etc.). Membership could increase or decrease as the MDT matures. Regardless of actual number, the involvement of multiple stakeholders means that success is less reliant on individuals. For example, if caregivers failed to manage hearing aids appropriately, this could still be identified and actioned by community teams or by a primary care professional.

MDT assembly should be driven by a stakeholder who is central to the issue and is affected by all other parties. Though this could potentially be the individual or their caregiver, they are unlikely to have the capability or resources to coordinate this. For those with hearing impairment and intellectual disability, Audiology seems to be a valid alternative. Shames and Simpson [60] suggest that Audiology is well placed to be at the heart of person-centered care. This would also increase the visibility and responsibility of the profession.

By having a robust core of assembly and awareness, good access, assessment and aftercare are more likely to be sustained. This would also mean that initiatives would not rely on individual stakeholders, as there would be shared ownership. By encouraging shared meaning and experience, values would align and mutual

Fig. 9.1 The 5 As model of multidisciplinary working in audiology services

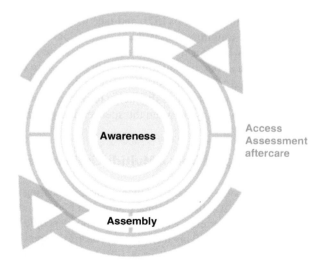

understanding would occur. The focus would then shift from service-centered to person-centered.

9.11 Conclusions

Great strides have been made in understanding the prevalence of hearing impairment in adults with intellectual disability, the implications of hearing problems as people age and the lack of general awareness by caregivers. With all of these, combined with understanding the impact of hearing on individuals' lives, the importance of assessment can be appreciated.

Hearing assessment is effective and informative, with an increasing variety of techniques that can be chosen and tailored to the individual's abilities, and with the audiology profession being increasingly skilled at person-centered approaches. It is our hope that content of this chapter has demonstrated the benefits of rehabilitation for all, especially when a joint, multi-professional approach is undertaken and implemented as a key component of an individual's support and care.

References

1. Uus K, Bamford J. Effectiveness of population-based newborn hearing screening in England: ages of interventions and profile of cases. Pediatrics. 2006;117:887–93.
2. World Health Organisation. WHO global estimates on prevalence of hearing loss. Geneva: World Health Organization; 2012.
3. Action on Hearing Loss. Facts and figures on hearing loss, deafness and tinnitus. London: Action on Hearing Loss; 2011.
4. Strydom A, Hassiotis A, Livingston G. Mental health and social care needs of older people with intellectual disabilities. J Appl Res Intellect Disabil. 2005;18:229–35.
5. Van Buggenhout GJ, Trommelen JC, Schoenmaker A, De Bal C, Verbeek JJ, Smeets DF, Ropers HH, Devriendt K, Hamel BC, Fryns JP. Down syndrome in a population of elderly mentally retarded patients: genetic-diagnostic survey and implications for medical care. Am J Med Genet. 1999;85:376–84.
6. Evenhuis HM. Medical aspects of ageing in a population with intellectual disability: II. Hearing impairment. J Intellect Disabil Res. 1995;39:27–33.
7. McShea L, Corkish C, McAnelly S. Audiology services: access, assessment and aftercare. Learn Disabil Pract. 2014;17:20–5.
8. National Institute for Health and Care Excellence (NICE). NICE guideline [NG98]. Hearing loss in adults: assessment and management. England: NICE; 2018.
9. Evenhuis HM, Theunissen M, Denkers I, Verschuure H, Kemme H. Prevalence of visual and hearing impairment in a Dutch institutionalized population with intellectual disability. J Intellect Disabil Res. 2001;45:457–64.
10. Neumann K, Dettmer G, Euler HA, Giebel A, Gross M, Herer G. Auditory status of persons with intellectual disability at the German Special Olympic Games. Int J Audiol. 2006;45:83–90.
11. Yeates S. The incidence and importance of hearing loss in people with severe learning disability: the evolution of a service. Br J Learn Disabil. 1995;23:79–84.
12. Meuwese-Jongejeugd A, Vink M, van Zanten B, Verschuure H, Eichhorn E, Koopman D, Bernsen R, Evenhuis H. Prevalence of hearing loss in 1598 adults with an intellectual disability: cross-sectional population based study. Int J Audiol. 2006;45:660–9.

13. Buchanan LH. Early onset of presbyacusis in Down Syndrome. Scand Audio. 1990;19:103–10.
14. Bent S, McShea L, Brennan S. The importance of hearing: a review of the literature on hearing loss for older people with learning disabilities. Br J Learn Disabil. 2015;43:277–84.
15. Kumar SA, Montgomery JK, Herer GR, McPherson DL. Hearing screening outcomes for persons with intellectual disability: a preliminary report of findings from the 2005 Special Olympics World Winter Games. Int J Audiol. 2008;47:399–403.
16. Hey C, Fessler S, Hafner N, Lange BP, Euler HA, Neumann K. High prevalence of hearing loss at the Special Olympics: is this representative of people with intellectual disability? J Appl Res Intellect Disabil. 2014;27:125–33.
17. Emerson E, Felce D, Stancliffe RJ. Issues concerning self-report data and population-based data sets involving people with intellectual disabilities. Intellect Dev Disabil. 2013;51:333–48.
18. Pryce H, Gooberman-Hill R. 'There's a hell of a noise': living with a hearing loss in residential care. Age Ageing. 2012;41:40–6.
19. Kiani R, Miller H. Sensory impairment and intellectual disability. Adv Psychiatr Treat. 2010;16:228–53.
20. Andersson E, Arlinger S, Magnusson L, Hamrin E. Audiometric screening of a population with intellectual disability. Int J Audiol. 2013;52:50–6.
21. Evenhuis H, van Splunder J, Vink M, Weerdenburg C, van Zanten B, Stilma J. Obstacles in large-scale epidemiological assessment of sensory impairments in a Dutch population with intellectual disabilities. J Intellect Disabil Res. 2004;48:708–18.
22. McShea L. Managing hearing loss in primary care. Learn Disabil Pract. 2015;18:18–23.
23. Learning disabilities observatory. People with learning disabilities in England 2015: main report. London: Public Health England; 2016.
24. Benova L, Grundy E, Ploubidis GB. Socioeconomic position and health-seeking behavior for hearing loss among older adults in England. J Gerontol B Psychol Sci Soc Sci. 2015;70:443–52.
25. Davis A, Smith P, Ferguson M, Stephens D, Gianopoulos I. Acceptability, benefit, and costs of early screening for hearing disability: a study of potential screening tests and models. Health Technol Assess. 2007;11:1–294.
26. Prasher VP. Screening of hearing impairment and its associated effects on adaptive behaviour in adults with down syndrome. Br J Dev Disabil. 1995;41:126–32.
27. Crandell CC, Roeser RJ. Incidence of excessive/impacted cerumen in individuals with mental retardation: a longitudinal investigation. Am J Ment Retard. 1993;97:568–74.
28. Smith WK, Mair R, Marshall L, Bilous S, Birchall MA. Assessment of hearing in persons with learning disabilities: the Phoenix NHS Trust, January 1997 to September 1998. J Laryngol Otol. 2000;114:940–3.
29. Fransman D. Can removal of back teeth contribute to chronic earwax obstruction. Br J Learn Disabil. 2006;34:36–41.
30. Sacks B, Wood A. Hearing disorders in children with Down syndrome. Down Syndrome News and Update. 2003;3:38–41.
31. Zigman WB. Atypical aging in Down syndrome. Dev Disabil Res Rev. 2013;18:51–67.
32. Pikora TJ, Bourke J, Bathgate K, Foley KR, Lennox N, Leonard H. Health conditions and their impact among adolescents and young adults with down syndrome. PLoS One. 2014;9:e96868.
33. Yeates S. Hearing impairment. In: Prasher V, Janicki M, editors. Physical health of adults with intellectual disabilities. 1st ed. Oxford: Blackwell; 2002. p. 111–32.
34. Admiraal RJ, Huygen PL. Causes of hearing impairment in deaf pupils with a mental handicap. Int J Pediatr Otorhinolaryngol. 1999;51:101–8.
35. Savarimuthu D, Bunnell T. The effects of music on clients with learning disabilities: a literature review. Complement Ther Nurs Midwifery. 2002;8:160–5.
36. Pagliano P. The multisensory handbook: a guide for children and adults with sensory learning disabilities. Milton Park, UK: Routledge; 2012.
37. Emerson E. Challenging behaviour: analysis and intervention in people with learning disabilities. Cambridge: Cambridge University Press; 1995.

38. Timehin C, Timehin E. Prevalence of hearing impairment in a community population of adults with learning disability: access to audiology and impact on behaviour. Br J Learn Disabil. 2004;32:128–32.
39. Sutton K, Thurman S. Challenging communication: people with learning disabilities who challenge services. Int J Lang Commun Disord. 1998;33(Suppl):415–20.
40. Kevan F. Challenging behaviour and communication difficulties. Br J Learn Disabil. 2003;31:71–80.
41. Miller H, Kiani R. Inter-relationships between hearing impairment, learning disability services and mental health: are learning disability services "deaf" to hearing impairments? Adv Ment Health Learn Disabil. 2008;2:25–30.
42. Carvill S. Sensory impairments, intellectual disability and psychiatry. J Intellect Disabil Res. 2001;45:467–83.
43. British Society of Audiology. Practice guidance: common principles of rehabilitation for adults in audiology services. UK: British Society of Audiology; 2016.
44. World Health Organisation. International classification of functioning, disability and health. Geneva: World Health Organization; 2001.
45. NHS England. Action plan on hearing loss. London: Department of Health; 2015.
46. Monitor. NHS adult hearing services in England: exploring how choice is working for patients. London: Monitor; 2015.
47. Krahn GL, Hammond L, Turner A. A cascade of disparities: health and health care access for people with intellectual disabilities. Ment Retard Dev Disabil Res Rev. 2006;12:70–82.
48. Meuwese-Jongejeugd A, Verschuure H, Evenhuis HM. Hearing aids: expectations and satisfaction of people with an intellectual disability, a descriptive pilot study. J Intellect Disabil Res. 2007;51:913–22.
49. Coppens-Hofman MC, Koch HH, Maassen BAM, Snik AFM. Evaluating the subjective benefit of hearing rehabilitation in adults with intellectual disability. Hear Bal Commun. 2013;11:24–9.
50. McShea L, Fulton J, Hayes C. Paid support workers for adults with intellectual disabilities; their current knowledge of hearing loss and future training needs. J Appl Res Intellect Disabil. 2016;29(5):422–32.
51. Hindhede AL. Disciplining the audiological encounter. Health Sociol Rev. 2010;19:100–13.
52. Gianopoulos I, Stephens D, Davis A. Follow up of people fitted with hearing aids after adult hearing screening: the need for support after fitting. Br Med J. 2002;325:471.
53. Kelly TB, Tolson D, Day T, McColgan G, Kroll T, Maclaren W. Older people's views on what they need to successfully adjust to life with a hearing aid. Health Soc Care Community. 2013;21:293–302.
54. Pryce H, Gooberman-Hill R. Foundations of an intervention package to improve communication in residential care settings: a mixed methods study. Hear Bal Commun. 2013;11:30–8.
55. Janicki MP. Toward a rationale strategy for promoting healthy ageing amongst people with intellectual disabilities. J Appl Res Intellect Disabil. 2001;14:171–4.
56. Newsam H, Walley RM, McKie K. Sensory impairment in adults with intellectual disabilities – an exploration of the awareness and practices of social care providers. J Policy Pract Intellect Disabil. 2010;7:211–20.
57. Ferguson MA, Brandreth M, Brassington W, Leighton P, Wharrad H. A randomized controlled trial to evaluate the benefits of a multimedia educational programme for first-time hearing aid users. Ear Hear. 2016;37:123–36.
58. McShea L. "I will make a difference" – training caregivers to improve the hearing of adults with learning disabilities. Brit J Healthc Assist. 2015;9:124–7.
59. McShea L. "I will make a difference"; using the 5As model to improve issues for adults with learning disabilities and hearing loss. In: Parsons R, editor. Learning disabilities: assessment, management and challenges. Hauppauge: Nova; 2016. p. 91–134.
60. Shames Y, Simpson J. Audiology's struggle for independence. Hear J. 2012;65:26–30.

Intellectual Disability and Epilepsy

10

Rohit Shankar, Lance Watkins, and Stephen Brown

10.1 Introduction

Epilepsy is a chronic disorder of the brain characterized by a predisposition to seizure activity, and associated with long term neurobiological, psychological, and social effects. A seizure can be defined as a transient occurrence of neurological symptoms associated with abnormal neuronal activity in the brain. The semiology of the seizure event will vary dependent upon the origin of the abnormal or excessive neuronal activity and may present with sensory, motor, emotional, or behavioral disturbance [1]. Two unproved seizures with at least a day apart were needed to diagnose epilepsy but The International League against Epilepsy (ILAE) Task Force has since refined this definition. Now clinicians are advised to consider an epilepsy diagnosis in individuals with *one* unprovoked seizure in association with other known risk factors [2].

10.2 Classification

The new Classification of the Epilepsies developed by the ILAE Commission for Classification and Terminology proposes a multilevel classification system. Clinician's should aim to make a diagnosis at all levels (dependent upon

R. Shankar (✉)
Cornwall Partnership NHS Foundation Trust, Bodmin, UK

Exeter Medical School, Truro, UK
e-mail: rohit.shankar@nhs.net

L. Watkins
Mental Health and Learning Disability Delivery Unit, Neath Port Talbot CLDT, Abertawe Bro Morgannwyg University Health Board, Swansea, Wales, UK

S. Brown
Professor (Retired) University of Plymouth Medical School, Cornwall, UK

© Springer Nature Switzerland AG 2019
V. P. Prasher, M. P. Janicki (eds.), *Physical Health of Adults with Intellectual and Developmental Disabilities*, https://doi.org/10.1007/978-3-319-90083-4_10

Table 10.1 ILAE (2017) classification of seizure types [4]

Focal Onset	Generalized onset	Unknown onset
Aware/Impaired awareness		
Motor	**Motor**	**Motor**
	Tonic-clonic Other motor (myoclonic, tonic, atonic, mixture)	Tonic-clonic Other motor (myoclonic, tonic, atonic, mixture)
Non-motor	**Non-motor** (absence)	**Unclassified**
Focal to bilateral tonic-clonic		

resources), while considering etiology of the epilepsy throughout the assessment process [3] (Table 10.1).

1. *Seizure type*—seizures are classified focal, generalized, and unknown onset.
2. *Epilepsy type*—as well as the seizure types above, good practice now considers combined generalized and focal epilepsy. Such diagnoses are likely to require investigations including characteristic findings on electroencephalogram (EEG).
3. *Epilepsy syndrome*—Cluster of symptoms including clinical history, seizure type, EEG changes, typical findings on neuroimaging (MRI), and genetic testing.

10.3 Epidemiology

The estimated prevalence of epilepsy in the general population may be anywhere between 0.6 and 1% [5]. In comparison, the prevalence of epilepsy in the intellectually disabled population ranges between 14 and 44% depending upon case ascertainment, with a proportional relationship with level of intellectual disability (Table 10.2) [6–11]. An overall prevalence of 22% has been shown based on a pooled meta-analysis of the data currently available [12].

Despite the clear relationship between epilepsy and intellectual disability understanding this association can be complex (Table 10.3). There may be a wide range of pathological processes influencing neurodevelopment at varying stages [25, 26]. This suggests multifactorial etiology which often results in multiple co-morbid conditions. People with intellectual disability and epilepsy have more physical co-morbidities than those with intellectual disability without epilepsy, which results in higher health costs and increased mortality rates [27]. Intellectual disability in combination with epilepsy significantly raises standardized mortality ratios and the highest rates of mortality are associated with a high frequency of generalized seizures and profound intellectual disability [28]. In a UK investigation seizures and epilepsy were the most frequent cause of potentially avoidable hospital admissions in people with intellectual disability, equating to 40% of all emergency admissions in adults with

Table 10.2 Prevalence of epilepsy and level of intellectual disability [12]

Mild	10%
Moderate, severe, profound	30%

Table 10.3 Epilepsy syndromes and epilepsy phenotypes associated with intellectual disability

Syndrome	Genetic abnormality	Epilepsy phenotype	Management
Dravet syndrome (severe myoclonic epilepsy)	SCN1A mutation	Febrile and non-febrile seizures in first 12 months of life Episodes of status epilepticus Intellectual decline in second year	Sodium channel blockers-Lamotrigine, phenytoin, and carbamazepine can aggravate seizures [13]
Tuberous sclerosis	TSC1, TSC2	69% epilepsy [14] Onset in infancy, 30% infantile spasms. Infantile spasms-typical hypsarrhythmia EEG pattern [15]	May respond well to Vigabatrin [16] Noval therapeutic options include mTOR inhibitors [17]
GLUT1 deficiency	SLC2A1	Seizures in first 4 months of life Dystonia-including exercise induced dyskinesia	Ketogenic diet [18]
Down syndrome	T21	Two peaks in seizure onset-first year of life after the age of 40 [19] Seizures may be associated with Alzheimer's dementia-generalized myoclonic seizures of high frequency and severity	Caution with AEDs with adverse cognitive profiles if dementia diagnosis present
Lennox-Gastaut syndrome (epileptic encephalopathy)		*Classic triad-* Seizures-multiple types, treatment resistant EEG findings-diffuse slow spike wave activity ($\leq$2.5 Hz), with fast activity during sleep ID and neuropsychiatric symptoms [20]	Rufinamide may offer most benefit [21] Lamotrigine-improved seizure control, mood, and sociability [22] Clobazam-useful adjunct [23] Topiramate-improvement in drop attacks [24]

intellectual disability [29]. Both epilepsy and intellectual disability are individually associated with psychiatric co-morbidities. In people with intellectual disability and active epilepsy there is further increased risk of mental illness [30]. The assessment of behavior and neuropsychiatric side effects in people with epilepsy and intellectual disability can be complex and require a multidisciplinary approach.

People with intellectual disability and epilepsy are more likely to experience treatment resistant seizures with up to two-thirds showing a poor response to

Table 10.4 Important aspects of Epilepsy history

Description of event—Pre-ictal, Ictal, Post-ictal (abnormal movements, abnormal tone, warning signs (aura), triggers, duration, day/nocturnal, frequency, any other events, injuries/complications—e.g., head injury, difficulty breathing.
Inter-ictal changes—mood, personality, behavior.
Past history—previous seizures/progression of epilepsy, history of febrile seizures as a child, previous history of head injury, history of significant medical conditions, genetics, family history of epilepsy or neurological disorder.

anti-epileptic medication [8]. The combination of intellectual disability, treatment resistant epilepsy, and neurological deficits is often associated with genetic abnormalities or underlying structural pathology [31]. Uncontrolled epilepsy can have serious negative consequences on both quality of life and mortality [32]. There is a limited evidence base to support the prescribing of anti-epileptic medication in this vulnerable population [33] Supporting people with intellectual disability and epilepsy especially those with poorly controlled epilepsy requires high levels of competence and confidence in staff in community settings [34].

10.4 Diagnosis

Epilepsy is primarily a clinical diagnosis and should be made by a medical practitioner with training and expertise in epilepsy. In order to establish a diagnosis of epilepsy a thorough history is required with good collateral information and witness reports of the event (Table 10.4). This is particularly important for people with intellectual disability who may have cognitive and communication deficits. It is preferable to obtain a detailed description of events including the pre-ictal, ictal, and post-ictal period. It is useful if this information is provided in a standardized way using validated seizure monitoring tools [35]. There may be benefit in video-recording events. This will require the consent of the patient, or if the individual lacks capacity a formal review should take place with all interested parties to assess whether it is in the individuals best interests.

10.5 Differential Diagnosis

There are a wide range of events that can mimic the presentation of a seizure (Table 10.5). Identifying a seizure disorder in the intellectual disabled population is further complicated by levels of cognitive impairment, communication difficulties, and associate co-morbidities. People with epilepsy and intellectual disability have higher rates of stereotyped motor behaviors often associated with neurodevelopmental disorders such as autism [36]. It has been shown that up to 25% persons with intellectual disability and epilepsy referred to a specialist center have been misdiagnosed [37].

Table 10.5 Differential diagnoses for seizures in people with intellectual disability

Cardiac—Syncope (vasovagal, orthostatic hypotension, arrhythmia)
Psychological—panic attack, dissociative disorder, psychosis, affective disorder, Non epileptic seizure
Behavioral disorder—stereotypies, sensory seeking behavior- including self-injurious behavior (SIB), compulsions
Vascular—migraine, transient ischemic attacks (TIA), transient global amnesia (TGA)
Metabolic—hypoglycemia, insulinoma, hypernatremia, hypocalcaemia
Sleep disorder—parasomnia, narcolepsy, enuresis, nightmares
Movement disorder—paroxysmal dyskinesia
Toxic state—alcohol, illicit substances, toxicity of prescribed medication

10.6 Epilepsy and Behavior

There are some key differences to be mindful of when considering the difference between a seizure and a behavioral disturbance. As a rule a seizure usually presents with similar behavior during each event. There is generally no clear precipitant and the individual will be unresponsive to attempts to communicate during the event. There is also the potential for behavioral or neuropsychiatric disturbance to occur as part of the complex epilepsy course. These symptoms may present during the peri-ictal (pre-ictal, ictal, post-ictal) or inter-ictal period. There are added complexities to consider in the pharmacological management of epilepsy including the potential neuropsychiatric effects of AEDs, and the impact of psychotropic medications on seizure control.

10.7 Investigations

A special report by the UK chapter intellectual disability working group of the ILAE has shown that people with epilepsy and intellectual disability wait longer for routine investigations including EEG and MRI brain imaging [35]. This may be a result of inequality in access to specialist care provision [34]. Services need to ensure that the reasonable adjustments required are put in place so that this vulnerable population have access to the relevant investigations required [35]. The use of video EEG alongside telemetry can be particularly helpful in differentiating seizures from other behaviors in this population. It has been shown that there is a high rate of abnormality detection on MRI brain in those individuals with intellectual disability who undergo investigation [38].

It is important to note that a normal EEG between seizures does not rule out epilepsy. The ideal scenario is to capture an event during the EEG recording. The presence of epileptiform activity on EEG is also possible in people without epilepsy, particularly people with intellectual disability [39]. MRI has essentially replaced CT as the imaging of choice for epilepsy because of its sensitivity and specificity in identifying structural lesions that could be the origin of epileptic discharges. However, MRI is not always widely available, and CT may be the most appropriate choice in an emergency. It is not uncommon for people with intellectual disability and associated co-morbidities to find it difficult to tolerate brain imaging. It may necessary to use sedation or even general anesthetic in order to complete investigations that require such an investigation in the person's best interest. If this is the case then capacity of the individual to consent must be assessed. Where the individual lacks the capacity to make an informed decision there should be a formal best interest's process as identified by the local legal processes weighing up the benefits and risks of such procedures and recorded accordingly. Electrocardiogram (ECG) and laboratory blood investigation are also an important part of the diagnosis process and will help rule out any potential other causes of events.

10.8   Treatment

A mainstay of epilepsy treatment is the prescription of AEDs. To date there is very little evidence-based research for AED prescribing in people with ID [33]. A Cochrane review into the pharmacological interventions for epilepsy in people with ID highlights the lack of evidence to support the efficacy, side-effect profile, and safety of AEDs for people with ID [40]. The treatment of epilepsy requires a person-centered approach with consideration to each stage of the ILAE classification of epilepsies [4]. This is perhaps more relevant to the ID population where there will be particular concerns over the potential cognitive and behavioral side effects of AEDs.

10.8.1 Pharmacological Management

A large proportion of people with intellectual disability and epilepsy experience a chronic refractory course, with up to 40% receiving multiple AEDs but still experiencing poor seizure control [41]. In the UK the Royal College of Psychiatrists (RCPsych) College Report CR206 (2017) is a technical paper advising on the prescription of AEDs for people with epilepsy and intellectual disability, based on current evidence. This paper explores the potential for drug interactions, AED formulation, and the management of neuropsychiatric co-morbidities. The College Report provides a simplified 'traffic light system' (first line, second line, and avoid) approach to AED prescription for people with intellectual disability.

The adverse effects of AEDs are more commonly observed when high doses are prescribed and dose titration is rapid [42]. Therefore it is recommended that AEDs are introduced at low dose and titration is slow, reducing the likelihood of dose related adverse effects. When adding a new drug it is recommended that a therapeutic dose is established before removing the old drug. This will help attribute any changes in efficacy or side effect profile more easily [43].

10.9 Lamotrigine (First Line)

Lamotrigine has been shown to be well tolerated in the intellectual disability population, with good efficacy in seizure control and improvement on a range of quality of life measures [44]. Lamotrigine is known to have mood stabilizing properties and a randomized open-label investigation not only showed improved seizure control but improvements in challenging behavior [45]. There is specific evidence to show that Lamotrigine improves seizure control and a wide range of quality of life and social measures in people with Lennox-Gastaut syndrome [46].

10.10 Sodium Valproate (First Line)

The evidence suggests that valproate is a broad spectrum treatment option that can be used for a variety of seizure types with a good safety profile [47]. It is a first-line treatment for primary generalized seizures and is recommended for use for people with treatment resistant seizures, and people with intellectual disability may be more responsive [33]. The main limitations to the widespread use of valproate are the side effect profile. Along with more common effect such as weight gain, valproate is known to have significant teratogenic effects and is therefore not recommended for women of child bearing age. This needs careful considerations in the intellectual disabled population for any women with borderline or mild intellectual disability who may be sexually active.

10.11 Topiramate (Second Line)

The efficacy of topiramate has been investigated through a number of randomized, placebo-controlled, add-on design trials. These investigations show good improvements in seizure control, however the power of the studies is too low to demonstrate statistically significant findings. Importantly no significant effect on behavior was observed [48]. There is evidence that topiramate may be effective against a wide range of seizure types, particularly dangerous atonic seizures observed in Lennox-Gastaut syndrome [49].

10.12 Levetiracetam (Second Line)

Levetiracetam appears to be generally well tolerated in the intellectual disabled population with improvement in seizure control and increased seizure freedom rates in open study designs [50]. An association between levetiracetam and neuropsychiatric side effects, particularly aggression has been observed, and these effects may be more common in people with intellectual disability [51]. As with most AEDs, the risk of neuropsychiatric side effects increases with a previous psychiatric history [52].

10.13 Carbamazepine (Second Line)

There is a very limited evidence base to support the efficacy of carbamazepine specifically in people with intellectual disability. There is evidence to suggest that slow release preparations may be better tolerated in the intellectual disabled population [53]. Carbamazepine in known to have a number of associated adverse effects including hyponatremia, sedation, dizziness, and bone marrow suppression. Carbamazepine also interacts with many other drugs which can significantly alter their efficacy and requires consideration before prescribing [43]. *Oxcarbazepine* has been investigated in on add on trial in children with good efficacy but relatively poor tolerability with the need for dose reduction or discontinuation in one fifth of cases [54].

10.14 Lacosamide (Second Line)

An open label retrospective investigation suggests that lacosamide may be a useful adjunct for people with intellectual disability and treatment resistant epilepsy. However, the evidence base is very limited and caution is therefore advised with interpretation [55].

10.15 Perampanel (Second Line)

In a multi-center retrospective case series perampanel was found to be safe and well tolerated, with good improvement in seizure control as an adjunctive agent [56]. However, there is evidence to suggest an increased risk of psychiatric side effects in people with intellectual disability. A cross sectional study identified that over half of the patients involved experience behavioral changes, most notably aggression [57]. It is therefore advise that caution is taken if prescribing for individuals with a previous history of behavioral disorder or psychiatric illness.

10.16 AEDs to Avoid

Older AEDs such as phenobarbitone and phenytoin should not be prescribed for people with intellectual disability without good reason and only if it is in that individuals best interests. Such medications are associated with significant side effect profiles including a detrimental impact upon cognition, behavioral disturbance, multiple drug interactions, and encephalopathy at toxic levels [58].

10.17 Other AEDs

Newer AEDs have little to no evidence base for prescribing for people with epilepsy and intellectual disability. AEDs such as pregabalin, brivaracetam, tiagabine, and zonisamide may be used more routinely in clinical practice as second/third/fourth line agents for treatment resistant seizures. However, efficacy, safety and tolerability have yet to be rigorously assessed in this population.

The UK Ep intellectual disabilities—research Register is a National Institute of Health Research adopted project undertaking a retrospective cohort study of real world outcomes, including tolerability and efficacy of AEDs in people with epilepsy and intellectual disability [33]. A recent investigation into perampanel by the Register has highlighted that people with moderate to profound intellectual disability are less likely to drop out- possibly due to their inability to report or communicate subjective side effects. This lower dropout rate was associated with higher rates of seizure improvement due to higher rates of retention and compliance [56]. Health care professionals have a role in educating patients, caregivers and families to understand epilepsy, the rationale for treatment, reduce stigma, and developing positive relationships. People with intellectual disability and their caregivers may not understand the importance of adhering to a treatment regime. A simple regime, the use of pictures and close liaison with the pharmacist all help. The use of pictures to communicate with people with intellectual disability can help such as the Books beyond words series [59].

10.18   Non-Pharmacological Interventions

10.18.1   Epilepsy Surgery

Intellectual disability is not, and should not be considered a contraindication for resective surgery [60]. In fact there is evidence to demonstrate that surgical intervention can improve both the behavioral and cognitive functioning of some people with epilepsy and ID [61]. For people with intellectual disability and treatment resistant epilepsy surgical intervention has been associated with improvement in seizure freedom compared to medical treatment, alongside improved quality of life measures [62].

10.18.2   Vagus Nerve Stimulation

Vagus nerve stimulation is indicated for use as an adjunctive therapy and can reduce the frequency of seizures in adults who remain refractory with AED treatment, and are not suitable for resective surgery [63]. Vagus nerve stimulation is a relatively safe surgical intervention for patients with intellectual disability [64]. There are some important short and long-term effects of vagus nerve stimulation to consider including the potential for impact upon normal cardiac conduction [65].

10.18.3   Ketogenic Diet

A Ketogenic diet is essentially high in fat and low in carbohydrates. There is evidence to support its efficacy in improving seizure control, specifically in Dravet syndrome and Glut1 deficiency [66]. However, a Cochrane review of non-pharmacological interventions for adults with epilepsy and intellectual disability shows the lack of evidence available in this population. One of the main drawbacks of the diet is its tolerability [67].

10.19 Risk Management

The risks associated with epilepsy can be complex and wide ranging. We have to consider the impact of seizures themselves upon mortality, injury, and hospitalization. We also have to appreciate the wider impact of a chronic epilepsy course upon psychological, emotional, and social functioning. The approach to risk assessment and management should be person centered and evidence based. This will usually involve assessing the patient's level of risk and depends on the individual, their environment, frequency and severity of epilepsy. There are certain risks that are increased with people with intellectual disability and it is important that healthcare professionals are aware of these higher risks and discuss them with the individual, their families and/or caregivers. Any assessment should also include a basic analysis of risk associated with bathing and showering, preparing food, using electrical equipment, managing prolonged or serial seizures, the impact of epilepsy in social settings, and the suitability of independent living [68, 69].

10.20 Sudden Unexpected Death in Epilepsy (SUDEP)

Sudden Unexpected Death in Epilepsy is the sudden and unexpected death of a person with epilepsy when no identifiable cause of death is made following post-mortem examination and toxicology [70]. The diagnosis of SUDEP is not straightforward and is essentially one of exclusion. The classification of SUDEP has more recently been further refined [71]. The incidence of sudden death appears to be 20 times higher in patients with epilepsy compared to the general population, and SUDEP is the most common cause of epilepsy related death [72]. The risk of SUDEP is increased for people with intellectual disability and treatment resistant epilepsy [73]. The UK NICE Clinical guidelines on the epilepsies [60] recommend that patient's, caregivers and families need to be counselled using information tailored to the patient's relative risk of SUDEP. The SUDEP and Seizure Safety Checklist is an evidence based tool that can be used to both assess and communicate risk with patient, their families and caregivers [72]. Effectively assessing and managing risk factors using a person centered approach can reduce the number of epilepsy relate deaths in people with intellectual disability (Table 10.6) [74–76].

Table 10.6   Desirable standards of care in the management of SUDEP [77]

- Seizure frequency: maximize seizure control (GTC and nocturnal seizures) with pharmacological and non-pharmacological treatment. <u>Aim for less than 3 seizures pre year.</u>
- Collateral risk: Work collaboratively with patient, families, and caregivers to deliver person centered risk reduction. Including advocating nocturnal supervision where indicated.
- Access to care: Ensure equitable access to specialist review and reasonable adjustments for people with intellectual disability.
- Comorbidities: Detailed assessment of physical and psychological co-morbidities including genetic testing, and liaison with relevant specialists.

10.21   Status Epilepticus

People with intellectual disability are more likely to experience status epilepticus and associated mortality rates are higher [78]. Status epilepticus is an emergency and may warrant the prescription of a rescue medication protocol to reduce the risk of potential harmful effects. Treatment should be given if the individual has a prolonged convulsive seizure that lasts for 5 min or more or if seizure occurs 3 or more times in an hour [60]. Rescue protocols can and should be adapted to ensure they are tailored specifically to an individual's needs and identified risks. Standardized guidelines on training standards and practice are available from the Joint Epilepsy Council of the United Kingdom and Ireland. Any rescue medication must be administered by an appropriately trained person. Training should include an overview of epilepsy and associated risk factors in order to help ensure safe administration of rescue medication by family members or care staff. Treatment options available in the community include buccal midazolam (first-line treatment) and rectal diazepam (if midazolam is not suitable).

Benzodiazepines can be used as both rescue medication and as an effective add-on treatment in refractory epilepsy. Clobazam in particular is recognized as being especially useful as intermittent rescue treatment, often used to manage cluster seizures. Clobazam is considered appropriate to use regularly as second line or adjunct therapy for all major seizure types. A major concern is the development of tolerance, however around 30% of people with epilepsy prescribed clobazam could continue without experiencing long-term tolerance [33].

10.22   Conclusion

The management of epilepsy in people with intellectual disability is complex, not least owing to the level of cognitive impairment and communication difficulties. Adults with intellectual disability are more likely to have treatment resistant epilepsy and multiple associated co-morbidities. Each case requires a person centered approach considering all aspects of epilepsy including seizures themselves, risk assessment, and the psychological and social impact of a multifactorial chronic disorder. The UK RCPsych has published two recent college reports detailing delivery of epilepsy care [79] and the approach to prescribing [43] for people with intellectual disability.

The delivery of epilepsy care to people with intellectual disability has been shown to be fragmented and at times inadequate due to inequalities in access to specialist care [34]. There is a need for improved collaboration between all professional bodies involved in the delivery of care to this population, with improvement in standards of assessment, information gathering, and the education and training of healthcare staff, families or caregivers [35].

References

1. Fisher RS, Boas WVE, Blume W, Elger C, Genton P, Lee P, Engel J. Epileptic seizures and epilepsy: definitions proposed by the International League Against Epilepsy (ILAE) and the International Bureau for Epilepsy (IBE). Epilepsia. 2005;46:470–2.
2. Fisher RS, Acevedo C, Arzimanoglou A, Bogacz A, Cross JH, Elger CE, Engel J, Forsgren L, French JA, Glynn M, Hesdorffer DC. ILAE official report: a practical clinical definition of epilepsy. Epilepsia. 2014;55:475–82.
3. Scheffer IE, Berkovic S, Capovilla G, Connolly MB, French J, Guilhoto L, Hirsch E, Jain S, Mathern GW, Moshé SL, Nordli DR. ILAE classification of the epilepsies: position paper of the ILAE commission for classification and terminology. Epilepsia. 2017;58:512–21.
4. Fisher RS, Cross JH, French JA, Higurashi N, Hirsch E, Jansen FE, Lagae L, Moshé SL, Peltola J, Roulet Perez E, Scheffer IE. Operational classification of seizure types by the International league against epilepsy: position paper of the ILAE commission for classification and terminology. Epilepsia. 2017;58:522–30.
5. De Boer HM, Mula M, Sander JW. The global burden and stigma of epilepsy. Epilepsy Behav. 2008;12:540–6.
6. Mariani E, Ferini-Strambi L, Sala M, Erminio C, Smirne S. Epilepsy in institutionalized patients with encephalopathy: Clinical aspects and nosological considerations. Am J Ment Retard. 1993;98(Suppl):27–33.
7. Matthews T, Weston N, Baxter H, Felce D, Kerr M. A general practice-based prevalence study of epilepsy among adults with intellectual disabilities and of its association with psychiatric disorder, behaviour disturbance and carer stress. J Intellect Disabil Res. 2008;52:163–73.
8. McGrother CW, Bhaumik S, Thorp CF, Hauck A, Branford D, Watson JM. Epilepsy in adults with intellectual disabilities: prevalence, associations and service implications. Seizure. 2006;15:376–86.
9. Morgan CL, Baxter H, Kerr MP. Prevalence of epilepsy and associated health service utilization and mortality among patients with intellectual disability. Am J Ment Retard. 2003;108:293–300.
10. Richardson SA, Koller H, Katz M, McLaren J. A functional classification of seizures and its distribution in a mentally retarded population. Am J Ment Defic. 1981;85:457–66.
11. Steffenburg U, Hagberg G, Kyllerman M. Active epilepsy in mentally retarded children. II. Etiology and reduced pre–and perinatal optimality. Acta Paediatr. 1995;84:1153–9.
12. Robertson J, Hatton C, Emerson E, Baines S. Prevalence of epilepsy among people with intellectual disabilities: a systematic review. Seizure. 2015a;29:46–62.
13. Guerrini R, Dravet C, Genton P, Belmonte A, Kaminska A. Lamotrigine and seizure aggravation in severe myoclonic epilepsy. Epilepsia. 1998;39:508–12.

14. Webb DW, Fryer AE, Osborne JP. On the incidence of fits and mental retardation in tuberous sclerosis. J Med Genet. 1991;28:395–7.
15. Saxena A, Sampson JR. Epilepsy in tuberous sclerosis: phenotypes, mechanisms, and treatments. In: Seminars in neurology, vol. 35. Germany: Thieme Medical Publishers; 2015. p. 269–76.
16. Curatolo P, Verdecchia M, Bombardieri R. Tuberous sclerosis complex: a review of neurological aspects. Eur J Paediatr Neurol. 2002;6:15–23.
17. Curatolo P, Bjørnvold M, Dill PE, Ferreira JC, Feucht M, Hertzberg C, Jansen A, Jóźwiak S, Kingswood JC, Kotulska K, Macaya A. The role of mTOR inhibitors in the treatment of patients with tuberous sclerosis complex: evidence-based and expert opinions. Drugs. 2016;76:551–65.
18. Klepper J, Scheffer H, Leiendecker B, Gertsen E, Binder S, Leferink M, Hertzberg C, Näke A, Voit T, Willemsen MA. Seizure control and acceptance of the ketogenic diet in GLUT1 deficiency syndrome: a 2-to 5-year follow-up of 15 children enrolled prospectively. Neuropediatrics. 2005;36:302–8.
19. Pueschel SM, Louis S, McKnight P. Seizure disorders in Down syndrome. Arch Neurol. 1991;48:318–20.
20. Berg AT, Berkovic SF, Brodie MJ, Buchhalter J, Cross JH, van Emde Boas W, Engel J, French J, Glauser TA, Mathern GW, Moshé SL. Revised terminology and concepts for organization of seizures and epilepsies: report of the ILAE Commission on Classification and Terminology, 2005–2009. Epilepsia. 2010;51:676–85.
21. Besag FM. Rufinamide for the treatment of Lennox–Gastaut syndrome. Expert Opin Pharmacother. 2011;12:801–6.
22. Motte J, Trevathan E, Arvidsson JF, Barrera MN, Mullens EL, Manasco P. Lamotrigine for generalized seizures associated with the Lennox-Gastaut syndrome. Lamictal Lennox-Gastaut Study Group. N Engl J Med. 1997;18:1807–12.
23. Ng YT, Conry JA, Drummond R, Stolle J, Weinberg MA. Randomized, phase III study results of clobazam in Lennox-Gastaut syndrome. Neurology. 2011;77:1473–81.
24. Sachdeo RC, Glauser TA, Ritter FO, Reife R, Lim P, Pledger G, Topiramate YL Study Group. A double-blind, randomized trial of topiramate in Lennox–Gastaut syndrome. Neurology. 1999;52:1882.
25. Bowley C, Kerr M. Epilepsy and intellectual disability. J Intellect Disabil Res. 2000;44:529–43.
26. Lhatoo SD, Sander JWAS. The epidemiology of epilepsy and learning disability. Epilepsia. 2001;42(s1):6–9.
27. Robertson J, Baines S, Emerson E, Hatton C. Service responses to people with intellectual disabilities and epilepsy: a systematic review. J Appl Res Intellect Disabil. 2015b;30:1–32.
28. Forsgren L, Edvinsson SO, Nyström L, Blomquist HK. Influence of epilepsy on mortality in mental retardation: an epidemiologic study. Epilepsia. 1996;37:956–63.
29. Glover G, Evison F. Hospital admissions that should not happen. Lancaster: Improving Health and Lives: Learning Disabilities Observatory; 2013.
30. Turky A, Felce D, Jones G, Kerr M. A prospective case control study of psychiatric disorders in adults with epilepsy and intellectual disability. Epilepsia. 2011;52:1223–30.
31. Busch RM, Najm I, Hermann BP, Eng C. Genetics of cognition in epilepsy. Epilepsy Behav. 2014;41:297–306.
32. Kerr M, Bowley C. Evidence-based prescribing in adults with learning disability and epilepsy. Epilepsia. 2001;42(s1):44–5.
33. Doran Z, Shankar R, Keezer MR, Dale C, McLean B, Kerr MP, Devapriam J, Craig J, Sander JW. Managing anti-epileptic drug treatment in adult patients with intellectual disability: a serious conundrum. Eur J Neurol. 2016;23:1152–7.
34. Kerr M, Linehan C, Thompson R, Mula M, Gil-Nagal A, Zuberi SM, Glynn M. A White Paper on the medical and social needs of people with epilepsy and intellectual disability: the task force on intellectual disabilities and epilepsy of the international league against epilepsy. Epilepsia. 2014;55:1902–6.

35. Kerr MP, Watkins LV, Angus-Leppan H, Goodwin M, Hanson C, Roy A, Shankar R. The provision of care to adults with an intellectual disability in the UK. A Special report from the intellectual disability UK chapter ILAE. Seizure. 2018;56:41–6.
36. Paul A. Epilepsy or stereotypy? Diagnostic issues in learning disabilities. Seizure. 1997;6:111–20.
37. Donat JF, Wright FS. Episodic symptoms mistaken for seizures in the neurologically impaired child. Neurology. 1990;40:156.
38. Andrews TM, Everitt AD, Sander JWAS. A descriptive survey of long-term residents with epilepsy and intellectual disability at the Chalfont Centre: is there a relationship between maladaptive behaviour and magnetic resonance imaging findings? J Intellect Disabil Res. 1999;43:475–83.
39. Gregory RP, Oates T, Merry RTG. Electroencephalogram epileptiform abnormalities in candidates for aircrew training. Electroencephalogr Clin Neurophysiol. 1993;86: 75–7.
40. Beavis J, Kerr M, Marson AG, Dojcinov I. Pharmacological interventions for epilepsy in people witH intellectual disabilities. Cochrane Database Syst Rev. 2007a;9:CD005399.
41. Espie CA, Gillies JB, Montgomery JM. Antiepileptic polypharmacy, psychosocial behaviour and locus of control orientation among mentally handicapped adults living in the community. J Intellect Disabil Res. 1990;34:351–60.
42. Kerr MP, Mensah S, Besag F, De Toffol B, Ettinger A, Kanemoto K, Kanner A, Kemp S, Krishnamoorthy E, LaFrance WC Jr, Mula M. International consensus clinical practice statements for the treatment of neuropsychiatric conditions associated with epilepsy. Epilepsia. 2011;52:2133–8.
43. Royal College of Psychiatrists. Prescribing anti-epileptic drugs for people with epilepsy and intellectual disability, College Report CR206. In: Royal College of Psychiatrists; 2017a. https://www.rcpsych.ac.uk/files/pdfversion/CR206.pdf.
44. Buchanan N. The use of lamotrigine in juvenile myoclonic epilepsy. Seizure. 1996;5(2): 149–51.
45. Crawford P, Brown S, Kerr M, Parke Davis Clinical Trials Group. A randomized open-label study of gabapentin and lamotrigine in adults with learning disability and resistant epilepsy. Seizure. 2001;10:107–15.
46. Trevathan E, Motte J, Arvidsson J, Manasco P, Mullens L. Safety and tolerability of adjunctive Lamictal for the treatment of the Lennox-Gastaut syndrome: results of multinational, double-blind, placebo-controlled trial. Epilepsia. 1996;37(Suppl 5):S202.
47. Marson AG, Al-Kharusi AM, Alwaidh M, Appleton R, Baker GA, Chadwick DW, Cramp C, Cockerell OC, Cooper PN, Doughty J, Eaton B. The SANAD study of effectiveness of valproate, lamotrigine, or topiramate for generalised and unclassifiable epilepsy: an unblinded randomised controlled trial. Lancet. 2007;369:1016–26.
48. Kerr MP, Baker GA, Brodie MJ. A randomized, double-blind, placebo-controlled trial of topiramate in adults with epilepsy and intellectual disability: impact on seizures, severity, and quality of life. Epilepsy Behav. 2005;7:472–80.
49. Kerr MP. Topiramate: uses in people with an intellectual disability who have epilepsy. J Intellect Disabil Res. 1998;42:74–9.
50. Kelly K, Stephen LJ, Brodie MJ. Levetiracetam for people with mental retardation and refractory epilepsy. Epilepsy Behav. 2004;5:878–83.
51. Helmstaedter C, Fritz NE, Kockelmann E, Kosanetzky N, Elger CE. Positive and negative psychotropic effects of levetiracetam. Epilepsy Behav. 2008;13:535–41.
52. Mula M, Trimble MR, Sander JW. Psychiatric adverse events in patients with epilepsy and learning disabilities taking levetiracetam. Seizure. 2004;13:55–7.
53. Kaski M, Heinonen E, Sivenius J, Tuominen J, Anttila M. Treatment of epilepsy in mentally retarded patients with a slow-release carbamazine preparation. J Intellect Disabil Res. 1991;35:231–9.
54. Gaily E, Granström ML, Liukkonen E. Oxcarbazepine in the treatment of epilepsy in children and adolescents with intellectual disability. J Intellect Disabil Res. 1998;42:41–5.

55. Flores L, Kemp S, Colbeck K, Moran N, Quirk J, Ramkolea P, von Oertzen TJ, Nashef L, Richardson MP, Goulding P, Elwes R. Clinical experience with oral lacosamide as adjunctive therapy in adult patients with uncontrolled epilepsy: a multicentre study in epilepsy clinics in the United Kingdom (UK). Seizure. 2012;21:512–7.

56. Shankar R, Henley W, Wehner T, Wiggans C, McLean B, Pace A, Mohan M, Sadler M, Doran Z, Hudson S, Allard J. Perampanel in the general population and in people with intellectual disability: Differing responses. Seizure. 2017a;49:30–5.

57. Andres E, Kerling F, Hamer H, Kasper B, Winterholler M. Behavioural changes in patients with intellectual disability treated with perampanel. Acta Neurol Scand. 2017;136: 645–53.

58. Livanainen M. Phenytoin: effective but insidious therapy for epilepsy in people with intellectual disability. J Intellect Disabil Res. 1998;42:24–31.

59. Bradley E, Hollins S. Books beyond words: using pictures to communicate. J Dev Disabil. 2013;19:24–32.

60. NICE clinical guideline 137 (2012) The epilepsies: the diagnosis and management of the epilepsies in adults and children in primary and secondary care. https://www.nice.org.uk/guidance/cg137.

61. Kerr M, Linehan C, Brandt C, Kanemoto K, Kawasaki J, Sugai K, Tadokoro Y, Villanueva V, Wilmshurst J, Wilson S. Behavioral disorder in people with an intellectual disability and epilepsy: a report of the intellectual disability task force of the neuropsychiatric commission of ILAE. Epilepsia Open. 2016;1:102–11.

62. Wiebe S, Blume WT, Girvin JP, Eliasziw M. A randomized, controlled trial of surgery for temporal-lobe epilepsy. N Engl J Med. 2001;345:311–8.

63. Englot DJ, Chang EF, Auguste KI. Vagus nerve stimulation for epilepsy: a meta-analysis of efficacy and predictors of response: a review. J Neurosurg. 2011;115:1248–55.

64. Prasher VP, Kerr M. Epilepsy and intellectual disabilities. 2nd ed. Cham: Springer; 2016.

65. Shankar R, Olotu VO, Cole N, Sullivan H, Jory C. Case report: vagal nerve stimulation and late onset asystole. Seizure. 2013a;22:312–4.

66. Hee Seo J, Mock Lee Y, Soo Lee J, Chul Kang H, Dong Kim H. Efficacy and tolerability of the ketogenic diet according to lipid: nonlipid ratios—comparison of 3: 1 with 4: 1 diet. Epilepsia. 2007;48:801–5.

67. Beavis J, Kerr M, Marson AG, Dojcinov I. Non-pharmacological intervention for epilepsy in people with intellectual disabilities. Cochrane Database Syst Rev. 2007b;9:CD005502.

68. Besag FM. Lesson of the week: tonic seizures are a particular risk factor for drowning in people with epilepsy. BMJ. 2001;322(7292):975.

69. Forjuoh SN, Guyer B. Injury prevention in people with disabilities: Risks can be minimised without unduly restricting activities. Br Med J. 2001;322:940–1.

70. Nashef L. Sudden unexpected death in epilepsy: terminology and definitions. Epilepsia. 1997;38(s11):S6–8. https://doi.org/10.1111/j.1528-1157.1997.tb06130.x.

71. Nashef L, So EL, Ryvlin P, Tomson T. Unifying the definitions of sudden unexpected death in epilepsy. Epilepsia. 2012;53:227–33.

72. Shankar R, Cox D, Jalihal V, Brown S, Hanna J, McLean B. Sudden unexpected death in epilepsy (SUDEP): development of a safety checklist. Seizure. 2013b;22:812–7.

73. Hesdorffer DC, Tomson T, Benn E, Sander JW, Nilsson L, Langan Y, Walczak TS, Beghi E, Brodie MJ, Hauser A. Combined analysis of risk factors for SUDEP. Epilepsia. 2011;52: 1150–9.

74. Shankar R, Jalihal V, Walker M, Laugharne R, McLean B, Carlyon E, Hanna J, Brown S, Jory C, Tripp M, Pace A. A community study in Cornwall UK of sudden unexpected death in epilepsy (SUDEP) in a 9-year population sample. Seizure. 2014;23:382–5.

75. Shankar R, Walker M, McLean B, Laugharne R, Ferrand F, Hanna J, Newman C. Steps to prevent SUDEP: the validity of risk factors in the SUDEP and seizure safety checklist: a case control study. J Neurol. 2016;263:1840–6.

76. Shankar R, Donner EJ, McLean B, Nashef L, Tomson T. Sudden unexpected death in epilepsy (SUDEP): what every neurologist should know. Epileptic Disord. 2017b;19:1–9.

77. Watkins L, Shankar R, Sander JW. Identifying and mitigating Sudden Unexpected Death in Epilepsy (SUDEP) risk factors. Expert Rev Neurother. 2018;18:265–74.
78. Pellock JM, Morton LD. Treatment of epilepsy in the multiply handicapped. Dev Disabil Res Rev. 2000;6:309–23.
79. Royal College of Psychiatrists. The management of epilepsy in adults with intellectual disability, College Report CR203. In: Royal College of Psychiatrists; 2017b. https://www.rcpsych. ac.uk/files/pdfversion/CR203.pdf.

Endocrinological Issues

11

Aidan McElduff and Neha Bansal

11.1 Introduction

Endocrinology is the study of one of the two systems which integrate function in complex organisms, including humans. The other is the nervous system. The endocrine system is characterized by special chemical mediators, classically called hormones, which are involved in every facet of human well-being including reproduction, growth and development, the maintenance of the internal milieu, and the utilization and storage of energy. These hormones can also affect brain function and behaviour, with some effects being temporary and others being permanent. Co-ordination of the endocrine system is controlled within the brain, particularly in the hypothalamus and surrounding areas. The system is complex and easily disrupted.

In times of stress and/or illness there are adaptive mechanisms which are beneficial in the short term but detrimental if they continue in the long term. Reproductive function and growth can be affected in this way. In times of stress it could be considered that the body does not want to waste resources on reproduction and/or growth, but rather conserve resources to deal with the immediate crises. At such times reproductive function is shut down and growth is inhibited. The relationship between life-stresses, such as examinations and amenorrhea in young, otherwise healthy women, is well known. Similarly, stress or disturbances of physical or emotional wellbeing have been identified as contributors to other disease states, including the insulin resistance syndrome, obesity, dyslipidemia, glucose intolerance, diabetes, and hypertension [1].

Given this, it is likely adults with intellectual disability, particularly those with dysfunctions involving the brain and/or multiple organs, will have some form of

A. McElduff (✉)
Discipline of Medicine, University of Sydney, Camperdown, NSW, Australia

N. Bansal
Greenfields, Birmingham Community NHS Trust, Birmingham, UK

© Springer Nature Switzerland AG 2019
V. P. Prasher, M. P. Janicki (eds.), *Physical Health of Adults with Intellectual and Developmental Disabilities*, https://doi.org/10.1007/978-3-319-90083-4_11

endocrine system disturbance to a greater or lesser extent. Endocrine disorders, which can result from the failure of the normal integration of complex physiological processes, include growth failure, hypogonadism, obesity and its complications, and/or osteoporosis.

11.2   Clinical Issues

Clinical endocrinology involves the study of the problems which result from disruption of the hormonal system (see Tables 11.1 and 11.2) either through deficient or excess biological activity. Endocrine disorders are common in the general population and one would predict they are very common in adults with intellectual disability [2]. There are also other reasons for a more likely occurrence. Firstly, endocrine disease can be an integral part of the syndrome responsible for the intellectual disability (syndrome-specific), either causally (e.g., congenital hypothyroidism) or a constant association (e.g., obesity in Prader-Willi syndrome). Secondly, endocrine disease may be more common in particular syndromes (e.g., hypothyroidism and diabetes in Down syndrome).

Table 11.1 Pituitary hormones

Hormone	Function
Adrenocorticotropic hormone	Controls adrenal glands
Thyroid stimulating hormone	Controls thyroid gland
Luteinizing hormone Follicle-stimulating hormone	Act in concert to control the gonads
Growth hormone	Growth via insulin-like growth factor (predominantly produced in the liver)
Prolactin	Breast milk production
Anti-diuretic hormone	Controls fluid status by inhibiting excess water loss from the kidneys

Table 11.2 Various hormones and their function

Gland	Hormone (S)	Function
Thyroid	Thyroxin Tri-iodothyronine	Widespread actions on multiple tissues
Adrenal	Cortisol Aldosterone Androgens	Stress responses Fluid and electrolyte balance ? Female libido
Testis Ovary (Gonad)	Testosterone Estrogens and Progesterone	Maleness Femaleness
Pancreas[a]	Insulin and others	Energy balance
Skin	Vitamin D then activated metabolites	Calcium and bone Homeostasis

[a]The islet of cells in the pancreas, which are the endocrine component of the pancreas secrete other hormones including glucagon, somatostatin, gastrin

11.3   Lifelong Care and Appropriate Stepping (Mile) Stones

A premise of this chapter is the role of the endocrine system in the integration of the human body. As we grow to maturity each milestone of development is used as a stepping-stone for the next stage of development. An error or fault in this process may have long lasting consequences that can never be fully corrected. In the usual course of events, growth and development leading to peak maturity is followed by early adult life with optimal health and then gradual, but inevitable decline, as one grows older. We are all aware that the decline can be accelerated by an unhealthy lifestyle.

Additional factors, which compound this decline or abnormal ageing, are the effects of age-related diseases. These also include the effects of disability/disabilities in adults with intellectual disability as such effects will be compounded over time, particularly if they are present from birth and thus during development. They will inevitably limit the attainment of peak potential and/or accelerate decline. Thus, every effort should be made to minimize the adverse consequences of the condition. Energy should be invested in optimizing the initial growth in an attempt to have adults reach their maximal potential even if this is restricted by the underlying developmental problems. This lifelong or lifespan approach, is recommended by the World Health Organization [3, 4]. Recommendation 2 of the WHO report on physical health issues states:

> "Health care providers caring for people with intellectual disability of all ages should adopt a life span approach that recognizes the progression of consequences of specific diseases and therapeutic interventions".

11.4   Risk Factors for Endocrine Problems

Several of the "disease" processes affecting people with intellectual disability may be the same as those affecting the general population although they may have a different spectrum of causes within a multifactorial etiology. Some of these contributing factors could be regarded as iatrogenic. Perhaps the simplest example of this concept is obesity. Basically, obesity relates to the imbalance between our energy intake (i.e., eating) and our energy output (i.e., activity). There are individual variations in the efficiency of this relationship, but overall an imbalance with more intake than output will result in weight gain. One hypothesis is that the people with intellectual disability are more prone to habitual overeating for complex societal reasons. On the other side of the energy balance, they are also likely to be under- active simply because of problems with motor activity, or more subtly, because of a cautious or neglectful approach by caregivers to their participation in physical activities. Thus, while the basic reasons for obesity are the same as the general population, that is, an imbalance between energy intake and energy output, the reasons for this imbalance may relate to the nature of the person's disability and/or the societal response to that disability.

Another example can be found in the use of some types of anticonvulsants. In individuals with restricted or limited access to sunlight the use of anticonvulsants can lead to Vitamin D deficiency. Anticonvulsant use is common in patients with intellectual disability and some more severely affected, immobile sub-groups may have restricted access to sunlight. Unless this potential problem is recognised, the long-term skeletal consequences of Vitamin D deficiency will occur in adults receiving some types of anticonvulsants (particularly phenytoin).

Finally, there is the difficult issue of pubertal development. In some children with intellectual disability, pubertal development will not occur. The reasons for this are varied and include: insidious undernutrition; diffuse non-specific damage to the hypothalamus resulting in secondary hypogonadism; a generalized non-specific abnormality relating to the stress of the illness; or a syndromic association (e.g., Turner's syndrome). Whatever the reasons, when puberty fails to occur in a child already diagnosed as having an intellectual disability, it is frequently not regarded as a problem, but may be seen as a blessing by some parents. In the general population, failure to undergo puberty is recognized as a reason to seek medical help. This does not happen in people with intellectual disability. For a number of reasons, this is a complex area. Some of the fears of pubertal development among adolescents with intellectual disability are more fanciful rather than factual. There may also be major consequences of failure of pubertal development, including lack of appropriate growth and development and lack of the normal ageing process. The decision whether or not to treat the failure of normal pubertal development needs to be taken as an active process rather than allowing pubertal non-development by default. This is an issue of some import and will be discussed more fully later.

11.5   Endocrine and Related Disorders

Obesity and under-nutrition are not strictly speaking endocrine disorders. Both are often seen by endocrinologists interested in metabolic disorders to exclude unusual underlying endocrine disorders and to supervise therapy. Both are associated with a range of endocrine complications. They will be discussed briefly again here but will be reviewed in more depth in Chap. 12.

11.5.1 Obesity

Obesity is increasingly common in developed nations and is a significant public health challenge due to its serious consequences. Whilst it was once thought to be largely age-related, increasingly obesity is showing no boundaries to age, with over 170 million children worldwide reported to be overweight [5]. Similarly, in those with intellectual disability, obesity is a serious concern and those with intellectual disability have been reported to be at increased risk in several studies [6–11]. In a recent study by Emerson et al. [12], it was reported that children with intellectual disability were significantly more likely to be obese compared to non- intellectually disabled children, accounting for 5–6% of all obese children.

Although, there may be other reasons for its prevalence in the intellectually disabled population. For example, some adults with intellectual disability, particularly those with Down syndrome appear to be more at risk for obesity for reasons discussed above [13]. People with intellectual disability may also be less conscious or aware of the risks associated with obesity and in some cases the degree of intellectual disability has been associated with the level of excess body weight, with those paradoxically being of more mild intellectual disability and having more independence being more at risk of obesity. Obesity is best managed by prevention since successful long-term correction of obesity is rare in the general population. People with intellectual disability may actually be advantaged in this regard. Experience with a structured intervention programme involving an experienced dietitian and an exercise physiologist suggests that people with intellectual disability are best compared with men who have never had health care advice. Relatively simple dietary advice and an attractive, organized and supervised group exercise programme can result in significant weight loss. Support from caregivers in weight management is also vital; particularly in terms of motivation, helping to set and achieve goals, and supporting the wider multidisciplinary team in tailoring interventions to suit individual needs [14]. As in the general population, loss of weight can lead to an obvious and marked improvement in the individual's self-esteem together with an improvement in cardiovascular risk factors and other positive health benefits including mobility.

11.5.2 Under-Nutrition

Under-nutrition commonly results from simple failure to provide nutrients to persons who cannot eat without the help of others. Adults with cerebral palsy and those with severe intellectual and physical disabilities have a high incidence of dysphagia and those with cerebral palsy may have poor oral-motor function, which places them in a high-risk group for severe under-nutrition. The consequences of this on their health, including an elevated risk of osteomalacia and fragility bone fractures, have been well documented [15]. There are various conflicting theories regarding metabolic needs of those with cerebral palsy. Some have suggested that those with cerebral palsy have increased metabolic needs due to hypertonia or movement disorders; whereas others report that these individuals have decreased metabolic needs due to adaptation as a result of chronic malnutrition [16]. Whatever the aetiology, all children with cerebral palsy are at risk of malnutrition. Therefore, a proactive approach by health care professionals and caregivers alike is necessary to bring about successful nutrition interventions for those people who suffer chronic under-nutrition.

On the flip side, under-nutrition during early years of life is reported to be associated with significantly impaired IQ, which persists into adulthood [17]. In this study, previously malnourished adults were compared to controls at different time points over four decades, with a key finding that the prevalence of intellectual disability was nine times greater compared to the control group. Specific vitamin and mineral deficiencies in children and mothers, such as Iodine and Iron, and their impact on cognitive development in the fetus and child are also well documented [18].

11.5.3 Thyroid Disease

Thyroid disease can occur at any age but is more common with increasing age and is particularly common in the Down syndrome population [19]. Compared to the general population, the prevalence of certain thyroid diseases such as Hashimoto's thyroiditis and Graves' disease has been found to be significantly higher in children with Down syndrome [20]. The pathophysiological mechanisms underlying why individuals with Down syndrome are more susceptible to developing autoimmune thyroid disease is not yet fully understood.

Thyroid disease can be difficult to diagnose in any group of patients and this is particularly so in persons with intellectual disability. Often the only symptom is reported by the caregiver, usually the mother, who observes that the patient's behaviour has changed in some nonspecific way. For this reason thyroid function tests should be performed on any unusual presentation and on a routine (preferably on an annual basis) in persons at high risk, such as those with Down syndrome. The management is usually straightforward but may also involve supervision of medication.

11.5.3.1 Hypothyroidism

Primary hypothyroidism (due to thyroid failure) is easily diagnosed if thyroid function tests (TFTs) are performed. The thyroid stimulating hormone (TSH) is elevated above the normal range and the measurement of free thyroxin (T4) is low. The changes from normal are a measure of the degree of hypothyroidism. The presence of thyroid autoantibodies suggests an autoimmune etiology. Investigation of the underlying etiology beyond measuring autoantibodies is rarely warranted. Rarely TSH is elevated with high or high-normal free T4. This requires specialist referral. Thyroid hormone resistance and TSH secreting tumours can produce these unusual findings.

Secondary hypothyroidism (due to pituitary/hypothalamic disorders) can be difficult to diagnose even with TFTs. The TSH can be low, normal or paradoxically slightly elevated. Free T4 is relatively low but usually only at the lower limit of normal. Other evidence of pituitary/ hypothalamic disturbances should be present, particularly secondary hypogonadism. If secondary hypothyroidism is suspected it requires specialist referral and investigation including imaging to determine the underlying pituitary/hypothalamic disorder.

In the absence of cardiac disease, hypothyroidism can be treated with an initial dose of 1.5 µg/kg/day thyroxine. Thyroid function tests should not be repeated for at least 8 weeks. Therapy is titrated to achieve a normal TSH. The most common error is to repeat thyroid function tests at too short an interval following a dose adjustment before a new equilibrium or steady state has been established. If cardiac disease is suspected or possible, thyroxin therapy should be introduced slowly. One possible regimen is to initiate therapy with thyroxin 25 μg per day, increasing by 25 μg per day at 6–12 weekly intervals provided the patient remains asymptomatic from a cardiac point of view. If symptoms are induced, cardiac intervention (either surgical or medical) will be required.

Thyroid dysfunction in adults with Down syndrome is well recognized, however the causes are not fully understood. Iughetti et al. [21] carried out a 10-year longitudinal study of thyroid function in children with Down syndrome and found that probability of acquired thyroid dysfunction increased from 30% at birth to 49% at 10 years. This highlights the need for careful monitoring in this high-risk group of people.

Congenital hypothyroidism (CH) is the most common congenital endocrine disorder and has an association with severe cognitive impairment and intellectual disability. Several studies have shown that in those adults with Down syndrome, there is a higher prevalence of CH and in particular, Cebeci et al. [22] showed that adults with Down syndrome have high prevalence of CH associated with hypoplasia of the thyroid gland. Thyroid dysgenesis is the most frequent cause of CH. Since the introduction of neonatal screening over the last 40 years, the prevalence of intellectual disability due to CH has declined as a result of earlier detection and initiation of treatment. The mean IQ is now about 20 points higher compared to patients born before screening began [23]. However, other studies of persons born after the introduction of screening show that cognitive impairments may still persist into adulthood [23]. This emphasizes the importance of continued new born screening and subsequent regular monitoring, even if treated early.

11.5.3.2 Hyperthyroidism (Thyrotoxicosis)

Thyrotoxicosis or hyperthyroidism is easily diagnosed in most situations. Free (triiodothyronine) T3 and free T4 are elevated with a suppressed (low) TSH. Elevated free T4 or free T3 in the presence of a normal TSH level requires specialist investigation as mentioned previously. TSH suppression should be in proportion to the elevation in the free T3 and free T4. The underlying cause of the hyperthyroidism must be identified. This may involve performing a thyroid scan and possibly measuring anti-TSH receptor antibodies.

There are some cases described where there have been reports of simultaneous onset of type 1diabetes mellitus and hyperthyroidism in children with Down syndrome, which was detected with TSH, positive anti-thyroid antibodies and an increase in thyroid gland size on ultrasound. This shows the importance of monitoring thyroid function in these patients, even if there are no apparent clinical symptoms [24].

The long-term treatment of hyperthyroidism will depend on the underlying etiology. Initial treatment of most thyrotoxicosis (i.e., Graves' disease or toxic nodular disease) consists of oral antithyroid medication (e.g., carbimazole. Propylthiouracil is no longer recommended for routine use due to rare but fatal liver failure). Thyrotoxicosis due to thyroiditis can be managed symptomatically with beta-blockers until the thyroiditis settles usually spontaneously. Antithyroid medications are ineffective in this situation. The dose of antithyroid medication is adjusted as the patient responds. This can be difficult under ideal circumstances. Compliance is an important issue as non-compliance can confuse dose titration. The initial dose of antithyroid medication is in proportion to the severity of the disease. A clinical response should become apparent within a few weeks. It is recommended to repeat the thyroid function tests at four weekly intervals with an appropriate dose adjustment until the tests are stable. Specialist referral should be considered particularly for more severe disease. Severe symptoms can be controlled with beta-blockers until the antithyroid medication has taken effect. Alternatively, a block and replace regimen can be utilised. This involves a dose of carbimazole which causes hypothyroidism with the introduction of thyroxine to return the TFTs to normal. This regimen also requires close supervision. Definitive therapy with radioactive iodine is a reasonable long-term option for Graves' disease, recognizing that hypothyroidism is almost inevitable. Lifelong follow up to detect hypothyroidism is mandatory after radioactive iodine treatment. Recall should be automatically initiated by the physician and not be dependent on the patient.

Thyrotoxicosis associated with multinodular thyroid disease may require investigation to exclude malignancy in one of the nodules (see below). Surgery may be preferable definitive treatment option in this situation. Malignancy is rare but not unknown in single toxic nodule. Thyroid biopsy should not be performed when the patient is thyrotoxic as the cytological findings in a toxic nodule cannot be distinguished from malignancy. Radioactive iodine should not be administered until the question of underlying malignancy has been settled.

11.5.3.3   Goiter

The discussion above has dealt with only functional thyroid disturbances. Structural problems can also arise and need not be associated with a disturbance in function. Thyroid enlargement can be generalized or nodular in nature. Thyroid nodules require investigation to exclude thyroid cancer. This involves a fine needle aspiration biopsy, which is frequently performed under ultrasound control and the biopsy sample is sent for cytological examination. A small (<1 cm) nodule found on ultrasound and impalpable on physical examination does not require a biopsy. Diffuse thyroid enlargement does not require separate investigation apart from thyroid function tests and the measurement of thyroid auto-antibodies. Thyroid auto-antibodies suggest the presence of thyroid auto-immunity and indicate a small (~2%/year) risk of hypothyroidism.

11.5.4 Diabetes

Diabetes mellitus is very common in the general population. An Australia-wide population study (AusDiab; [25]) found a prevalence of 7.5% in the adult population (age over 25). Shaw and colleagues noted that the prevalence increased dramatically with age, such that in 80-year-olds, 1 in 4 had Type 2 diabetes. One half of the individuals identified with diabetes had not been diagnosed. The prevalence is increasing in both the developed and the developing world. Lifestyle factors (such as obesity and inactivity) are believed to be responsible for this increased prevalence. Since obesity and inactivity are common in adults with intellectual disability, it seems reasonable to assume that diabetes will also be common and that at least a similar proportion goes undiagnosed. A recent Swedish register-based study found that people with intellectual disability are 20% more likely than the general population to have a diagnosis of diabetes mellitus and 26% more likely to have prescription of drugs for diabetes mellitus compared to the general population [26]. Strategies designed to prevent obesity and increase activity should reduce the frequency of diabetes. An increased awareness of this problem and routine testing of at risk sub-groups should lead to an increased rate of diagnosis and the introduction of appropriate management.

Since we now have strong Level 1 evidence that the micro and macrovascular complications of Type 2 diabetes can be reduced with appropriate early treatment, it is important that diabetes is diagnosed as early as possible. For Type 2 diabetes, which can be asymptomatic, this will require screening. The gold standard diagnostic test is the measurement of glycosylated haemoglobin, which has now been validated by WHO in [27]. Risk factors for diabetes include obesity, immobility, age and a positive family history.

A large component of the management of diabetes involves screening for the specific microvascular (i.e., retinopathy, nephropathy and neuropathy) and macrovascular (i.e., cardiac, cerebral and peripheral) complications. This may be difficult in adults with intellectual disability. Sensory neuropathy can be difficult to detect as clinical examination is subjective. Eye examination for retinopathy may require general anaesthetic. Similarly, for macrovascular disease, patients may not report symptoms and a high degree of clinical suspicion may be required to detect problems. As people with intellectual disability live to an older age, macrovascular disease will become a more common problem.

On a more positive note, experience has shown that adults with Down syndrome do not develop retinopathy at a rate expected from their degree of glycaemic control. This may be due to the fact that they almost universally have low/normal blood pressures. The United Kingdom Prospective Diabetes Study [28, 29] demonstrated that retinopathy was prevented by treatment directed toward lowering blood pressure. Thus, adults with Down syndrome and diabetes may be at less risk of retinopathy because of typically low blood pressure. This is an example of how, in some situations, specific features of people with intellectual disability may provide benefit rather than adverse effect.

The current management strategies for people with diabetes are to promote self-care and responsibility, aiming for tight glycaemic control. The risk of this strategy is hypoglycaemia with all its potentially devastating consequences. Major, potentially life threatening, hypoglycaemia is relatively common. As a general rule adults with intellectual disability are not capable of assuming appropriate self-care. This may be due to limitations in understanding of this condition, which is not helped by poor communication between health professionals and people with intellectual disability. Where patients are asymptomatic and understanding of diabetes is limited, this may contribute towards a lack of motivation and low mood due to feelings of loss of independence in making food and lifestyle choices [30]. The treatment targets for adults with intellectual disability who have diabetes will almost certainly be modified from that of the general population because of the dangers of hypoglycemia. The target for glycaemic control should be to make them feel well and free of symptoms, whereas in the general population the target is a tighter degree of glycaemic control aiming to prevent or delay the progression of diabetic complications. My own experience differs from that reported by Anwar et al. [31], who observed that adults with Down syndrome and diabetes had similar degrees of glycaemic control to the general population. However, these data may reflect poor controls from the general population. In our diabetic clinic the mean glycosylated haemoglobin in patients with Type 1 or Type 2 diabetes is less than 7.5%. Experience has shown that this is not the case in adults with diabetes and intellectual disability, most of whom have Down syndrome. In our clinic, we have accepted glycosylated haemoglobin values of 9–10% in this group (in an assay with an upper limit of normal of 6%).

Patients with type 1 or insulin-requiring diabetes are more difficult to manage than those with type 2 diabetes. Assistance with insulin administration and home glucose monitoring is almost always required. Diabetes should be treated in collaboration with a diabetic clinic. One uncommon condition which is more prone to diabetes where diabetic control is extremely difficult is Prader-Willi syndrome. The difficulties in controlling diet in this disorder is the most obvious reason for this difficulty.

Several studies [32, 33] have reported that lifestyle modification involving increased activity and diet to obtain modest weight loss (~5% of body weight) significantly reduced the occurrence of type 2 diabetes in high-risk groups. This benefit should be extended to high-risk individuals with intellectual disability. This would include individuals with obesity, inactive individuals, those with a family history of type 2 diabetes and those with any previous abnormality in glucose tolerance, including high glucose levels during an illness. Metformin therapy was also useful in preventing deterioration to diabetes in some subgroups in the DPP. Metformin's role in those high risk individuals with intellectual disability is not clear at this time.

11.5.5 Vitamin D Deficiency

Over the decade the role of Vitamin D in maintaining health has become less clear. Although low vitamin D status is associated with a variety of adverse health outcomes, However, the role of maintaining optimum serum concentration levels of Vitamin D to prevent bone disease remains clear. As people with intellectual disability may be more likely to stay indoors and therefore have insufficient exposure to sunlight, they are at risk of Vitamin D deficiency [34, 35]. Many adults with intellectual disability may also have epilepsy for which they are managed with anticonvulsant therapy, which may also put them at higher risk of developing Vitamin D deficiency. In the past, there has been controversy over the role of anticonvulsants in producing low Vitamin D levels and subsequently osteoporosis [36]. In more recent studies, similar results have been reported ([37–39] [40];) and as a result, prophylactic administration of vitamin D and Calcium supplements have been recommended for adults taking anticonvulsants. In people who receive low sun exposure, some anticonvulsant therapy increases the risk of becoming vitamin D deficient in the absence of supplementation. Vitamin D status is best reflected by the measurement of 25 Hydroxy Vitamin D. This should be measured annually at the end of winter.

11.5.6 Hypogonadism

There are various definitions of hypogonadism. The gonad (testis or ovary) has two separate but interlinked functions: gamete production and sex hormone production. In males the testis constantly produce sperm, while in females the ovary releases eggs which have been present since embryological ovarian formation. Sperm production requires adequate levels of testosterone. A man may produce normal levels of testosterone but have abnormal or sub-normal sperm production. Testicular volume is an acceptable surrogate for the sperm producing function of the testis because most of the volume of the testis is made up of sperm producing cells. A small volume testis is very likely to have impaired sperm production, although the reverse is not true (i.e., there is no guarantee that a normal testis has normal sperm production). The normal adult testis is 24 +/− 4 ml in volume (mean +/− SD) [41]. Testes greater than 15 ml in volume are usually considered normal. Testicular volume should be measured by comparison to an orchidometer.

The normal pre-menopausal ovary contains eggs and a woman is not regarded as hypogonadal unless the ovary contains no eggs. Thus a woman who does not have regular menstruation in the presence of ovaries which contain eggs is only considered hypogonadal if the circulating estradiol level is low. Hypogonadism in a premenopausal woman is usually secondary to low gonadotrophins due to a disturbance in the hypothalamic/pituitary region of the brain. This is often precipitated by under-nutrition. Thus, hypogonadism can be defined in relationship to gamete production/presence, sex hormone production, or the combination of both. The broader definition of hypogonadism, including impairment in either function, is adopted in this discussion unless otherwise stated.

Hypogonadism is particularly common in adults with intellectual disability and management of the condition is fraught with difficulty on a number of levels [42] Among some parents, there is often spoken joy at the gentle, childlike qualities of the hypogonadal (no sex hormone production) adult male because there is an underlying fear that testosterone at puberty will be associated with aggressiveness. Among parents the fear for adult women is that menstruation will be difficult to manage and the risk of pregnancy is often an unspoken concern. However, the risk of pregnancy is very low if gonadal function is impaired enough to require sex hormone replacement therapy. Hormone replacement therapy in this situation can be tailored in both men and women to provide contraception if fertility is an issue. Infertility has no direct medical consequences.

Hypogonadism (no sex hormone production) does have destructive medical consequences not the least of which are an increased risk of osteoporosis and probably obesity. The decision not to treat is usually made passively rather than actively discussed. Any decision to provide a different standard of care than in the general population should be explicitly communicated to family and caregivers and clearly documented.

The possibility of hypogonadism should be considered if physical changes of puberty are not clearly evident by the age of 14–16 years. The threshold for girls should be towards the lower end of this range and for boys towards the upper end. The possibility of pubertal delay can be confirmed by a combination of physical examination and special investigations including measuring of luteinising hormone, follicle stimulating hormone and the specific gonadal steroid, either testosterone or estradiol. This assessment should be made by a specialist. In some circumstances gonadal failure is inevitable (e.g., Turner's syndrome) and is something that should be anticipated and planned.

As noted above, the testes fulfil two functions. The majority of the volume of the testes is composed of sperm producing cells. A man with small testes will not necessarily have decreased circulating testosterone, whereas all males with small testes will have at a minimum, impaired sperm production. This latter abnormality will not require treatment if fertility is not desired and should be thought of separately from a deficiency in androgen production.

11.5.7 Cryptorchidism

Cryptorchidism (or undescended testes or testes not in the scrotum) is one of the most common congenital abnormalities in male infants, affecting about 6% of full term male newborns [43]. It is also more common in hypogonadal males. Cryptorchidism carries a3–4 times increased lifetime risk of testicular cancer. This risk is further increased in certain chromosomal disorders [44] and possibly in Down syndrome [45]. Previous studies have also suggested that there is a high prevalence of cryptorchidism in individuals with profound and severe intellectual disability, and particularly in those having cerebral palsy [46, 47]. In clinical practice, if two testes are not identified, a search for the undescended testes should be undertaken. Given the late identification of undescended testes in males with intellectually disabilities as reported in Haire's study [47], routine screening and regular monitoring has been suggested. Ultrasound examination is probably the first step in most individuals if on clinical examination there is no evidence of testes. In adults, intra-abdominal testes are usually removed and at the very least should be brought into the scrotum to allow routine regular surveillance. Testicular examination should be part of routine physical examination in adults with intellectual disability as they may be at increased risk of a relatively common cancer and are unlikely to perform self-examination. Men, particularly those over 50 years of age, receiving testosterone therapy require assessment for prostatic cancer.

11.5.8 Menopause

The other aspect of hypogonadism is the natural hypogonadism which occurs in women at the time of the menopause. In the general population there is vigorous discussion about the need to treat all post-menopausal women with hormone replacement therapy (HRT). There is a general consensus that younger women with ovarian failure do require therapy. There are clear cut benefits of HRT in the prevention or minimization of post-menopausal symptoms and in the prevention of osteoporosis. Many women have no or few symptoms and many will not develop osteoporosis, although our ability to predict who is at risk has not yet been perfected. On this basis, not all women will require treatment. There are side effects of HRT; the biggest fears are breast cancer, (uterine cancer if progesterone is not included in the HRT regimen) and venous thrombosis. Is HRT warranted in post-menopausal women with intellectual disability? As in the general population, this decision must be individualized. Either a plethora of symptoms, which might not be spontaneously reported, would tend to push the decision towards administration of HRT at least for a relatively short time period. If that decision is made, then careful monitoring is required. People with intellectual disability have been found to have generally lower levels of knowledge and understanding of menopause in relation to what it is, when it happens and what it means for their physical and mental health [48]. It is therefore important to monitor and be vigilant of any symptoms and try to explain in terms that are best understood in order to encourage patient autonomy. There are also studies which report that the age of onset of menopause is lower in females with Down syndrome compared to those without Down syndrome [49, 50]. As a result, these individuals are at an increased risk for post-menopausal health disorders such as osteoporosis.

There is increasing evidence that continuous HRT in women five years or more past the menopause is effective. In the immediate post-menopause, cyclic therapy is more appropriate. In the immediate post-menopause, therapy could be with Premarin 625 μg per day and cyclical medroxyprogesterone, 10 mg for the last 12 days of each month. This should result in an appropriate withdrawal bleed, although either therapy may require individual adjustment. For continuous therapy in patients who have been hypogonadal for several years, it is more reasonable to start with a smaller dose of Premarin and increase slowly to 625 μg per day, in an attempt to minimize the breast tenderness which many women report. Established therapy of Premarin (625 μg per day) and medroxyprogesterone (5 mg per day) results in appropriate hormone replacement with the absence of menstruation in the majority of women. All women receiving HRT require annual surveillance for breast cancer and endometrial hypertrophy. Men, particularly those over 50 years of age, receiving testosterone therapy require assessment for prostatic cancer.

11.5.9 Osteoporosis

As outlined previously, the achievement and maintenance of normal bone mineral density is a complex integrated process which relies on normal growth and development, the normal timing of puberty, the maintenance of adult sex hormone concentrations, normal activity and nutrition and the absence of other diseases. Osteoporosis [defined as a disease characterized by low bone mass and micro-architectural deterioration in bone tissue leading to enhanced bone fragility and a consequent increase in fracture risk [51]] can result from a failure to achieve peak bone mass and/or accelerated bone loss with age. Severe or established osteoporosis is defined as osteoporosis in the presence of a fragility or minimal trauma fracture. Factors which may impair the achievement of peak bone mass and/or result in rapid bone loss are frequent in people with intellectual disability. Thus adults with intellectual disability are more likely to be osteoporotic. This has been confirmed in a relatively young (mean age 35 years) sample of adults with intellectual disability [52]. In a more recent review by Srikanth et al. [53], increased prevalence of risk factors for osteoporosis in adults with intellectual disability population were identified which included; antiepileptics, immobility, history of falls and fractures. Other risk factors include vitamin D deficiency which people with intellectual disability may be more prone to (see above). Other studies have identified that there may be a specific problem in people with Down syndrome due to their disproportionate smaller body size [52, 54, 55]. However, as a group, adults with intellectual disability are generally at high risk of osteoporosis, not only due to the above risk factors outlined, but also the increasing longevity of this group.

Age and small body size are the best clinical predictors of low bone mineral density. Other predictive factors include Down syndrome and hypogonadism. In one population, low bone mineral density was associated with a history of fracture among females, although this was not the case with males [52].

To minimise the possibility of low bone density, individuals with intellectual disability should receive adequate nutrition and be encouraged to achieve maximal mobility. Those with no regular exposure to sunlight or no routine vitamin D supplementation, will need careful monitoring of their vitamin D status. Medical surveillance of people with intellectual disability will need to include an explicit approach to the assessment and treatment of osteoporosis [56].

11.5.9.1   Fractures and Osteoporosis

Fractures can occur with minimal trauma. Minimal trauma is defined as the force Involved in a fall from standing height or less. Factors that contribute to these minimal trauma fractures are a propensity to fall and the change in the strength of the bones, reducing their ability to withstand fracture. The latter has two components that can occur individually or together. The first is a decrease in bone density so that there is less bone per unit volume (osteoporosis). The second component is a change in the quality of the bone, but at this time this is difficulty to measure (although ultrasound may address this in the future).

Some sub-groups of adults with intellectual disability are at increased risk of fracture compared with the general population [57]. This increased risk appears to be associated with an increased risk of falling [58, 59]. In the study by Hsieh and colleagues, 25% of adults were reported to have had a fall over the preceding 12 months. Several risk factors for falls in adults with intellectual disability were identified in this study, including; being female, having arthritis, having a seizure disorder, taking more than four medications, using walking aids and difficulties in lifting greater than 10 lb. Fractures in this population are associated with increased morbidity [59].

Measurement of Bone Mass and Fracture Risk
There are several non-invasive low radiation techniques for measuring bone mass loosely termed bone mineral density (BMD), including dual photon absorptiometry [60]. These techniques have been shown to measure BMD precisely and accurately although technical artefacts can and do occur particularly with commonly performed spinal measurements. The bone mineral density of groups with and without fracture overlap, consistent with the idea that other factors (i.e., propensity to fall) must be involved. Reduced bone mineral density is a continuous risk factor for fracture similar to hypercholesterolemia and heart disease. Dreyfus et al. [61] looked at BMD screening in adults with intellectual disability and disappointingly, found that overall screening rates were lower than screening rates in the general population, despite the increased risk in this group.

Treatment
In the general population there are a number of available treatment options [62, 63]. These treatments have generally been validated as reducing the risk of minimal trauma fracture based on changes in vertebral shape (i.e., the so-called sub-clinical vertebral wedge fractures). Fewer of the treatments have been validated as reducing the risk of clinical peripheral fractures. Treatments which have been shown to reduce peripheral fractures, such as treatment with alendronic acid, require a large number of patients to be treated to prevent one clinically relevant fracture. Treatments are not without side-effects. Alendronic acid can result in esophageal reflux and esophagitis. If the person already had any signs of dysphagia they are already very vulnerable to esophageal reflux. Ideally before these are widely used in patients with intellectual disability there should be specific studies demonstrating their safety and efficacy. It would be reasonable to postulate that adults with Down syndrome who may have a particular abnormality related to their poor muscle function might have a different response to these therapies than the general population. However, this remains to be seen.

The overall approach to reducing the risk of fractures should be broad based rather than a traditional single therapy approach. It should be lifelong, aiming at prevention and should include attention to life style factors. Physicians who treat patients with intellectual disability will understand this approach particularly well. A multifactorial approach to falls reduction has been shown to reduce the number of falls and consequent fractures [64]. One component of this multifactorial approach is a reduction in the number of drugs which aggravate falling. Many psychotropic medications fit into this category. Care should be taken in balancing this risk with the benefits obtained from such therapies.

11.5.10 Dyslipidemia

This is a relatively uncommon cause for endocrinological referral. Treatment for adults with intellectual disability is the same as in the general population. Lifestyle factors, particularly diet, should be addressed. Persistent predominant hypercholesterolemia can be treated with the 3-hydroxl-3-methylglutaryl coenzyme A (HMG CoA) reductase inhibitors (the statins). Other agents such as the acid resins and nicotinic acid are less well tolerated. Gemfibrozil or other fibric acid derivatives can be used in this hypercholesterolemia and are preferred for predominant hypertriglyceridemia.

With life expectancy for people with intellectual disability becoming more comparable to the general population, the prevalence of age related cardiovascular disease is also becoming more comparable. This emphasises the need to monitor for development of metabolic syndrome, which is becoming increasingly prevalent in those adults with intellectual disability, particularly in the mild range where independent living is promoted. De Winter et al. [65] reported in a Dutch population of 412 adults with intellectual disability, a prevalence of 25.1% of metabolic syndrome, which is significantly higher than the general Dutch adult population (15.7%). In the same population of Dutch intellectually disabled adults, De Winter et al. [66] found that 98.9% had unhealthy diet, 63% lack of exercise, 13.6% were smokers, 70.4% had increased abdominal weight, 31.8% had hypercholesterolemia, 36.8% had hypertension and 8.7% had diabetes. Preventive screening programs and education on healthy lifestyle choices need to be more focused on adults with intellectual disability.

11.6   Screening

Medical problems among adults with intellectual disability are significantly under-diagnosed [2]. Reasons for this are discussed in Chaps. 17 and 18. It seems entirely reasonable to recommend routine screening for all adults with intellectual disability for a range of common conditions, including those listed above. In some cases, this will require only a physical examination. In the event of economic constraints, screening could be restricted to high-risk patients. It is easy to justify annual thyroid function tests in adults with Down syndrome. Similarly, as diabetes is so common in the population, routine screening, could also be easily justified. For simplicity, it is recommended to use glycosylated hemoglobin. This is not a sensitive test for the detection of diabetes but it is specific (apart from those with some underlying haemoglobinopathies). Furthermore, since the goal of treatment is to normalize glycosylated haemoglobin, provided the patient has a normal glycosylated hemoglobin, no further action need be taken. This will avoid the difficult problem of interpreting plasma glucose in relation to meals or ensuring that the patient is fasting. A diagnosis of diabetes suspected on glycosylated haemoglobin screening should be confirmed by appropriate glucose measurements. Vitamin D status should certainly be assessed annually in patients on anticonvulsant therapy by measuring 25 hydroxy Vitamin D concentration.

11.7 Therapeutic Approaches

Efforts to optimize nutritional care and bring about healthy eating habits should be a priority. This is necessary to prevent both over and under-nutrition, both of which are significant problems in this at-risk group and both of which can have long-term, wide spectrum consequences later in life, leading to several easily identified problems such as obesity, diabetes, osteoporosis or gonadal dysfunction. Similarly, when self-initiated activity is restricted, programs to promote maximum use of motor skills are required. This has an immediate benefit for the person involved and in the longer term will prevent or minimize limitations in motor skills. In addition, where known interactions of drug therapy (for example, phenytoin and an environment lacking sun exposure) are known to have deleterious effects these need to be counteracted. The identification of specific endocrine disorders is part of this approach, which is in keeping with the approach recommended by the WHO [3, 4] where it is proposed that "People with intellectual disability, and their caregivers, need to receive appropriate and ongoing education regarding healthy living practices in areas such as nutrition, exercise, oral hygiene, safety practices and the avoidance of risky behaviour, such as substance abuse and unprotected or multiple partner sexual activity" (Recommendation 6. Report 1-Physical Health Issues).

11.8 Access to Health Care in the Usual Paradigm of Health Care Delivery

As a general principle, endocrine disease should be managed as in the general population but the current paradigm for the delivery of health care is often not optimized to deal with this special subgroup of the population. Chapter 18 discusses in detail barriers in accessing appropriate health care services but for endocrinological disorders problems can include:

1. Many endocrine diseases present with a predominance of symptoms rather than physical signs. Adults with intellectual disability generally cannot verbally communicate their symptoms and so they often present in an atypical fashion. Recommendation 9 by WHO [4] states "Functional decline in older adults with intellectual disability warrants careful medical evaluation; undiagnosed mental health and medical conditions can have atypical presentations in people with limited language capabilities. Regular screening for visual and hearing impairment

should be implemented for people with intellectual disability during the child-hood and late adulthood years". Further, Recommendation 11 highlights possible deficiencies in service providers, by stating "Carers need training in assessing and communicating the basic health status of the adults with intellectual disability".

2. Physical signs in endocrine disease are often subtle and are potentially eas-ily masked by dysmorphic features particularly to an examiner who does not see a significant number of adults with intellectual disability. "Health care providers serving older adults with intellectual disability should recog-nize that adult and older-age onset medical conditions are common in this population and may require a high index of suspicion of clinical diagnosis". (Recommendation 8-[4]).

3. Physical examination is difficult in the uncooperative patient.

4. Endocrine test results can be influenced by medications frequently used in this population, although these problems are increasingly well recognized and newer laboratory methodologies often overcome the difficulties.

5. Current management of chronic diseases involves a significant component of self-care or self-management. The management of diabetes can be regarded as a prototype. Patients with intellectual disability as a group are almost always unable to assume the increased responsibility involved in self-care. This results in suboptimal management. People with intellectual disability require increased supervision of care including assistance to ensure compliance with medication.

Often patients with intellectual disability do not readily fit into our current model of health care delivery. This is exacerbated if the system is time constrained in any way. A different method of delivering health care to this subgroup is needed to deal with these problems. This has been highlighted by WHO in recommendation 10 [4]. Health care providers and policy makers need to eliminate attitudinal, architectural, and health care reimbursement barriers, that interfere with the provision of high quality health services for people with intellectual disability. More general prob-lems and deficiencies in the provision of appropriate heath care to people with intel-lectual disability are discussed in Chaps. 17 and 18.

11.9 Conclusion

Endocrine problems are common in people with intellectual disability for the same reasons as in the general population and for reasons specifically associated, directly or indirectly, with the condition itself. Some of the indirect associations may be cor-rectable. All efforts to maximize an individual's potential will have long-term ben-efit. This is true for all aspects of the person's mental and physical state and not limited to the endocrine system. Nevertheless as the endocrine system has a wide-spread coordinating role, many of the failures to achieving maximal potential will occur through failure of integration via the endocrine system. Once the diagnosis of intellectual disability is made, the pitfalls that can lead to problems in the future need to be recognized and avoided [4].

Common endocrine problems, which occur among adults with intellectual disability include, obesity and diabetes with its associated coronary artery disease risk, hypogonadism, osteoporosis and hypothyroidism. These diseases can have additive, compounding, long-term effects on the individual. For an individual to achieve their maximum potential and to maintain this potential for as long as possible, these disease processes need to be anticipated and prevented if at all possible or detected early and treated vigorously. Only in this way will the health and longevity of people with intellectual disability be improved.

References

1. Chrousos GP. Stress, chronic inflammation, and emotional and physical well-being: concurrent effects and chronic sequelae. J Allergy Clin Immunol. 2000;106(Suppl 5):S275–91.
2. Beange H, McElduff A, Baker W. Medical disorders in adults with intellectual disability: a population study. Am J Ment Retard. 1995a;99:595–604.
3. Evenhuis H, Henderson CM, Beange H, Lennox N, Chicoine B. Healthy ageing—Adults with intellectual disabilities: Physical health issues. Geneva: World Health Organization; 2001.
4. World Health Organisation. Healthy ageing adults with intellectual disabilities. Background reports on physical and mental health, women's health and ageing and social policy. physical health issues. Geneva: World Health Organization; 2000.
5. World Health Organisation. Population-based approaches to childhood obesity prevention. Geneva: World Health Organisation; 2012.
6. De Winter CF, Bastiaanse LP, Hilgenkamp TI, Evenhuis HM, Echteld MA. Overweight and obesity in older people with intellectual disability. Res Dev Disabil. 2012;33(2):398–405. https://doi.org/10.1016/j.ridd.2011.09.022. PubMed PMID: 22119687
7. Gawlik K, Zwierzchowska A, Rosolek B, Celebanska D, Moczek K. Obesity among adults with moderate and severe intellectual disabilities. Adv Rehabil. 2016;30:17–25. https://doi.org/10.1515/rehab-2015-0040.
8. Hsieh K, Rimmer JH, Heller T. Obesity and associated factors in adults with intellectual disability. J Intellect Disabil Res. 2014;58:851–63. https://doi.org/10.1111/jir.12100. PubMed PMID: 24256455
9. Krause S, Ware R, McPherson L, Lennox N, O'Callaghan M. Obesity in adolescents with intellectual disability: Prevalence and associated characteristics. Obes Res Clin Pract. 2016;10:520–30. https://doi.org/10.1016/j.orcp.2015.10.006.
10. Phillips KL, Schieve LA, Visser S, Boulet S, Sharma AJ, Kogan MD, Boyle AC, Yeargin-Allsopp M. Prevalence and impact of unhealthy weight in a national sample of US adolescents with autism and other learning and behavioral disabilities. Matern Child Health J. 2014;18:1964–75. https://doi.org/10.1007/s10995-014-1442-y.
11. Rimmer JH, Yamaki K. Obesity and intellectual disability. Ment Retard Dev Disabil Res Rev. 2006;12:22–7. Review
12. Emerson E, Robertson J, Baines S, Hatton C. Obesity in British children with and without intellectual disability: cohort study. BMC Public Health. 2016;16:644. https://doi.org/10.1186/s12889-016-3309-1.
13. Prasher VP. Overweight and obesity amongst down syndrome adults. J Intellect Disabil Res. 1995;39:437–41.
14. Spanos D, Melville CA, Hankey CR. Weight management interventions in adults with intellectual disabilities and obesity: a systematic review of the evidence. Nutr J. 2013;12:132. https://doi.org/10.1186/1475-2891-12-132. Review
15. Beange H, Gale L, Stewart L. Project Renourish: a dietary intervention to improve nutritional status in people with multiple disabilities. Aust N Z J Dev Disabil. 1995b;20:165–74.

16. Kuperminc MN, Stevenson RD. Growth and nutrition disorders in children with cerebral palsy. Dev Disabil Res Rev. 2008;14:137–46. https://doi.org/10.1002/ddrr.14.
17. Waber DP, Bryce CP, Girard JM, Zichlin M, Fitzmaurice GM, Galler JR. Impaired IQ and academic skills in adults who experienced moderate to severe infantile malnutrition: a forty-year study. Nutr Neurosci. 2014;17:58–64. https://doi.org/10.1179/1476830513Y.0000000061.
18. Groce N, Challenger E, Berman-Bieler R, Farkas A, Yilmaz N, Schultink W, Clark D, Kaplan C, Kerac M. Malnutrition and disability: unexplored opportunities for collaboration. Paediatr Int Child Health. 2014;34(4):308–14. https://doi.org/10.1179/2046905514Y.0000000156.
19. Prasher VP. Down syndrome and thyroid disorders: a review. Down Syndr Res Pract. 1999;6:105–10.
20. Aversa T, Lombardo F, Valenzise M, Messina MF, Sferlazzas C, Salzano G, De Luca F, Wasniewska M. Peculiarities of autoimmune thyroid diseases in children with Turner or Down syndrome: an overview. Ital J Pediatr. 2015;41:39. https://doi.org/10.1186/s13052-015-0146-2.
21. Iughetti L, Predieri B, Bruzzi P, Predieri F, Vellani G, Madeo SF, Garavelli L, Biagioni O, Bedogni G, Bozzola M. Ten-year longitudinal study of thyroid function in children with Down syndrome. Horm Res Paediatr. 2014;82:113–21. https://doi.org/10.1159/000362450.
22. Cebeci AN, Güven A, Yildiz M. Profile of hypothyroidism in Down's syndrome. J Clin Res Pediatr Endocrinol. 2013;5(2):116–20. https://doi.org/10.4274/Jcrpe.884.
23. Léger J. Congenital hypothyroidism: a clinical update of long-term outcome in young adults. Eur J Endocrinol. 2015;172:R67–77. https://doi.org/10.1530/EJE-14-0777.
24. Marques I, Silva A, Castro S, Lopes L. Down syndrome, insulin-dependent diabetes mellitus and hyperthyroidism: a rare association. BMJ Case Rep. 2015. pii: bcr2014208166. doi: https://doi.org/10.1136/bcr-2014-208166. PubMed PMID: 26123455; PubMed Central PMCID: PMC4488676.
25. Shaw JE, Dunstan DW, Zimmet PZ, Cameron AJ, de Courten MP, Welborn TA. Epidemic glucose intolerance in Australia. Proceedings of the 37th Annual Meeting of the European Association for the Study of Diabetes. 2001. Abstract 9.
26. Axmon A, Ahlström G, Höglund P. Prevalence and treatment of diabetes mellitus and hypertension among older adults with intellectual disability in comparison with the general population. BMC Geriatr. 2017;17:272. https://doi.org/10.1186/s12877-017-0658-2.
27. World Health Organisation. Use of glycated haemoglobin (HbA1c) in the diagnosis of diabetes mellitus: Abbreviated report of a WHO consultation. Geneva: World Health Organization; 2011.
28. Adler AI, Stratton IM, Neil HA, Yudkin JS, Matthews DR, Cull CA, Wright AD, Turner RC, Holman RR. Association of systolic blood pressure with macrovascular and microvascular complications of type 2 diabetes (UKPDS 36): prospective observational study. Br Med J. 2000;321:394–5.
29. UK Prospective Diabetes Study Group. Efficacy of atenolol and captopril in reducing risk of macrovascular and microvascular complications in type 2 diabetes: UKPDS 39. Br Med J. 1998;317:713–20.
30. Cardol M, Rijken M, van Schrojenstein Lantman-de Valk H. People with mild to moderate intellectual disability talking about their diabetes and how they manage. J Intellect Disabil Res. 2012;56:351–60. https://doi.org/10.1111/j.1365-2788.2011.01472.
31. Anwar AJ, Walker JD, Frier BM. Type 1 diabetes mellitus and Down's syndrome: prevalence, management and diabetic complications. Diabet Med. 1998;15:160–3.
32. Diabetes Prevention Program (DPP) [missing title]. 2001. Accessed from www.nih.gov/news/pr/aug2001/niddk-08.htm.
33. Tuomilehto J, Lindstrom J, Eriksson JG, Valle TT, Hamalainen H, Ilanne-Parikka P, Keinanen-Kiukaanniemi S, Laakso M, Louheranta A, Rastas M, Salminen V, Aunola S, Cepaitis Z, Moltchanov V, Hakumaki M, Mannelin M, Martikkala V, Sundvall J, Uusitupa M, the Finnish Diabetes Prevention Study Group. Prevention of type 2 diabetes mellitus by changes in lifestyle among subjects with impaired glucose tolerance. N Engl J Med. 2001;344:1343–50.
34. Frighi V, Morovat A, Stephenson MT, White SJ, Hammond CV, Goodwin GM. Vitamin D deficiency in patients with intellectual disabilities: prevalence, risk factors and management strate-

gies. Br J Psychiatry. 2014;205:458–64. https://doi.org/10.1192/bjp.bp.113.143511. PubMed PMID: 25257061
35. Grant WB, Wimalawansa SJ, Holick MF, Cannell JJ, Pludowski P, Lappe JM, Pittaway M, May P. Emphasizing the health benefits of vitamin D for those with neurodevelopmental disorders and intellectual disabilities. Nutrients. 2015;7:1538–64. https://doi.org/10.3390/nu7031538.
36. Wark JD, Larkins RG, Perry KD, Peter CT, Ross DL, Sloman JG. Chronic diphenylhydantoin therapy does not reduce plasma 25hydroxyvitamin D. Clin Endocrinol (Oxf). 1979;11: 267–74.
37. Meier C, Kraenzlin ME. Antiepileptics and bone health. Ther Adv Musculoskelet Dis. 2011;3:235–43. https://doi.org/10.1177/1759720X11410769.
38. Menon B, Harinarayan CV. The effect of anti-epileptic drug therapy on serum 25hydroxyvitamin D and parameters of calcium and bone metabolism–a longitudinal study. Seizure. 2010;19:153–8. https://doi.org/10.1016/j.seizure.2010.01.006. Epub 2010 Feb 7
39. Mintzer S, Boppana P, Toguri J, DeSantis A. Vitamin D levels and bone turnover in epilepsy patients taking carbamazepine or oxcarbazepine. Epilepsia. 2006;47:510–5.
40. Pack AM, Morrell MJ, Randall A, McMahon DJ, Shane E. Bone health in young women with epilepsy after one year of antiepileptic drug monotherapy. Neurology. 2008;70:1586–93.
41. Santen FJ. Male hypogonadism. In: SSC Y, Jaffe RB, editors. Reproductive endocrinology. 3rd ed. Philadelphia, PA: WB Saunders Co.; 1991. p. 745–000.
42. McElduff A, Center J, Beange H. Hypogonadism in men with intellectual disabilities: a population study. J Intellect Dev Disabil. 2003;28:163–70.
43. Lip SZL, Murchison LED, Cullis PS, Govan L, Carachi R. A meta-analysis of the risk of boys with isolated cryptorchidism developing testicular cancer in later life. Arch Dis Child. 2013;98:20–6.
44. Cortes D, Visfeldt J, Moller H, Thorup J. Testicular neoplasia in cryptorchid boys at primary surgery: case series. Br Med J. 1999;319:888–9.
45. Satge D, Sasco AJ, Cure H, Leduc B, Sommelet D, Vekemans MJ. An excess of testicular germ cell tumors in Down's syndrome: three case reports and a review of the literature. Cancer. 1997;80:929–35.
46. Cortada X, Kousseff BG. Cryptorchidism in mental retardation. J Urol. 1984;131:674–6.
47. Haire AR, Flavill J, Groom WD, Dhandapani B. Unidentified undescended testes in teenage boys with severe learning disabilities. Arch Dis Child. 2015;100:479–80. https://doi.org/10.1136/archdischild-2014-307155. Epub 2015 Feb 2. Review
48. McCarthy M. Going through the menopause: perceptions and experiences of women with intellectual disability. J Intellect Dev Disabil. 2002;27:281–95.
49. Ejskjaer K, Uldbjerg N, Goldstein H. Menstrual profile and early menopause in women with Down syndrome aged 26-40 years. J Intellect Dev Disabil. 2006;31:166–71.
50. Seltzer GB, Schupf N, Wu H-S. A prospective study of menopause in women with Down's syndrome. J Intellect Disabil Res. 2001;45:1–7. https://doi.org/10.1111/j.1365-2788.2001.00286.
51. Consensus Development Conference. Diagnosis, prophylaxis and treatment of osteoporosis. Am J Med. 1993;94:646–50.
52. Center J, Beange H, McElduff A. People with mental retardation have an increased prevalence of osteoporosis: a population study. Am J Ment Retard. 1998;103:19–28.
53. Srikanth R, Cassidy G, Joiner C, Teeluckdharry S. Osteoporosis in people with intellectual disabilities: a review and a brief study of risk factors for osteoporosis in a community sample of people with intellectual disabilities. J Intellect Disabil Res. 2011;55:53–62. https://doi.org/10.1111/j.1365-2788.2010.01346.x.
54. Kao CH, Chen CC, Wang SJ, Yeh SH. Bone mineral density in children with Down syndrome detected by dual photon absorptiometry. Nucl Med Commun. 1992;13:773–5.
55. Sepúlveda D, Allison DB, Gomez JE, Kreibich K, Brown RA, Pierson RN, Heymsfield SB. Low spinal and pelvic bone mineral density among individuals with Down syndrome. Am J Ment Retard. 1995;100:109–14.
56. Petrone LR. Osteoporosis in adults with intellectual disabilities. South Med J. 2012;105:87–92. https://doi.org/10.1097/SMJ.0b013e3182427042. Review

57. Tannenbaum TN, Lipworth L, Baker S. Risk of fractures in an intermediate care facility for persons with mental retardation. Am J Ment Retard. 1989;95:444–51.
58. Hsieh K, Rimmer J, Heller T. Prevalence of falls and risk factors in adults with intellectual disability. Am J Intellect Dev Disabil. 2012;117(6):442–54. https://doi.org/10.1352/1944-7558-117.6.442.
59. Spreat S, BakerPotts JC. Patterns of injury in institutionalized mentally retarded residents. Ment Retard. 1983;21:23–9.
60. Johnston CC, Slemenda CW, Melton LJ. Clinical use of bone densitometry. N Engl J Med. 1991;324:1105–9.
61. Dreyfus D, Lauer E, Wilkinson J. Characteristics associated with bone mineral density screening in adults with intellectual disabilities. J Am Board Fam Med. 2014;27:104–14. https://doi.org/10.3122/jabfm.2014.01.130114.
62. Eastell R, Boyle IT, Compston J, Cooper C, Fogelman I, Francis RM, Hosking DJ, Purdie DW, Ralston S, Reeve J, Reid DM, Russell RGG, Stevenson JC. Management of male osteoporosis: report of the UK Consensus Group. Q J Med. 1998;91:71–92.
63. Meunier PJ, Delmas PD, Eastell MR, Papapoulos S, Rizzoli R, Seeman E, Wasnick RD. Diagnosis and management of osteoporosis in postmenopausal women: Clinical guidelines. Clin Ther. 1999;21:1025–39.
64. Tinetti ME, Baker DI, McAvay G, Claus EG, Garrett P, Gottschalk M, Koch ML, Trainor K, Horwitz RI. A multifactorial intervention to reduce the risk of falling among elderly people living in the community. N Engl J Med. 1994;331:821–7.
65. De Winter CF, Magilsen KW, van Alfen JC, Willemsen SP, Evenhuis HM. Metabolic syndrome in 25% of older people with intellectual disability. Fam Pract. 2011;28(2):141–4. https://doi.org/10.1093/fampra/cmq079. PubMed PMID: 20937662
66. De Winter CF, Magilsen KW, van Alfen JC, Penning C, Evenhuis HM. Prevalence of cardiovascular risk factors in older people with intellectual disability. Am J Intellect Dev Disabil. 2009;114:427–36. https://doi.org/10.1352/1944-7558-114.6.427. PubMed PMID: 19792058

Part III

Oral and Dental Health

12

Evan Spivack, Mark D. Robinson, and Tomas J. Ballesteros

12.1 Introduction

Advances in medical science have led to dramatic increases in the survivability of newborns previously considered nonviable and in the life span of individuals who, in the past, experienced shorter lives [1]. Similarly, advances in dental knowledge and awareness have led to marked decreases in edentulism [2] and a greater desire for teeth that are not only functional but esthetically pleasing. Evidence has been presented that demonstrates strong links between oral and systemic health [3], highlighting the importance of oral care in persons with complex medical profiles.

It is broadly recognized that oral health care must be integrated into the overall care plan developed for persons with intellectual and developmental disabilities. The concept of professional dental care has shifted from an episodic to a comprehensive care model and dental schools are now incorporating clinical and didactic training in "special care dentistry" into their doctoral curricula [4]. Additionally, increasing attention has been given to utilizing a multidisciplinary and interprofessional approach to patient care.

This chapter highlights the need for dental care among persons with intellectual and developmental disabilities, explores the oral and dental findings common in this population, outlines basic dental treatment planning concerns, and discusses approaches to providing this care.

E. Spivack (✉) · M. D. Robinson · T. J. Ballesteros
Department of Pediatric Dentistry, Special Care Treatment Center, Rutgers School of Dental Medicine, Newark, NJ, USA

© Springer Nature Switzerland AG 2019
V. P. Prasher, M. P. Janicki (eds.), *Physical Health of Adults with Intellectual and Developmental Disabilities*, https://doi.org/10.1007/978-3-319-90083-4_12

12.2   Epidemiology of Dental Disease

Intellectual disability is the most common developmental disorder that inhibits full participation in society for many people [5]. In a study of over 4700 people with intellectual disability, it was noted that this population faces significant challenges in receiving treatment for dental disease. The study included participants in a diverse range of living arrangements, and exhibiting various medical conditions and levels of cooperation. Nearly 88%of the participants had caries experience; 32.2% had untreated dental caries; 80.3% were diagnosed with periodontitis; and 10.9% were edentulous [6]. A literature review of oral health and intellectual disability reported that persons with intellectual disability had poorer oral health, greater numbers of tooth extractions, more caries, fewer fillings, greater gingival inflammation, and greater rates of edentulism and had less access to preventative dentistry and poorer services when compared to the general population [7].

Many characteristics associated with intellectual disability may contribute to an increased risk of experiencing oral disease. These include cognitive, physical and behavioral limitations that make it difficult to perform daily oral care and cooperate during dental visits [6]. Several U.S. government reports have called attention to the disproportionate impact of oral disease on people with disabilities, including persons with intellectual disability. In each report, lack of information about the complex issues involved in meeting the needs of this group was identified as a significant barrier to efforts to understand and improve their oral health [6].

12.3   Management of Individuals with Systemic Health Concerns

Individuals with intellectual disability often present with significant comorbidities that may impact the provision of dental care. Dentists must be aware of these conditions and understand their ramifications for treatment. In some cases, consultation with other health care professionals, or modification of the dental care plan, may be indicated. Dentists may often collect bloodwork, medical test results, reports and assessments allowing greater insight into the potential medical issues necessary for consideration in the development of a dental treatment plan. In consulting with other healthcare providers, dentists must understand risk stratification for patients who will need invasive dental treatment. These concerns include post-operative healing, bleeding control, and long-term care. As the body changes, the oral cavity will change as well; the oral needs of these individuals must keep pace with systemic change.

Considerable research has linked the health of the oral cavity with overall health. In 2012, the American Heart Association (AHA) released a scientific statement indicating that while the current literature does not support a causative relationship between periodontal disease and vascular disease, these two entities do share common risk factors [8]. This relationship between oral and systemic health has been understood for many years and the importance of this linkage for those with intellectual disability is particularly important. Most often noted are the correlations between periodontal health and cardiovascular disease, diabetes, and pulmonary disease.

Periodontal disease is an inflammatory process occurring due to the colonization of pathologic bacteria, resulting in alveolar bone loss in the mandible and maxilla. High-risk bacteria, including aggregatibacter, porphyromonas, treponema and fusobacterium species are periodontal pathogens also implicated in increasing arterial endothelial dysfunction. Endothelial injury and dysfunction as a result of *P. gingivalis* demonstrate proinflammatory cytokines and chemokines [9]. Studies illustrate the concept of infectious burden (a culmination of many bacteria including those associated with periodontal disease) resulting in atherosclerotic disease [10]. Prevention and management of cardiovascular disease, particularly for those individuals at increased risk for these conditions, must include an oral care component.

Studies have shown that the prevalence of atherosclerotic heart disease in those with intellectual disability is similar to that in the general population. However, specific developmental conditions are known to be associated with a higher degree of cardiac anomalies. Individuals with Down syndrome have an incidence of up to 40% of cardiac cushion defects (ASD and VSD). These individuals, as well as others with unrepaired cyanotic congenital cardiac defects, repaired defects with valvular regurgitation and/or residual shunting, may require antibiotic administration prior to dental treatment as prophylaxis against possible infective endocarditis. Guidelines for antibiotic use have been crafted and updated by joint committees of the American Medical Association (AMA) and the American Dental Association (ADA) [11].

The geriatric individual with intellectual disability may have an implanted pacemaker, which may be subject to electromagnetic interference (EMI) from dental equipment. While advances in pacemaker technology have significantly reduced the incidence of perioperative EMI, dental providers are encouraged to seek detailed information about a person's pacemaker. Individuals will often have information regarding the device model and activation date that should be recorded by the dentist. Discussion with the patient's cardiologist regarding considerations for treatment planning is appropriate and advised [12].

The strong association between diabetes and periodontal disease is well known, with scientific documentation of a bi-directional relationship between the diseases existing since the 1990s. Numerous studies show an improvement in glycemic control after treatment of diabetes, while additional evidence has confirmed that poor glycemic control is a contributing factor to worsening periodontal disease. Persons with Down syndrome may have difficulties maintaining glycemic control and may also have problems maintaining proper oral hygiene. Difficulties in maintaining proper oral hygiene arise from noncompliant behavioral issues or from a severe decline in health. Impaired immune function is a potential consequence of poor glycemic control. Resulting exacerbation of oral health problems such as candidiasis, xerostomia and impaired wound healing may lead to worsening periodontal disease and an increase in dental caries [13].

Difficulties in maintaining oral hygiene are often noted in individuals with intellectual disability. These difficulties often manifest in the form of indivdual refusal and defiance, compromised positioning from spastic muscle movement, or lack of proper assistance from family caregivers or group home staff. Combined with impaired immune function that may be a result of poor glycemic control, this resultant increase in oral pathogens may lead to or exacerbate existing oral health problems. Additionally, some studies suggest that edentulous participants exhibit worse glycemic control than those with teeth, placing those without teeth at higher risk for complications associated with type 2 diabetes [14]. Through improvement in oral health and maintenance of the dentition, persons with intellectual disability can reduce the risk of developing complications associated with poor glycemic control.

Periodontal disease may increase the risk for lung diseases including chronic obstructive pulmonary disease (COPD) and pneumonia. COPD and periodontitis are both long term chronic conditions characterized by systemic inflammation and destruction of connective tissues. While studies have not solidified a causal relationship, bacteria common in periodontal disease have also been implicated in pulmonary conditions. It has been posited that these bacteria are responsible for infection when inhaled into the lower respiratory tract, increasing the risk of developing or exacerbating pulmonary conditions. One meta-analysis found that those with COPD demonstrated higher levels of circulating cytokines and destructive mediators than those without COPD, consistent with long term bacterial insult [15]. Individuals with long-term chronic lung conditions can benefit greatly by improving oral hygiene, thus removing harmful bacteria and reducing the overall exposure to harmful inflammatory insult.

Oropharyngeal dysphagia is a significant complicating finding in many individuals with cerebral palsy as well as in other individuals with airway and neuromuscular concerns. Some studies note the incidence of dysphagia in children with cerebral palsy to be 43–100% [16]. Individuals who are unable to ambulate and therefore use wheelchairs for mobility will often have decreased diaphragmatic strength and decreased strength in other muscles assisting with respiration. Additionally, these individuals may have compromised postures forcing anatomical positioning leading to unfavorable pressure on the lungs. Restricting lung volume in this manner will decrease capacity and lead to inefficient oxygen exchange. In some cases, these individuals will require ventilators or positive pressure airflow to maintain oxygenation. Such conditions will significantly limit the provision of dental care in the routine office setting and can be a risk factor for increased periodontal inflammation. In order to treat these individuals, dentists must often limit appointment times, increase use of suction to prevent aspiration, be aware of changes in the individuals' oxygen saturation and assure a readily available oxygen supply throughout treatment.

12.4 Common Oral Diseases

Dental caries and periodontal disease are the two most common oral diseases affecting dentate adults. While adults with intellectual disability are prone to these diseases just as are age-peers in the general population, there are often differences in disease presentation and prevalence due to the medical, anatomic and cognitive differences noted in these populations.

12.4.1 Dental Caries

By definition, dental caries is an infectious and transmissible disease caused by bacteria colonizing the tooth surfaces. Unlike most infectious diseases affecting humans, caries is the result of an imbalance of the indigenous oral biota rather than that of a nonindigenous, exogenous pathogen [17]. The predominant bacteria colonizing initial lesions are streptococcus mutans. Lactobacillus microorganisms are associated with advanced lesions that have already progressed through the enamel surface into the dentin layer, even perhaps advancing to the pulp chamber. Recent evidence also has supported the role of yeast (candida albicans) as a member of the mixed oral microbiota involved in caries causation [18].

The entire tooth is susceptible to caries. Coronal caries affects the crown of the tooth, which is protected by a hard enamel layer and is visible above the gum line. This portion of the tooth is involved with a majority of normal tooth function (mastication) and parafunction (bruxism). The occlusal aspect of the crown is characterized by the presence of pits and fissures which may retain plaque and become susceptible to dental caries. The root of the tooth ordinarily lies below the gumline. It does not have an enamel layer for protection, thus increasing caries susceptibility when exposed to the oral environment containing cariogenic food and liquids.

Diet plays a major role in the incidence of dental caries. Consuming a diet high in fermentable carbohydrates and sugars will significantly increase caries risk. Persons with intellectual disability tend to have poorer diets than do other adults due to their living situations and being dependent upon others for the provision of meals. Caregivers must be made aware of the individual's nutritional needs and dietary issues, and asked to strive to provide healthy and balanced meals, low in sugars and fermentable carbohydrates.

Food consistency plays a significant role in caries susceptibility. A diet higher in roughage and of a firmer, mechanical consistency will allow for greater self-cleansing of the teeth and soft tissues. Conversely, the individual who consumes a prescribed puree-consistency diet due to swallowing difficulties and/or a history of aspiration will often have food debris clinging to his or her teeth, thus increasing the likelihood of caries development and progression. For these individuals, maintenance of high-quality oral homecare and close professional follow-up is critical. Xerostomia will also contribute to difficulties in cleansing the mouth and in increasing the risk of dental caries.

The modality of feeding will also influence an individual's caries susceptibility. Individuals with poor or non-functional swallowing mechanisms are at a high risk for aspiration of food or liquids and are often fed parenterally via a gastric or nasogastric feeding tube. When maintained completely without oral intake, where sugars and fermentable carbohydrates are not introduced to the oral environment, these individuals present a much lower caries risk than those individuals who are fed orally.

Once dental caries has been diagnosed, the decision must be made whether to restore or extract the affected tooth. A number of determinants will factor into this decision, with the potential for restorability generally the primary concern. If a tooth is deemed to have adequate structure once the decayed portion is removed, the dentist may develop a restorative plan to support and augment this remaining natural tooth structure. A variety of materials are available from which the dentist will choose the one best suited to meet the various anatomic, structural, and environmental changes to which the restoration will be subjected.

Dental amalgam is a mixture of silver, tin, copper, and mercury. In use internationally for over 150 years, amalgam has been studied more extensively than any other dental restorative material. It is often the material of choice for use in posterior tooth restorations as its strong material properties allow it to withstand heavy masticatory forces as well as parafunctional stresses. Amalgam has cariostatic properties as well, and it is not rare to find amalgam restorations having endured for several decades even under challenging oral conditions. Amalgam is the least technique-sensitive of the existing dental restorative materials, allowing for satisfactory results even in poorly cooperative individuals or in situations where proper isolation from saliva contamination during placement is difficult or impossible.

Resin-based composite restorative materials are dramatically different from dental amalgam. Primarily composed of Bis-GMA, other monomers and assorted fillers, the composite materials bond to tooth structure and are both tooth-colored and highly polishable, making them attractive choices for restorations in the more esthetic anterior dentition. While a number of studies have compared the longevity of resin-based materials to amalgam, the durability of these restorations is greatly affected by heavy functional and parafunctional forces such as bruxism. Unlike amalgam, these materials are not cariostatic and are subject to polymerization shrinkage and marginal leakage that can lead to dentinal sensitivity and recurring decay. Additionally, tooth restoration with resin-based materials is highly technique sensitive, making these materials less appropriate for use in individuals with challenging behaviors.

Glass ionomer restorative materials offer the dentist an attractive option for use in difficult restorative situations, such as those frequently encountered in individuals with intellectual disability. Several formulations of these materials are available, some of which are metal-reinforced or otherwise appropriate for use in posterior teeth, while others are tooth colored and provide good esthetics in the anterior region. Glass ionomers are less technique sensitive than composite resin materials and are more forgiving during placement in the mouth's moisture-containing environment. Perhaps the most compelling property these materials offer is the significant cariostatic effect resulting from the material's capacity for fluoride release. This property makes glass ionomer materials a strong choice for use in individuals who are highly caries-prone due to poor oral hygiene, xerostomia, or other factors.

Silver diamine fluoride (SDF) is a clear, odorless liquid that can be placed directly on carious tooth structure and used to arrest dental caries. It has been used successfully across the globe in children and as part of the atraumatic restorative treatment (ART) technique, a minimally-invasive procedure in which injections of

local anesthesia and the use of rotary instrumentation of teeth is limited or elimi-
nated. The ability to halt dental caries in a less traumatic way makes SDF a valuable
component of the dental armamentarium when caring for individuals with limited
ability to tolerate traditional dental restorative techniques.

As dental caries advance deeper into the tooth, involvement of the pulp becomes
more likely. The resulting pulpitis may quickly progress from reversible (if the
decay is removed and the tooth restored) to irreversible, declining towards pulpal
necrosis and the risk of pain and abscess formation. At this point, endodontic therapy (root canal treatment or advanced endodontic procedures) will be required if the
tooth is to be restored. For individuals who are unable to cooperate for these length-
ier procedures or in those situations where the combination of pulpal involvement
and structural tooth loss leads to a poorer prognosis, extraction of the offending
tooth may be the option of choice.

12.4.2   Periodontal Disease

Periodontal disease is the inflammatory process affecting the soft and hard structures that support the teeth: the gingiva, periodontal ligaments and the alveolar
bone. In its early stage (gingivitis), the gingiva will become swollen and red, the
natural inflammatory response to the presence of harmful bacteria present around
the teeth in the form of plaque and calculus. Gingivitis can progress to become periodontitis, a condition in which the gingiva pull away from the tooth and supporting
tissues are destroyed. Bone can be lost, and the teeth may loosen and eventually
exfoliate or require extraction due to the presence of infection and/or pain [19].
While inflammation resulting from bacterial infection is the cornerstone of periodontal disease, numerous factors can influence disease progression and severity.
Prominent risk factors include inherited or genetic susceptibility, smoking, lack of
adequate home care, advancing age, diet, history of systemic disease, and medications [19]. In a study of over four thousand dentate persons with intellectual disability, over eighty percent were diagnosed with periodontitis. Prevalence was
highest in those 60 years and older (92.6%) and lowest in the youngest age range of
20 through 39 years (55.8%) [6].

Periodontal attachment will deteriorate when challenged by inflammation of the
tissues and deepening of the pockets surrounding the dentition. Eventually, this will
lead to destruction of the bone supporting the teeth. In general, loss of alveolar bone
is a painless and silent process. As the disease process advances, tooth mobility
increases and individuals may develop acute infections of the periodontium leading
to painful abscesses. The severity of periodontitis is, in part, dependent upon anatomic location. Affected posterior teeth will often have a better prognosis due to the
larger root surface area: these teeth often have large, broad roots and often are multi-
rooted, allowing for greater anchorage in the alveolus. Diet has a great bearing upon
periodontal health. Vitamins, minerals and trace elements are directly related to
gingival and periodontal health and regeneration as well as to bone formation.
Understanding the individual's medical history is necessary in addressing the

systemic impact of periodontal disease. Numerous studies have suggested that periodontal disease is linked to a variety of medical conditions including heart disease, diabetes, and rheumatoid arthritis [19].

Poorly controlled diabetes may contribute to increased severity of periodontal disease and more rapid progression of attachment loss and clinical symptoms. Conversely, poorly controlled periodontitis has been implicated as a factor in the diabetic individual's glycemic control. Poor oral hygiene leading to increased inflammation may result in serum glucose elevation and hyperglycemia.

Prevention is the cornerstone of any plan to improve and maintain periodontal health. Education of the individual and caregiver is necessary if the progression of periodontal disease is to be slowed. Such education must emphasize home oral care strategies including proper tooth brushing, flossing and mouth rinsing. The implementation of these strategies must be customized to meet the specific needs and abilities of the individual, taking into account degree of cognitive and physical limitations as well as numerous oral factors. The dentist should also guide the individual and/or caregiver towards the selection of mechanical oral hygiene aids that are best suited to meet individual needs. A variety of toothbrushes and flossing aids are available, and will complement the choice of dentifrice, floss and oral rinse.

An equally important component of the preventative plan is assessment of the individual's diet and guidance towards a healthier and more orally-friendly nutritional scheme. Such diet planning should seek to minimize refined sugars, carbohydrates and acidic food and drink and emphasize fruits, vegetables, and proteins that will support healthier dentition and periodontium [20]. Often, referral of the individual to a nutritionist may prove valuable, particularly if the implementation of a healthy diet is made difficult by individual variables.

12.4.3 Edentulism

Edentulism can be defined as the physical state of the jaws following removal of all erupted teeth and the condition of the supporting structures available for reconstructive or replacement therapies [1]. The past several decades have seen an overall general decline in edentulism. According to one study, there has been a downward trend in edentulism between 1999 and 2008, although significant variations exist across racial/ethnic groups [2]. Adults with intellectual disability generally have fewer financial resources which may affect the treatment decision regarding keeping or extracting their teeth.

Resorption of the alveolar ridges begins as soon as teeth are extracted and continues over time until the bony ridges lose anatomic form. Due to this resorption, prosthetic replacement of teeth with complete dentures becomes extremely difficult and sometimes impossible without the performance of complex, difficult and expensive surgical procedures to replace lost bone.

The completely edentulous individual may have options other than complete dentures for replacing teeth. Implant-supported prosthetics, involving surgical placement of titanium dental implants into the jaws followed by prostheses custom-fabricated to attach to the implants, may be a viable option. The prosthesis may be permanently attached to the implants or may be removable, utilizing the implants to provide increased stability and improved functionality.

Partial edentulism, in which the individual still retains some teeth, leaves several options for tooth replacement. The fixed partial denture consists of precision-fabricated crowns attached to pontics replacing the missing teeth. This bridge, or fixed partial denture, is cast as a single unit, with the abutment crowns cemented to the natural teeth adjacent to the edentulous space. While offering some advantages over the use of removable partial dentures, the fixed option is often more costly, requires more cooperation from the individual during the fabrication process and is significantly more difficult to maintain, possibly leading to early loss of the prosthesis and additional teeth.

Removable partial dentures will usually have clasps that rest on and hold onto the existing teeth, creating a more stable and retentive prosthesis. Advantages of the removable prosthesis include lower cost, easier (but often longer) process of fabrication and perhaps most importantly, the denture may be removed for daily cleaning. Once fabricated, a number of considerations factor into the success of removable prostheses. Foremost is the individual's ability to tolerate a foreign object in the mouth. Wearing dentures involves a learning curve and becoming comfortable with them may take several weeks or even months of practice. The person with intellectual disability may have difficulty adapting to a prosthesis as both cognitive and physical limitations will prolong the adaptation process. The oral structures must "learn" how to tolerate dentures and the oral soft tissues and musculature develop "memory", allowing the prosthesis to properly rest on the oral structures. This may often be a difficult and time consuming learning process and adult with intellectual disability.

Ill-fitting complete dentures cause several problems for an edentulous adult with intellectual disability, as poorly adapted dentures may shift in the mouth, traumatizing the soft tissues and causing abrasions and lacerations which may in turn become secondarily infected by bacteria or candida species. Soft tissue concerns that may arise include denture stomatitis, ulcerations, mucosal hypertrophy and epulis formation, all of which may contribute to pain and decreased masticatory ability. These conditions will persist and progress unless the dentures are either adjusted, relined, or even re-fabricated. Partial dentures, as they are supported by the remaining teeth, are less likely to shift and cause the problems noted above.

Denture maintenance maybe problematic in adults with intellectual disability. Oral prostheses must be properly cleaned and maintained to prevent bacterial and fungal growth. Both the adult and his or her caregivers need to be properly instructed on how to clean and maintain the prosthesis. Due to their cognitive and physical limitations, many persons with ID must rely on a caregiver to carry out denture hygiene tasks, so all members of the caregiving team should be made aware of the care procedures for the dentures. Caregivers may also need instruction in placement and removal of the dentures and should be alerted to report any signs that may indicate problems in their use.

Adequate salivary flow is essential to the proper and comfortable functioning of a denture. In general, denture retention, especially with complete dentures, becomes severely compromised with the reduction of salivary flow. Decreased saliva production is a byproduct of disease, medication use, and gland damage secondary to radiation and other causes, and is often a feature of the aging process. In addition to causing decreased denture retention, xerostomic conditions may lead to fungal overgrowth, most often presenting as erythematous candidiasis.

Xerostomia and other anatomic and mechanical factors may cause dentures to easily dislodge and lead to frequent intraoral movement. Other than causing soft tissue pathology as previously discussed, this will inhibit chewing efficiency. By not being able to chew as they once did, an adult with intellectual disability may begin to reduce oral food intake, eventually leading to significant weight loss and malnutrition.

Due to the concerns over denture sores and denture-related pathology, regular follow-up by the individual's dentist should be strongly encouraged. Oral hygiene, denture hygiene and the maintenance of a caries-free and periodontally healthy mouth are all critical components of denture success.

12.5   Oral Pain

Oral and dental pain are common reasons for dental office visits by people with intellectual disability [21]. Often, the person experiencing pain is nonverbal or of limited verbal ability, and the report of pain is made by a caregiver. While objective physical signs may be present and the cause of the pain obvious (e.g., dental caries, periodontal abscess), an inability to elicit subjective signs and symptoms due to communication limitations will significantly complicate the process of reaching a diagnosis.

Pain is an important indicator of the presence of a pathological condition requiring evaluation and treatment. Many people with intellectual disability experience a diminished sensitivity to painful stimuli (such as in familial dysautonomia) or may have a high threshold to pain [22]. It is incumbent on the dentist to inquire about possible signs and symptoms of pain that might otherwise go unrecognized in this population.

12.5.1 Eliciting the Complaint

Individuals with expressive language limitations will often be unable to directly report pain. Instead, caregivers may report behavioral changes that should serve as cues to the existence of pain or discomfort. The most common behavioral changes often revolve around eating and may include: holding one side of the face; grimacing; avoidance of food (particularly those of harder consistency); eating at a slower pace than usual; and swallowing food without chewing. Caregivers may also report guarding during tooth brushing, sleep disturbances, increasingly aggressive behaviors, self-injury (particularly biting), and weight loss. Specific, targeted questions may include how long the behavior has persisted, what specific triggers there are for these behaviors, the duration of the behaviors after stimulation, and what measures lead to amelioration of symptoms [23]. Based on the responses to these questions, and in concert with clinical examination and diagnostic testing, it may be determined that the cause of the presenting signs and symptoms is oral/dental in origin. Possible odontogenic and orally-based causes of pain may include dental caries, erupting teeth, impacted teeth, periodontal infection, aphthous ulcers, sialadenitis and candidiasis. Pain may also be caused by periodontal ligament damage secondary to bruxism, as well as by temporomandibular joint disorders of multifactorial etiology.

While reported pain may be of oral or dental origin, extraoral possibilities must also be considered. Questioning and examination must explore and where possible rule out sinus concerns, ear infections, and headache. Radiating jaw pain may be indicative of acute cardiac concerns requiring immediate action. Other possible causes of pain include trigeminal neuralgia and atypical neuralgias [24]. Often, despite signs of discomfort seeming to indicate a dental or cephalic origin, the actual cause of the pain may be far removed from the head and neck region. The dentist should consider other causes of pain, including constipation and other gastrointestinal disorders, joint and bone pain, and other musculoskeletal concerns—as well as other possibilities as suggested by the individual's medical history [25].

After exhaustively ruling out possible organic origins of pain, the dentist may consider psychological causes of behaviors being interpreted as pain. Mimicry, attention-seeking behavior, manifestations of stress and depression and dementia may present as behaviors consistent with pain. If pain is suspected and no clear dental source is identified, the dentist should refer the individual to other appropriate medical professionals for further evaluation. If the individual has not previously been seen for this complaint by the primary care physician, such a referral is an obvious first step. Other suggested referrals, depending on the presenting symptoms, would include ENT, GI, neurology, orthopedic, and psychiatric services. In select cases, referral to a dental or medical pain service may be warranted.

12.5.2 Self-Injurious Behaviors (SIs)

Some adults with intellectual disability may exhibit self-injurious behaviors (SIBs) of various types [26]. While study findings differ, prevalence rates of SIBs are reported to range from 8 to 23% [27]. Several factors commonly seen in persons with intellectual disability are linked to increased SIB incidence, including decreased communication ability, limited cognitive functioning, and psychological stress. Self-injury is also a signal feature of a number of genetic disorders and medical conditions including Lesh-Nyhan syndrome, Riley-Day syndrome, Cornelia de Lange syndrome, and autism spectrum disorder.

Oral self-injury includes biting of the lips, inner cheeks, and tongue, as well as biting the arms, hand and fingers. The severity of biting may vary widely between individuals and over time. It should be noted that damage to the soft tissues may be severe, leading to pain, infection, scarring and tissue destruction. The dentist should routinely inquire as to the presence of any such behaviors and their triggers and manifestations.

Psychological and pharmacologic approaches, many times used in combination, vary in effectiveness. Often, damage to oral soft tissues can be prevented or minimized by the fabrication of oral devices such as mouthguards of various design. In more extreme cases where self-injurious behaviors cannot be controlled through other means and there is marked risk of soft tissue damage, extraction of teeth must be considered [28].

12.6   Other Common Oral Concerns

While dental caries and periodontal disease are the prevalent oral concerns faced by a majority of individuals, other conditions may exacerbate and complicate the dentist's ability to provide effective care. An individualized and comprehensive treatment plan must take into account all medical and dental diagnoses, behavioral issues, oral and craniofacial anomalies and effects of diet and medications. Among the primary concerns with which the dentist must contend are xerostomia, acid erosion of tooth structure and overgrowth of gingival tissues.

12.6.1 Xerostomia

Xerostomia, or dry mouth, results from a reduction in, or absence of, salivary flow [29]. This condition, which is often found in persons with intellectual disability, is not a disease state in and of itself. Instead, xerostomia is most commonly noted as a side effect of many types of medications [30], a side effect of head and neck radiation treatment, or as a symptom of other disease entities. Data on the prevalence of xerostomia is limited, but recently reported estimates in the general population range from 10 to 46% [29].

The most common cause of xerostomia is decreased or altered salivation as a side effect of medications. Over 400 prescription and over-the-counter (OTC) medications have been implicated as causes of hyposalivation. Antihistamines, antihypertensives, antiseizure medications, muscle relaxants, analgesics, inhaled corticosteroids and antidepressants (specifically tricyclics), which are prevalent among some adults with intellectual disability are known agents having anticholinergic effects that may increase the risk of xerostomia. Adults with intellectual disability who take multiple medications are also at an increased risk for dry mouth [30].

Adults with intellectual disability undergoing cancer chemotherapy treatment may suffer from acute toxicities to the salivary gland tissues that will lead to decreased saliva production. Often, salivary flow will return to normal sometime after the cessation of these chemotherapeutic agents. Head and neck radiation treatment, on the other hand, will often lead to permanent tissue damage causing a lifelong risk of xerostomia.

Numerous disease states have been linked to xerostomia [29]. Sjogren disease, the autoimmune condition affecting connective tissues, has long been associated with salivary gland dysfunction. Other disorders, including poorly controlled diabetes, poorly controlled hypertension, stroke, cystic fibrosis, Alzheimer's disease, and Parkinson's disease have also been associated with xerostomia.

Signs and symptoms of xerostomia include difficulty in speaking, chewing and, swallowing; alteration in taste; hoarseness, and sore throat, as well as dry, cracked lips and a dry tongue. The dental implications of xerostomia are considerable as well. Adults with intellectual disability with inadequate salivary flow will retain greater amounts of plaque, demonstrate more friable gingival and mucosal tissues, suffer from greater degrees of gingivitis and periodontitis, experience a significant increase in caries rate (particularly at the cervical and root surfaces), and be at increased risk for traumatic oral lesions and oral candidiasis [31].

12.6.2 Acid Erosion

Despite dental enamel being the hardest substance in the human body, the teeth are susceptible to the destructive effects of acid-induced erosion [32]. Acidic assault on the dentition may come from the citric and phosphoric acids in soft drinks and fruit drinks, the effects of a high-carbohydrate diet, and the reduction in pH buffering caused by xerostomia. Another major factor is the possible presence of gastroesophageal reflux disease (GERD).

GERD is a chronic digestive disorder in which weakness of the lower esophageal sphincter (LES) permits antegrade movement of acidic stomach contents into the esophagus. While there is a genetic predisposition towards acid reflux, ingestion of certain foods and beverages, as well as obesity, may also worsen the symptoms of GERD [33]. Many people with intellectual disability take one or more medications known to potentially worsen gastric reflux. These include commonly prescribed alpha, beta and calcium channel blockers; anticholinergic agents; benzodiazepines and barbiturates [34]. Untreated, GERD may result in esophagitis, esophageal ulceration and lead to Barrett's esophagus, increasing the risk of esophageal cancer. Extraesophageal manifestations of GERD include sinusitis, asthma, bronchitis, chest pain and sinus arrhythmia. Several researchers have noted links between GERD and obstructive sleep apnea (OSA) [33].

From a dental perspective, GERD and other causes of acid erosion may lead to significant loss of tooth structure, weakening the teeth, and causing an increased likelihood of breakdown. The classic dental manifestations of GERD include thinned, smooth enamel on the lingual surfaces of anterior teeth and cupping of the cusp tips of posterior teeth. When compounded with the effects of bruxism often seen in persons with intellectual disability, GERD may have a devastating effect on the adult's occlusion and result in functional and esthetic deficits [35].

12.6.3 Gingival Overgrowth

Commonly seen in persons with intellectual disability, gingival overgrowth (also referred to as gingival hyperplasia and gingival hypertrophy) may arise from a variety of causes [36]. Most commonly, this enlargement of gingival tissues is a localized or generalized response to the presence of plaque on the teeth. Systemic causes, including pregnancy and hormonal imbalances, as well as disease entities such as leukemia, may also cause this condition. Hereditary gingival fibromatosis is a rare condition causing gingival enlargement most often, but not exclusively, noted during childhood.

Medication-induced gingival hyperplasia is commonly seen among those adults with seizure disorders who may be taking phenytoin and other antiepileptic drugs; those with hypertension managed by calcium channel blockers; and post-transplant individuals prescribed the immunosuppressant cyclosporine. Partial and in some cases complete resolution of tissue overgrowth may be noted upon cessation of the medications; however, removal of excess gingival tissue (gingivectomy) is often warranted. Oral hygiene efforts reducing the amount of plaque will reduce the severity of gingival hyperplasia and slow the recurrence of tissue overgrowth following gingivectomies [37].

12.7 Providing Oral Care

12.7.1 Assessing the Medical and Behavioral Status

Dental patients with intellectual disability are often likely to demonstrate significant chronic health problems [38]. A thorough familiarity with the individual's medical history, including a list of current medications, is critical prior to initiating dental treatment. Medical conditions commonly noted include hypertension, diabetes, osteoarthritis, epilepsy, gastroesophageal reflux disease (GERD) and cardiac and pulmonary diseases. Psychiatric diagnoses may include depression and anxiety.

At the initial dental visit, a thorough medical history should be obtained, noting current and past diagnoses, details of these diagnoses including any pertinent sequelae, a listing of prior hospitalizations and surgeries, a list of all current medications (prescription, over the counter and herbal/nutritional supplements) and a list of any allergies or adverse reactions to food or drugs. Many individuals with intellectual disability report sensitivities to latex [39], a factor often relevant in dental care.

A review of the medical history may lead the dentist to consult with the person's primary care physician to clarify the history or provide further information necessary for the provision of dental care. In some cases, the dentist will find that consultation with other medical specialists active in the individual's care is necessary prior to initiating treatment. A behavioral history should be obtained, detailing the adult's past interactions with dentists and other health care providers. An understanding of the individual's specific positive and negative behavioral triggers, as well as routine daily behaviors may prove helpful. Knowledge of these factors may allow for the development of an individualized office routine and offer insights that may influence oral home care regimens.

12.7.2 The Office Visit Experience

Persons with intellectual disability will often view the dental office environment, with its unfamiliar sights, sounds, smells and personnel, as both threatening and anxiety-producing. This may lead to heightened agitation and resistance, delaying or even completely preventing the provision of needed care. Adults with intellectual disability who adapt well to consistency will often benefit from being seen at the same time of day, in the same treatment room, and by the same dental team members for each visit. The routine may also extend to the operatory environment (music, lighting, etc.) and to the routines for seating the individual and utilizing stabilization adjuncts. For those adults with higher cognitive function, acclimatization to the dental office and treatment operatory prior to the initial appointment date may prove beneficial in reducing anxiety. This may be done in-person, through the use of a "virtual office tour" or using photographs. Visiting the dental office prior to treatment may also help familiarize the individual and reduce anxiety. Anxiety during appointments may be alleviated by allowing the adult to be accompanied into the treatment area by a family member or caregiver. Often, the caregiver will be able to provide both reassurance to the adult and valuable information and assistance to the health care provider that may significantly improve the course and outcome of the visit.

Mild oral anxiolytic or sedative medications may significantly decrease anxiety and adverse behaviors in select individuals. Prior to the use of these medications, it is imperative that the prescriber be thoroughly familiar with the adult's health status and has reviewed the medical history and list of current medications and allergies. The benzodiazepines have a long history of safe and successful use in the intellectually disabled population when utilized judiciously [40]. Non-benzodiazepines may prove successful in those adults who are either allergic to or have demonstrated resistance to these drugs [41]. Nitrous oxide is a commonly used and safe agent that has a long history of use in dental practice [42]. It can be an effective adjunct to individual care, with the primary limiting factor in its use being the adult's ability to accept the presence of the mask and breathe through the nose as directed. Behavioral and/or anatomic considerations may limit the use of this anxiolytic modality of care.

Protective stabilization may be a helpful adjunct in some individuals and situations [43]. Prior to treatment, the need for and type of adjuncts to be used should be discussed with the adult's guardian and consent obtained. Devices such as mouth props to maintain oral opening can allow for improved visualization and safer access for examination and treatment. Papoose-style stabilization systems are available in pediatric and adult sizes as well, with some practitioners believing that the swaddling effect of the wrap is soothing for some individuals. Medical conditions, including pulmonary issues and osteoporosis or other musculoskeletal concerns, may contraindicate the use of these stabilization systems.

Treatment under deep sedation or general anesthesia may be appropriate for adults who have either medical or behavioral issues that preclude the safe and effective provision of dental care in the outpatient setting [44]. A thorough assessment of relevant risks and benefits must be made, in concert with medical consultation and an in-depth discussion of the process, procedures, and possible sequelae with the adult and his or her family or guardian.

The provision of dental care in the operating room setting under general anesthesia presents the opportunity for multidisciplinary care where the individual may be unable to otherwise tolerate such procedures. Coordination of services, including ENT, gynecology, podiatry and other medical specialties, while it involves significant planning, can help to increase efficiency and minimize the risks associated with multiple rounds of general anesthesia.

12.8 Oral Care at Home

The mouth is a dynamic environment that can be significantly affected by changes in diet and nutritional status. Many children and adults with intellectual disability maintain specific diets calling for the eliminations or additions of certain nutrients. These dietary modifications must be considered in an assessment of risk for dental caries and periodontal diseases. Treatment recommendations made by the dentist will also often be influenced by dietary patterns and eating habits, particularly in those instances where increased exposure to sugars is anticipated.

Diets commonly followed by persons with intellectual disability may include increases in fiber, healthy oils, vitamins, and protein. Specifically, the gluten-free, casein free (GFCF) diet and ketogenic diet offer many food choices which contain short-chain sugars. Recent literature supports the contention that diets such as GFCF may improve symptoms associated with long term gastrointestinal inflammation by alleviating the overall chronic inflammatory insult to individuals with intellectual disability [45, 46]. Although naturally-sourced, the sugars and grains present in these diets pose the same risks for dental disease as do other food choices.

Fiber is less likely to contribute to the dental disease process since these long-chain sugars are often not easily fermentable to oral bacteria. Similarly, protein, oils, and vitamins are not fermentable by bacteria and therefore pose little cariogenic risk.

Adequate water intake is essential and offers significant benefit to both systemic and oral health. Water plays a critical role in cleansing the mouth, with frequent rinsing providing one of the easiest ways to remove food debris from tooth surfaces. The oral anatomy allows for fluids to access areas that most tooth brushes cannot reach. This is particularly beneficial to those individuals who are more prone to developing very thick plaque and calculus. As adults at risk for thick plaque development may be taking medications that cause xerostomia, require constant oxygen flow or the use of CPAP, have a feeding tube, or are aggressively defiant to oral hygiene, water intake is important to the overall oral care plan.

Many adults with intellectual disability consume beverages that are acidic and high in sugar content. Over time, consumption of these drinks may place teeth at risk for acid erosion and demineralization. It is recommended that low-sugar drinks be substituted for drinks high in sugar. If it is not possible to eliminate these drinks from the diet, diluting the drinks with water can reduce the effects of the sugar.

Behavior prompting is a commonly used technique meant to elicit specific responses through verbal, auditory and tactile stimuli. In some cases, food is used as a prompt in order to maintain the individual's focus and attention. Food and drink high in sugar content is often used as a prompt for specific behaviors. Alternate food groups should be encouraged that can provide the same benefits in behavior prompting while also serving as a source for proper nutritional health. Examples of foods that may be substituted include sugar-free flavored waters or seltzer (replacing sodas, iced tea, and coffee), vegetables (in place of candy) and pretzels (in place of cookies or chips)—although consideration should be given to the salt content on pretzels.

12.8.1 Developing a Proper Home Care Regimen

The development of a proper regimen of oral home care will yield significant benefits in overall systemic health. The specific needs and challenges faced in developing such a regimen are as unique as the person with intellectual disability for whom such a regimen is being prepared. A successful home care program will be effective in removing food and plaque, maintaining the health of the hard and soft tissues of the mouth and will not prove so onerous that it cannot be maintained by either the adult or caregiver.

The standard oral hygiene maintenance program recommended by dental professionals is the mechanical removal of food particles through tooth brushing, flossing, and rinsing. Many individuals with intellectual disability will require modifications of this standard. If an individual cannot maintain an attention span or show compliant behavior sufficient to allow for all three components of this regimen, the focus should be on effective tooth brushing. For individuals with intellectual disability who can tolerate routine oral hygiene, the classic method of toothbrushing recommended by most dental professionals is known as the modified Bass technique (MBT). This approach to plaque and debris removal calls for the toothbrush bristles to angle towards the gum line, effectively cleaning both the teeth and gingival tissues [47]. While the American Dental Association recommendation is to brush twice daily, adults with special needs who are at higher risk for oral disease may benefit from brushing after each meal. For adults who will not allow or tolerate the MBT, caregivers can attempt to grossly debride tooth surfaces using towels, Toothette® oral swabs, or oral irrigation tools such as a Waterpik®.

There is a broad variety of toothbrush types easily available for purchase in pharmacies, supermarkets, and other venues. Studies have demonstrated the superiority of powered toothbrushes over manual brushes [48]. The vibrations caused by power brushes, however, may be unsettling to those adults with autism or other sensory sensitivities. For those individuals who require or prefer manual brushes, it is important to note that the brush purchased should have soft nylon bristles. These bristles are the gentlest when contacting oral hard and soft tissues, and will be least likely to produce damage. To maintain the bristles at their most effective, brushes should be changed every few months, or when the bristles begin to fray. The toothbrush should also be changed after an illness.

Dental flossing is critical in removing food and plaque from between the teeth and from the gum tissues. The ADA recommends flossing once per day. While dental floss is commonly wrapped around the fingers for use in the mouth, there are a wide variety of flossing aids available for purchase. These devices hold the floss in place and provide handles that make the floss easier to manipulate, whether it is done by the adult or a caregiver. To prevent injuring the gum tissues, it is important that the person whose teeth are being flossed remains cooperative and still throughout the procedure. If this is not the case, it may be preferable to forego flossing and devote greater attention to toothbrushing and the use of mouth rinses.

The total surface area of the mouth far exceeds the total surface area of teeth, and a proper oral care regimen will assure that the entire area is maintained. Mouth rinses offer a way to reach those areas of the mouth that are not cleaned with brushing and flossing alone [49]. There are many mouth rinse products available, each having their own directions for use. Alcohol-containing mouth rinses have dominated the marketplace for decades and while the alcohol content of these rinses is safe when used appropriately, complications can result when large quantities of these products are swallowed against manufacturer recommendations. Many non-alcoholic mouth rinses have been developed that provide comparable benefits to alcohol-containing rinses [50]. For those individuals who cannot use the mouth rinses as suggested by manufacturers, a positive effect may still be obtained by applying the mouth rinse to the gingiva with a toothbrush, Toothette® oral swabs, or even a towel. Most mouth rinses on the market are sold as over the counter (OTC) products, and these are effectively used for the vast majority of individuals. For adults with intellectual disability with advanced periodontal conditions, a prescription strength mouth rinse may prove necessary. In these cases, a 0.12% chlorhexidine gluconate rinse is prescribed for its antibacterial properties.

The dental provider must be diligent in assuring that structured recall appointments are in place to assist in maintaining adequate plaque removal. During an appointment the dental provider will need to minimize aspirants created from instrument use and will work with dental assistants to provide adequate suction. In some cases, aggressive dental therapy may not be possible, and the dental provider may be limited to using hand instruments and conservative techniques. Plaque removal is important to reduce the risk of individuals aspirating oral bacteria which may worsen existing respiratory problems. Additionally, parents, group home staff, and caregivers must be educated and counselled in oral hygiene maintenance at the adult's residence.

12.9   Fluoride and Toothpastes

Fluoride is readily available in many countries. Many communities have access to fluoridated water. Dentists and hygienists also use topical fluoride gels and varnishes after dental cleaning to help strengthen and protect the teeth. Fluoride not only has antimicrobial properties but can also remineralize areas of the tooth that are weaker and prone to damage and cavitation [51]. Many toothpastes, mouth rinses, and dental products contain fluoride. These should be used for individuals who are at risk for dental decay. Those individuals who are at a severe risk of dental decay, due to either medical issues or poor oral hygiene, may be prescribed toothpastes which have a much higher concentration of fluoride. When using these prescription strength toothpastes, the recommended dosage of fluoride should not be exceeded.

12.10   Conclusion

Many individuals with intellectual and developmental disabilities present with significant comorbidities that may impact the provision of dental care. When treating oral health, practitioners should be cognizant of these conditions and appreciate the ramifications of these conditions in treatment. As such, consultation with other health care professionals, or modification of the dental care plan, is the best course of action. Even though dental practitioners may focus on dental health, assessing bloodwork, medical test results, reports and assessments will provide a framework for greater insight into the potential medical issues necessary for consideration in the development of a dental treatment plan. In consulting with other healthcare providers, dental personnel will consider risk stratification for individuals with intellectual disability who will need invasive dental treatment. Such considerations need to include post-operative healing, bleeding control, and long-term care—and adding value to the adult's overall program plan. With aging, just as there are body changes, the oral cavity will change as well; the oral needs of these individuals must keep pace with systemic change and be part of the overall medical care plan.

References

1. Zahedi C. Treatment of orally handicapped edentulous older adults using dental implants. Dent Clin N Am. 2016;60:663–91.
2. Slade GD, Akinkugbe AA, Sanders AE. Projections of U.S. edentulism prevalence following five decades of decline. J Dent Res. 2014;93:959–65.
3. Cullinan MP, Ford PJ, Seymour GJ. Periodontal disease and systemic health: current status. Aust Dent J. 2009;54(s1):s62–9.

4. Krause M, Vainio L, Zwetchkenbaum S, Inglehart MR. Dental education about patients with special needs: a survey of U.S. and Canadian dental schools. J Dent Educ. 2010;74:1179–89.
5. Hughes MJ, Gazmararian JA. The relationship between income and oral health among people with intellectual disabilities: a global perspective. Spec Care Dentist Assoc. 2015;35:229–35.
6. Morgan JP, Minihan PM, Stark PC, Finkelman MD, Yantsides KE, Park A, Nobles CJ, Tao W, Must A. The oral health status of 4,732 adults with intellectual and developmental disabilities. J Am Dent Assoc. 2012;143:838–46.
7. Wilson NJ, Lin Z, Villarosa A, George A. Oral health status and reported oral health problems in people with intellectual disability: A literature review. J Intellect Dev Disabil. 2018;17:1–3.
8. Lockhart PB, Bolger AF, Papapanou PN, Osinbowale O, Trevisan M, Levison ME, Taubert KA, Newburger JW, Gornik HL, Gewitz MH, Wilson WR, Smith SC Jr, Baddour LM, American Heart Association Rheumatic Fever, Endocarditis, and Kawasaki Disease Committee of the Council on Cardiovascular Disease in the Young, Council on Epidemiology and Prevention, Council on Peripheral Vascular Disease, and Council on Clinical Cardiology. Periodontal disease and atherosclerotic vascular disease: does the evidence support an independent association? a scientific statement from the American Heart Association. Circulation. 2012;125:2520–44. https://doi.org/10.1161/CIR.0b013e31825719f3. Epub 2012 Apr 18
9. Rodrigues P, Reyes L, Chadda A, Belanger M, Wallet S, Akin D, Dunn W, Progulske-Fox A. Porphyromonas gingivalis strain specific interactions with human coronal artery endothelial cells: a comparative study. PLoS One. 2012;7:1–10.
10. Sessa R, Di Pietro M, Filardo S, Turriziani O. Infectious burden and atherosclerosis: a clinical issue. World J Clin Cases. 2014;2:240–9.
11. American Association of Endodontists (AAE). Antibiotic prophylaxis 2017 Update: AAE Quick Reference Guide. 2017. Accessed from: aae.org/specialty/wp-content/uploads/sites/2/2017/06/aae_antibiotic-prophylaxis-2017update.pdf.
12. Tom J. Management of patients with cardiovascular implantable electronic devices in dental, oral and maxillofacial surgery. Anesth Prog. 2016;63:95–104.
13. Mark A. For the patient: diabetes and oral health (editorial). JADA. 2016;147(10):852.
14. Taboza Z, Costa K, Silveira V, Furlaneto F, Montanegro R, Russell S, Dasanayake A, Rego R. Periodontitis, edentulism, and glycemic control in patients with type 2 diabetes: a cross-sectional study. BMJ Open Diabetes Res Care. 2018;6:e000453. https://doi.org/10.1136/bmjdrc-2017-000453.
15. Shi Q, Zhang B, Xing H, Xu J, Liu H. Patients with chronic obstructive pulmonary disease suffer from worse periodontal health - evidence from a meta-analysis. Front Physiol. 2018;9:1–12.
16. Lagos-Guimaraes H, Teive H, Celli A, Santos R, Abdulmassih E, Hirata G, Gallinea L. Aspiration pneumonia in children with cerebral palsy after videofluoroscopic swallowing study. Int Arch Otorhinolaryngol. 2016;20:132–7.
17. Caufield PW, Li Y, Dasanayake A. Dental caries: an infectious and transmissible diseases. Compend Contin Educ Dent. 2005;26(5 Suppl 1):10–6.
18. Zero DT, Fontana M, Angeles Martinez-Mier E. The biology, prevention, diagnosis and treatment of dental caries, scientific advances in the United States. J Am Dental Assoc. 2009;140:26S–34S.
19. American Academy of Periodontology (AAP). Periodontal disease fact sheet. 2017. Accessed from: https://www.perio.org/newsroom/periodontal-disease-fact-sheet
20. Ritchie CS, Kinane DF. Nutrition, inflammation, and periodontal disease. Nutrition. 2003;19:475–6.
21. Anders PL, Davis EL. Oral health of patients with intellectual disabilities: a systematic review. Spec Care Dentist. 2010;30:110–7.
22. Duerden EG, Oatley HK, Mak-Fan KM, McGrath K, Taylor P, Szatmari M, Roberts P. Risk factors associated with self-injurious behaviors in children and adolescents with autism spectrum disorders. J Autism Dev Disord. 2012;42:2460–70.
23. Herr K, Coyne PJ, McCaffrey M, Manworren R, Merkel S. Pain assessment in the patient unable to self-report: position statement with clinical practice recommendations. Pain Manag Nurs. 2011;12:230–50.

24. Scully C, Felix DH. Oral medicine—update for the dental practitioner: orofacial pain. Br Dent J. 2006;200:75–83.
25. Vogtle LK. Pain in adults with cerebral palsy: impact and solutions. Dev Med Child Neurol. 2009;51:113–21.
26. Poppes P, van der Putten AJJ, Vlaskamp C. Frequency and severity of challenging behaviour in people with profound intellectual and multiple disabilities. Res Dev Disabil. 2010;31:1269–75.
27. Cooper SA, Smiley E, Allan LM, Jackson A, Finlayson J, Mantry D, Morrison J. Adults with intellectual disabilities: prevalence, incidence and remission of self-injurious behaviour, and related factors. J Intellect Disabil Res. 2009;53:200–16.
28. Limeres J, Feijoo JF, Baluja F, Seoane JM, Diniz M, Diz P. Oral self-injury: an update. Dent Traumatol. 2013;29:8–14.
29. Hopcraft MS, Tan C. Xerostomia: an update for clinicians. Aust Dent J. 2010;55:238–44.
30. Shetty SR, Bhowmick S, Castelino R, Babu S. Drug-induced xerostomia in elderly individuals: an institutional study. Contemp Clin Dent. 2012;3:173–5.
31. Guggenheimer J, Moore PA. Xerostomia: etiology, recognition and treatment. J Am Dental Assoc. 2003;134:61–9.
32. Lussi A, Jaeggi T, Zero D. The role of diet in the aetiology of dental erosion. Caries Res. 2004;38(suppl):34–44.
33. Rosemurgy AS, Donn N, Luberice K, Ross SB. Gastroesophageal reflux disease. Surg Clin North Am. 2011;91:1015–29.
34. DeVault KR, Castell DO. Updated guidelines for the diagnosis and treatment of gastroesophageal reflux disease. Am J Gastroenterol. 2005;100:190–200.
35. Barron RP, Carmichael RP, Marcon MA, Sandor GK. Dental erosion in gastroesophageal reflux disease. J Can Dent Assoc. 2003;69:84–9.
36. Doufexi A, Mina M, Ioannidou E. Gingival overgrowth in children: epidemiology, pathogenesis and complications: a literature review. J Periodontol. 2005;76:3–10.
37. Mavrogiannis M, Ellis JS, Thomason JM, Seymour RA. The management of drug-induced gingival overgrowth. J Clin Periodontol. 2006;33:434–9.
38. Oeseburg B, Dijkstra GJ, Groothoff JW, Reijneveld SA, Jansen DE. Prevalence of chronic health conditions in children with intellectual disability: a systematic literature review. Intellect Dev Disabil. 2011;49:59–85.
39. Peixhino C, Tavares-Ratado P, Tomas MR, Taborda-Barata L, Tomaz CT. Latex allergy: new insights to explain different sensitization profiles in different risk groups. Br J Dermatol. 2008;159:132–6.
40. Ogle OE, Hertz MB. Anxiety control in the dental patient. Dent Clin N Am. 2012;56:1–16.
41. Donaldson M, Gizzarelli G, Chanpong B. Oral sedation: a primer on anxiolysis for the adult patient. Anesth Prog. 2007;54:118–29.
42. American Academy of Pediatric Dentistry (AAPD) Council on Clinical Affairs. Guideline on appropriate use of nitrous oxide for pediatric dental patients. [Clinical Practice Guidelines: Reference Manual, 37(6)]. Pediatric Dent. 2013;30(7 supp):140–2. 2008-2009. Accessed from http://www.aapd.org/media/policies_guidelines/g_nitrous.pdf
43. Romer M. Consent, restraint, and people with special needs: a review. Spec Care Dentist J. 2009;29:58–66.
44. Dougherty N. The dental patient with special needs: a review of indications for treatment under general anesthesia. Spec Care Dentist. 2009;29:17–20.
45. Lira-Junior R, Figueredo CM. Periodontal and inflammatory bowel disease: is there evidence of complex pathogenic interactions? World J Gastroenterol. 2016;22(35):7963–72.
46. Niland B, Cash B. Health benefits and adverse effects of a gluten-free diet in non-celiac disease patients. Gastroenterol Hepatol. 2018;14:82–91.
47. Schleuter N, Klimek J, Saleschke G, Ganss C. Adoption of a toothbrushing technique: a controlled, randomized clinical trial. Clin Oral Investig. 2010;14:99–106.
48. Kurtz B, Reise M, Klukowska M, Grender J, Sigusch BW. A randomized clinical trial comparing plaque removal efficacy of an oscillating-rotating power toothbrush to a manual toothbrush by multiple examiners. Int J Dent Hyg. 2016;14:278–83.

49. Araujo M, Charles C, Weinstein R, McGuire J, Parikh-Das A, Du Q, Zhang J, Berlin J, Gunsoly J. Meta-analysis of the effect of an essential oil-containing mouthrinse on gingivitis and plaque. J Am Dent Assoc. 2015;146:6110–622.
50. Marchetti E, Tecco S, Caterini E, Casalena F, Quinzi V, Mattei A, Marzo G. Alcohol-free essential oils containing mouthrinse efficacy on three-day supragingival plaque regrowth: a randomized crossover clinical trial. Trials. 2017;18:1–8.
51. Thurnheer T, Belibasakis GN. Effect of sodium fluoride on oral biofilm microbiota and enamel demineralization. Arch Oral Biol. 2018;89:77–83.

Nutrition and Physical Health

13

Dawna Torres Mughal

13.1 Introduction

Diet and nutrition are important to the health of adults with intellectual disability throughout their life course. Foods and nutrition, however, cannot effectively work alone; they should be viewed in a holistic framework among other factors that together influence health, especially the health of persons with complex diet-related needs. Framing food and nutrition issues in people's social context and environment can help service providers better realize that optimal nutrition care goes beyond providing food but rather requires a multifactorial approach [1] and systems solution. This framework serves as a context for discussing the nutrients and their applications to individuals with intellectual disability and their families and other caregivers.

This chapter covers select nutrients, their key functions, recommended intakes, deficiencies and excesses and major food sources, highlighting principles relevant to persons with intellectual disability. The nutrients include protein, carbohydrates, lipids, water, fat-soluble vitamins (vitamins A, D, E and K), water-soluble vitamins (vitamins C, B-12 and folate) and minerals (calcium, iron, and iodine). While knowledge of these nutrients contributes to food choices, it is insufficient to drive changes in eating behavior which is complex and influenced by physiological, psychosocial, emotional, environmental, and cultural factors [2]. The literature describes various behavior-oriented models for facilitating behavior changes. Guiding adults with intellectual disability and their families change behaviors is not just giving information and expect them to heed and use the advice [2]. Theory guides practice. Interventions can be more effective if they are grounded in theories that deal with health-related behaviors [3]. Theoretical models and constructs chosen should be relevant to the needs and goals of the intervention in a given practice

D. T. Mughal (✉)
Gannon University, Erie, PA, USA
e-mail: MUGHAL001@gannon.edu

© Springer Nature Switzerland AG 2019
V. P. Prasher, M. P. Janicki (eds.), *Physical Health of Adults with Intellectual and Developmental Disabilities*, https://doi.org/10.1007/978-3-319-90083-4_13

setting. A model can be eclectic, combining features of different theories to guide the intervention in a more systematic and holistic way [4]. Using appropriate theory-guided behavior-oriented strategies, providers can guide individuals or groups translate nutrients to a healthy flexible eating pattern that meets their preferences and needs.

Mindful of the social context, dietary guidelines emphasize healthy eating patterns, the total diet, consisting of a variety of foods and not individual nutrient or food or meal [5]. When we teach adults with intellectual disability skills in food selection and preparation, they may think more about "This food tastes good. I like it. It's good for me." Taste comes first as studies have shown that many people choose food primarily for the taste and not for nutrition. Cost is the second most important reason. Time, convenience and marketing (advertisements in various media) and the environment affect food choices as well [2]. However, delicious and affordable foods that meet an individual's personal and cultural preferences and a positive eating experience are a practical tool for teaching healthy food choices and their contribution to the person's health goals.

13.2 Select Diet-Related Characteristics of Individuals with Intellectual Disability

Adults with intellectual disability are a nutritionally vulnerable group. Feeding problems, poor oral health, polypharmacy and drug-nutrient interactions, metabolic disorders, decreased mobility, gastrointestinal problems and altered growth patterns affect food intake and put these individuals at risk for malnutrition [6]. Table 13.1 shows select nutrition problems that are often associated with certain conditions of intellectual disability and that can contribute to malnutrition [6] (Chap. 14 discusses these in more detail). Reports have noted that as more people with intellectual disability live longer, they are likely to develop the same disabling chronic diseases (see Table 13.2) which are prevalent in the general aging population [6–9]. Superimposing the syndrome-specific morbidity and other concurrent illnesses on the age-related physiologic and physical changes magnifies the risk for malnutrition and its secondary health problems. Achieving and maintaining good nutritional health poses a challenge because adults with intellectual disability have conditions that can interfere with eating a balanced diet and maintaining proper nutrition. Malnutrition is preventable. Timely nutrition screening can identify persons who are at risk for malnutrition and who can benefit from nutrition assessment and intervention or medical nutrition therapy. Nutrition assessment is a systematic process that collects and evaluates anthropometric measurements, laboratory values, nutrition-focused physical examination data, dietary and other relevant information. Person-centered, it is designed to identify the problems, develop a nutrition care plan and implement it, monitor the person, and evaluate the effectiveness of the plan in achieving therapeutic goals [6].

Table 13.1 Common nutrition-related issues in individuals with intellectual disabilities

Syndrome or developmental disability and list of resources	Nutrition diagnosis	Etiology and/or signs and symptoms
Autism spectrum disorder (ASD) ASD is a developmental disorder that affects communication and behavior. Autism spectrum disorder https://www.nimh.nih.gov/health/topics/autism-spectrum-disorders-asd/index.shtml	Inadequate energy intake	Inadequate food intake Medication side effects affecting appetite
	Limited food acceptance	Sensory processing issues Avoidance of foods/food groups
	Inadequate intake of calcium/vitamin D/iron and other nutrients	Limited food choices, avoidance of foods/food groups Complementary and alternative medicine treatment such as vitamin B-6 supplements, following a gluten-free, casein-free diet may place a child at risk for nutritional deficiencies
	Overweight	BMI >85th percentile for children aged age 2–20 years Use of food for behavioral intervention Estimated excessive energy intake Medication side effects affecting appetite Sedentary activity level Limited food choices that are excessive in calories
Cerebral palsy https://www.ninds.nih.gov/Disorders/Patient-Caregiver-Education/Hope-Through-Research/Cerebral-Palsy-Hope-Through-Research	Increased energy expenditure	Unintended weight loss
	Excessive energy intake	Increased body adiposity Reduced energy intake secondary to treatment with medication to decrease muscle tone Hypotonia Changes in mobility status Feeding/diet provides more calories than estimated energy requirement

(continued)

Table 13.1 (continued)

Syndrome or developmental disability and list of resources	Nutrition diagnosis	Etiology and/or signs and symptoms
	Inadequate oral intake	Unintended weight loss Inability to self-feed lack of coordination Poor dentition, presence of cavities or abscesses Gastroesophageal reflux disease Oral motor dysfunction/dysphagia Medications affecting appetite Failure to thrive Malnutrition
	Inadequate fluid and fiber intake	Constipation Inability to consume fluid and food independently Dysphagia altered taste perception, inability to communicate thirst
		Abnormal swallow study showing aspiration and/or oral/pharyngeal dysphagia Coughing, choking, prolonged chewing, pocketing of food, regurgitating, and facial expression changes during eating Reduced food intake Unintended weight loss Prolonged feeding times, lack of interest in food, food avoidance, mealtime resistance
	Food medication interactions	Constipation related to antispasticity medications Increased risk of osteopenia/osteoporosis related to antiseizure and antigastroesophageal reflux disease medications Risk of B-12 deficiency related to antigastroesophageal reflux disease medications
Cystic fibrosis https://ghr.nlm.nih.gov/condition/cystic-fibrosis https://rarediseases.org/rare-diseases/cystic-fibrosis/	Increased energy expenditure	Unintended weight loss Malnutrition
	Inadequate fat-soluble vitamin intake	Reduced vitamin levels

Table 13.1 (continued)

Syndrome or developmental disability and list of resources	Nutrition diagnosis	Etiology and/or signs and symptoms
	Altered GI function	Abnormal digestive enzyme and fecal fat studies Growth stunting or failure Evidence of vitamin and/or mineral deficiency Steatorrhea Constipation Gastroesophageal reflux disease
Down syndrome https://www.ndss.org/ about-down-syndrome/ down-syndrome/ https://www.cdc.gov/ncbddd/ birthdefects/downsyndrome. html	Inadequate oral intake	Dementia Swallowing difficulty Unintended weight loss
	Breastfeeding difficultly	Feeding difficulty with weak suck Poor weight gain
	Altered GI function	Feeding difficulty with weak suck Poor weight gain
	Overweight/obesity	Increased body adiposity Estimated excessive energy intake Reduced energy needs related to hypotonia BMI >85th percentile/age for age 2–20 years
Genetic disorder that results in a deficiency or defective enzyme action in a metabolic pathway: Phenylketonuria https://ghr.nlm.nih.gov/ condition/phenylketonuria https://rarediseases.org/ rare-diseases/phenylketonuria/ https://www.genome. gov/25020037/ learning-about- phenylketonuria/	Imbalance of nutrients Impaired nutrient utilization Altered nutrition related laboratory values	Food and nutrition knowledge deficit of dietary changes related to new diagnosis Nutrient restriction due to metabolic disorder
	Unintended weight loss	Poor appetite due to metabolic disorder Inadequate energy intake Lack of adequate insurance coverage for low protein foods/ special metabolic formulas, limited access to formula Food and nutrition knowledge deficit of dietary changes related to new diagnosis

(continued)

Table 13.1 (continued)

Syndrome or developmental disability and list of resources	Nutrition diagnosis	Etiology and/or signs and symptoms
Prader-Willi syndrome https://ghr.nlm.nih.gov/ condition/ prader-willi-syndrome https://rarediseases.org/ rare-diseases/ prader-willi-syndrome/ http://pwsaofwi.org/ wp-content/uploads/2014/10/ Nutritional-Strategies-in-the-Management-of-PWS-HANDOUT.pdf	Breastfeeding difficulty Inadequate oral intake	Feeding difficulty with weak suck Poor weight gain
	Excessive energy intake Overweight/obesity	Increased body adiposity BMI >85th percentile/age at age 2–20 years Reduced energy needs Self-monitoring deficit
	Limited adherence to nutrition-related recommendations	Inability to limit or refuse foods offered Lack of social support for Implementing changes
	Undesirable food choices	Intake inconsistent with diet quality guidelines Unable to independently select foods consistent with food quality and energy controlled guidelines
	Intake of unsafe food	Food obsession Hyperphagia Eating serves a purpose other than nourishment Pica
Spina bifida (myelomeningocele) https://www.cdc.gov/ncbddd/ spinabifida/facts.html https://www.ninds.nih.gov/ Disorders/Patient-Caregiver-Education/Fact-Sheets/ Spina-Bifida-Fact-Sheet https://www.nchpad. org/777/4145/Nutrition~Spotli ght~~~Nutritional~Considerati ons~for~Adults~with~Spina~B ifida	Increased protein needs	Chronic, nonhealing wounds

Table 13.1   (continued)

Syndrome or developmental disability and list of resources	Nutrition diagnosis	Etiology and/or signs and symptoms
	Swallowing difficulty	Abnormal swallow study showing aspiration and/or oral/pharyngeal dysphagia Frequent respiratory infections/ pneumonias Coughing/choking with foods/ liquids Presence of Arnold Chiari II malformation of the brain
	Altered GI function	Low fluid and fiber intake Neurogenic bowel Constipation
	Overweight/obesity Unintended weight gain	Increased body adiposity BMI >85th percentile/age for age 2–20 years Estimated excessive energy intake Self-monitoring deficit Limited mobility Reduced energy needs related to altered body composition, short stature

This article was published in the Journal of the Academy of Nutrition and Dietetics, Vol 115, Ptomey LT & Wittenbrook W, Position of the Academy of Nutrition and Dietetics: Nutrition Services for Individuals with Intellectual and Developmental Disabilities and Special Health Care Needs. Pages 593–608, copyright The Academy of Nutrition and Dietetics (2015)
Used with permission Copyright Elsevier

    The nutrients that adults with intellectual disability need are the same as those of the general population. The amounts and the dietary composition vary with individual needs. Nutrition-related problems frequently observed in certain disabilities (see Tables 13.1 and 13.2) require individualization of energy and nutrient requirements and dietary modifications. For adults with intellectual disability who live at home and depend on their family or other caregivers, nutrition education of their caregivers is critical to ensure that caregivers know how to meet the adult's nutritional needs that will likely change over time.

13.3   Macronutrients: Carbohydrate, Protein and Lipid

The energy-yielding macronutrients (carbohydrate, protein, and lipid) not only yield energy (through ATP), but also perform other vital biological functions. To a certain extent, they are interconvertible in their integrated metabolism so that glucose can be formed from protein and vice versa. For example, if calorie intake is inadequate to meet a person's needs, the body will catabolize protein to yield

Table 13.2 Health issues of individuals with intellectual disabilities and underutilized health promotion programs

Cardiovascular	Endocrine	Gastrointestinal	Musculoskeletal	Pulmonary
Cerebral hemorrhage	Diabetes, type 1 and type 2	Constipation	Osteoarthritis	Asthma
Heart attack	Hyper/ hypothyroidism	Gastric/duodenal ulcer	Osteoporosis	Chronic bronchitis
Hypertension	Obesity	Gastroesophageal reflux disease		Emphysema
Stroke	Thyroid problems	Stomach/ gallbladder Some type of cancer		

Other health issues

Addiction	Sensory
Aging-related issues	Vision/cataracts
Epilepsy	Hearing difficulty
Mental health problems	Dental health
Migraines/frequent headaches	Tumor, malignant
Poor nutrition	

Underutilized preventive programs for health promotion

Health education/information

Health promotion programs: Healthy eating, weight reduction, physical activity, and exercise classes

Health screening programs: Health checks, *Helicobacter pylori* screening, sexual health (e.g., contraception), women's health (e.g., breast and cervical cancer screening), men's health (e.g., testicular cancer screening), and dementia screening

Data from: Davis et al. [7] and Haveman et al. [8]

glucose for energy. Energy production, however, is not the primary function of protein. In fact, carbohydrate and lipid, the main energy sources, protect it from being used up for energy. Excess carbohydrate (glucose) and protein above the body's needs are converted to fat and stored in the fat depot. The body will catabolize the stored fat for energy when needed; however, because lipids (triglycerides) produce only a small amount of glucose from the glycerol part of the triglycerides and the fatty acids cannot be used to form glucose, they cannot correct hypoglycemia. Certain molecules from carbohydrate oxidation can be used to synthesize amino acids, the building blocks of protein [10]. It is helpful to think of the metabolic events that occur when the body is feasting or fasting and of energy balance that prevents chronic feasting or fasting and their consequences. Uncontrolled diabetes mellitus illustrates this important concept of integrated metabolism. Impaired carbohydrate metabolism, due to absolute or relative insulin lack, accelerates fat and protein catabolism to provide glucose (from protein, not from fat) for energy when the body cannot properly use carbohydrates. Starvation and low-calorie diet illustrate the same concept [10]— see Chap. 14, this text, on malnutrition.

13.3.1 Proteins

Proteins are made up of amino acids as building blocks linked in a chain and have variable structures, shapes, and physiological functions. They are distributed throughout the body and are essential to life. The name protein was derived from the Greek word "Proteos" which means "primary" or "taking first place" and which aptly describes the critical importance of protein to life [11].

Functions. Although they reside largely in the skeletal muscles, proteins perform many other functions and are therefore called the "body's worker molecules" [12]. They function as enzymes; hormones; structural parts of bones; antibodies for warding off infection; transporters of fats, other nutrients and medications in circulation; carrier of oxygen in the red blood cells; and fluid and pH balance regulator. They also provide materials for the synthesis of RNA and DNA and other nitrogen-containing molecules such as creatine, choline, serotonin, and carnitine. As an alternate energy source, they provide 4 kcal/g [10–12].

Recommmended intake. The recommended dietary allowance (RDA) for healthy adults is 0.8 g/kg/day. The acceptable macronutrient distribution range (AMDR) is 10–35% of the day's calories, which accommodates variations in protein intake. Growth, pregnancy and lactation; hypermetabolic conditions like fever, infection, injury, burns, fractures, and cancer; inadequate calorie intake; and low protein quality and digestibility increase need [10, 13]. It is important for adults with intellectual disability (ID), especially as they age, to meet their protein needs. Protein deficiency and malnutrition increase susceptibility to infection, delay wound healing, impair function, increase hospital admissions and health care costs and lessen quality of life [14]. It is helpful to remember that protein and energy are linked together; i.e., insufficient calorie intake induces protein breakdown for energy and diverts it from its vital primary functions [10].

Some experts assessed the RDA as insufficient for older adults and recommended 1.0 g/kg [15], 1.0–1.5 g/kg for treating sarcopenia [16] and 1.0–1.3 g/kg, combined with weekly (two times) progressive resistance exercise [17]. Sarcopenia, which is an age-associated progressive loss of skeletal muscle mass and function, is prevalent in older adults. Fat infiltrates the muscles reducing muscle quality [18]. Some people gain fat while losing muscles. This condition known as sarcopenic obesity has worse outcomes than sarcopenia alone [16]. Muscle wasting leads to frailty, impaired activities of daily living, falls, fractures, hospitalizations and mortality [19, 20]. As a survey reported, the prevalence of sarcopenia in adults with intellectual disability (N = 884, age 54 years plus) was 14.3% and sarcopenia was positively associated with mobility impairment and inflammation and negatively associated with body mass index (BMI) [21]. Progress has been made to better define, recognize, and diagnose sarcopenia using various screening and diagnostic tools. A short questionnaire (SARC-F) has been developed and validated as a quick screening tool [18]. Older adults with intellectual disability who have risk factors for sarcopenia can benefit from timely screening and intervention. Many have the risk factors such as impaired mobility, lack of physical activity, poor diet, low BMI (although obese individuals may have sarcopenic obesity), and chronic conditions that can contribute to sarcopenia. In September 2016 sarcopenia was given an ICD-10-CM (M62.84) code recognizing it as a disease entity. This should lead to more improvement in clinicians' awareness and interests in the disease, screening and diagnostic tools, prevention and treatment, and outcomes for adults with intellectual disability [22]. Current treatment consists of adequate energy and protein intake (supplementation if needed), leucine-enriched essential amino acids, adequate vitamin D status, and resistance exercise [16, 18].

Food sources. It is helpful to choose, as much as possible, high-biologic value proteins that include meat, poultry, fish and sea foods, eggs, soybeans and the milk group. Lean proteins are recommended [5]. Plant proteins have lower biological value compared to animal-derived proteins. Vegans and vegetarians should eat a variety of plant proteins, including nuts and seeds, to improve the quality of their protein mix [23]. Information on protein food sources is available at https://www.choosemyplate.gov/protein-foods.

13.3.2 Carbohydrates

Carbohydrates include complex carbohydrates (starches, glycogen and dietary fibers) and simple carbohydrates (sugars intrinsic in foods, such as fructose in fruits and lactose in milk, and sugars added to foods) [24]. Simple sugars are made up of one or two single sugar units and complex carbohydrates are made up of many sugar units. Select examples of simple sugars include the monosaccharides glucose and fructose and the disaccharides sucrose (table sugar) and lactose. Select examples of complex carbohydrates include starch (stored in plants for energy) and glycogen (stored in animal liver and skeletal muscles) [25]. Starch, a long chain of glucose units, yields glucose when completely digested. Glycogen, via glycogenolysis, yields glucose to raise blood glucose level when needed [25]. Carbohydrates provide the largest proportion of the calories in the diet. Majority of the carbohydrates consumed consist of starch, sucrose, and lactose [24].

Functions. Carbohydrate has various physiological functions and diverse uses in the food industry and in home cooking. As the body's chief energy source, it provides 4 kcal/g and energy (from ATP) to the cells for cellular metabolic processes. Quickly absorbed, glucose from foods is important for maintaining normal blood glucose level and supporting the brain's energy needs [24], although the brain can adapt to lower levels by using ketones during prolonged fasting or starvation [25]. The brain is the only organ that is truly glucose-dependent but it is fully capable of using ketones for energy [13]. In addition to sparing protein from being used for energy, carbohydrates also promote the complete oxidation of lipids, preventing the formation of ketones, which are intermediate products of lipid oxidation. Ketones can accumulate in the blood leading to ketonemia and ketosis. A low-carbohydrate diet, starvation, and uncontrolled diabetes mellitus cause breakdown of lipids and protein for energy and ketone formation. In type 1 diabetes mellitus, metabolic acidosis is one of the serious short-term complications which should be treated promptly [11].

Although an integration of the metabolism of carbohydrates, protein, and lipids occurs, carbohydrates can follow different metabolic pathways depending on the body's physiological needs. Note the physiological reactions in feasting or fasting states. Hormones (insulin, glucagon, epinephrine, and glucocorticosteroids), enzyme systems, and integrated metabolism play an important regulatory role. The B vitamins (thiamin, riboflavin, niacin and pantothenic acid) and proteins, as enzymes, assist in carbohydrate metabolism and energy production. This illustrates the collaboration among the nutrients in a system [11]. The body aims to maintain normoglycemia [11] because either hypoglycemia or hyperglycemia perturbs normal body functions. Hormonal imbalance is disruptive as seen in the consequences of hyperglycemia in poorly controlled diabetes mellitus. It is helpful to remember that impaired carbohydrate metabolism adversely affects protein and lipid metabolism [11]. Adults with intellectual disability, because of their exposure to risk factors (obesity, physical inactivity, and unhealthy diet), are predisposed to developing type 2 diabetes mellitus [6]. Taggart and his colleagues [26] indicated that many of the respondents to their survey had poor diabetes control and that the standards of care were not followed. Receiving proper treatment and management can prevent or at least delay the long-term microvascular and macrovascular complications of diabetes including heart disease and stroke [27] which are risk factors for dementia [28].

Recommended intake. The RDA for healthy adults is 130 g/day which is the minimum amount to provide glucose for the brain. The AMDR is 45–65% of the day's total calories, giving individuals flexibility in planning their diet [13, 25]. It is helpful to visualize the plate ½ of which is filled with colorful vegetables and fruits and about ¼ with grains. Legumes (beans, peas, and lentils) also provide protein; milk supplies not only lactose but also calcium and high-quality protein [29]. Complex carbohydrates (grains, legumes and vegetables) are recommended because they provide fiber and other nutrients. At least half of the grain selections should be whole grains and whole fruits are recommended over juices [5]. Added sugars (sweeteners and syrups) should be limited to 10% of the day's calories as they add energy with no or few nutrients [5]. Other ingredients to consider are available at https://www.choosemyplate.gov/other-ingredients-consider. Additional information on the grain group is available at https://www.choosemyplate.gov/grains.

13.3.3 Dietary Fiber

Fiber is a group of heterogeneous molecules that have diverse chemical composition, structure and physiological effects. Although they are nondigestible to humans, their physiological actions in the gastrointestinal tract confer health benefits [13]. Despite the campaign to eat more fiber-rich foods, "fiber gap" is prevalent globally as most people's fiber intakes are far below the recommended amount [5, 30–32]. It affects children in many countries, causing chronic constipation [31]. Low consumption of fruits and vegetables (including legumes) and whole grains and the differences in the definition of dietary fibers in various countries contribute to the fiber gap. Because of the health benefits of these food groups and of fiber, fiber gap poses a public health concern [5]. People with intellectual disability have barriers to eating healthy foods, including fruits and vegetables which affect fiber intake [33]. To address this gap, in 2009 CODEX published its comprehensive definition of dietary fiber, aiming for worldwide acceptance by member countries. Since then several countries have adopted the definition which acknowledges the role of both intrinsic fiber and fiber added to foods in the context of "all fibers fit" [31].

Recommended intake. The Adequate Intake (AI) for healthy adults is 14 g/1000 calories per day or 38 g and 25 g for men and women, respectively. Since it is based on calorie needs, people with intellectual disability who need more or fewer than 2000 calories can adjust their fiber intake [13]. When enjoyed as a family affair, eating more vegetables, fruits, and whole grains can encourage them to eat more of these wholesome foods. A helpful guide to remember is that in the food groups, only the vegetables; fruits; grains (especially whole grains); and legumes, nuts and seeds (protein group) contain dietary fiber. Whole fruits and vegetables are better than juices [29]. Fiber supplements do not provide the nutrients that fiber-rich foods deliver [34]. It is better to eat real food to fill the fiber gap. Additional information on food sources of dietary fiber is also available at https://health.gov/dietaryguidelines/2015/guidelines/appendix-13/.

Functions. Various articles have been published describing the types of fiber, their food sources, and physiological functions. Reported health benefits relate to weight management, diabetes mellitus control, blood lipid reduction in cardiovascular diseases and gastrointestinal disorders. Refer to these extensive reviews for details [30, 32, 34–42].

Constipation is prevalent among adults with intellectual disability, especially among those with profound intellectual disability and cerebral palsy. Immobility, poor diet, lack of physical activity and use of antipsychotics and anticonvulsant are contributory factors [43, 44], Constipation is also prevalent in older adults in the general population [45, 46]. The complications of chronic constipation are serious and can adversely affect quality of life. Individuals with intellectual disability who cannot verbally communicate their pain and discomfort may express them through behavioral changes and aggression [44]. A thorough assessment to identify the causes can help determine the intervention which often includes lifestyle modifications (more fiber- rich foods and fluid, regular toileting schedule, and physical activity). They should increase fiber gradually to prevent any adverse gastrointestinal effects [45]. If they need fiber supplement, it is important to know the appropriate supplement to use as dietary fibers behave differently in the gut which affects the therapeutic outcomes [38].

Consumers need more education on food sources and fiber content of foods [31]. Clear and relevant messages about the amount of fiber to eat; use of nutrition facts panel information; practical ways for increasing intake of fruits, vegetables, and whole grains; and focus on food and flavor rather than on fiber per se can reduce consumers' confusion [47]. Health literacy, cognitive and functioning ability, needs and resources of adults with intellectual disability and their families should be considered in planning an educational conversation with them.

13.3.4 Lipids

Lipids include diverse compounds whose structures and physiological functions range from relatively simple short-chain fatty acids to more complex structures. For example, the group includes fatty acids, triglycerides, phospholipids, cholesterol, fat-soluble vitamins, corticosteroid hormones and lipoproteins [11]. Lipids in foods include fats and oils. Fats are solid at room temperature and oils are liquid. Solid fats are high in saturated fats while oils are high in unsaturated with exceptions (coconut, palm, and palm kernel oils). Fats are" invisible", hidden in many foods (e.g. Avocado, nuts and seeds, dairy products, baked products, and many others), or are "visible", easily seen and identified (e.g. butter, cream cheese, lard, margarine, oils, salad dressings and shortening) [48]. Consumers are often advised to "watch out" for the invisible fats. It takes great effort even for those who use food labels to ascertain the amount of fats hidden in foods.

Functions. Lipids are a multipurpose nutrient. As a concentrated source of calories (9 kcal/g), they can boost energy intake of underweight adults with intellectual disability who need to gain weight; they store energy reserve, cushion vital organs, transport fat-soluble vitamins, provide essential fatty acids, and protect protein from being catabolized for energy [13, 49, 50]. Additionally, cholesterol is a precursor of vitamin D and bile acids. Bile acids aid in lipid digestion [11]. In cooking, lipids contribute to the sensory appeal of foods [13] and can enhance people's enjoyment of their meals.

Lipids have been demonized as a nutrient to avoid; however, they have a place in a healthy eating pattern. People who strictly limit their fat intake consequently limit their fat-soluble vitamin intake. The key message to the public is around total diet quality that includes a variety of foods and energy intake that is balanced with physical activity to maintain healthy weight. It does not set a specific limit for total fat intake as this can vary widely within a person's estimated energy requirement. It does recommend that, because of their established adverse health effects, saturated fats should be limited to 10% of the day's calories [5]. There is no RDA for lipids. The AMDR (20–35% of the day's calories) offers flexibility in the amount of dietary fat but also controls excess fat or carbohydrate [13].

Confusion about lipids, with unintended consequences, is so widespread [51] that it is worth a deep dive if space in this chapter allows. Given the nutrition confusion among consumers [51, 52], nutrition education is critical to persons with intellectual disability and their families. Nutrition science is complex and the media tend to report research in sound bites which, out of context, can be misinterpreted. It is best to seek information from qualified professionals. Results of a survey indicated that instead of seeking qualified professionals, majority of the responders rely on their friends and families for at least a little for both nutrition and food safety information, but yet only 29% of them have high trust in these sources [52].

Omega-polyunsaturated fatty acids. The omega-3 and omega-6 fatty acids have been hot topics in nutrition. The discussion here oversimplifies the complex biochemistry of lipids and focuses primarily on their select features, using as examples the families of omega-3 and omega-6 polyunsaturated fatty acids (PUFAs). These PUFAs, because of their health claims, have attracted all-around interest. This section briefly describes their structure, conversion of the precursors to the more unsaturated fatty acids within their respective family, and select health benefits and food sources.

Linoleic acid (LA), an omega-6 or n-6 PUFA, and alpha –linolenic acid (ALA), an omega-3 or n-3 PUFA, are essential fatty acids because the body cannot synthesize them and must obtain them from the diet. They are precursors for the other long-chain PUFA within their respective family. They occur as triglycerides in foods [50]. From here on, the terms n-6 PUFA and n-3 PUFA will be used.

An n-3 PUFA is made up of a long chain of carbon atoms (18–22) that has a certain number of double bonds in specific positions, a methyl group at the terminal carbon (or omega) and carboxylic acid group head at the other end. The number of carbon-to-carbon double bonds indicates the degree of unsaturation. Saturated fats have no double bond, monounsaturates and polyunsaturates have one and more than one double bonds, respectively. The first double bond is between carbon atoms 3 and 4 from the methyl end, thus omega-3 [11]. It is important to note that the structure, chain length, and degree of unsaturation affect the performance of lipids in cooking and their physiological role. The n-3 family includes alpha-linolenic (ALA), eicosapentaenoic acid (EPA) and docosahexaenoic acid (DHA). ALA has 18 carbons and 3 double bonds; EPA, 20 carbons and 5 double bonds; and DHA, 22 carbons and 6 double bonds [50, 53]. ALA, found in plants, is the parent n-3 PUFA which the body converts to EPA and DHA by lengthening and desaturating the carbon chain. This conversion, however, is low [50, 53] and is slowed down by transfats [54] and an excessive amount of linoleic acid (LA) [54, 55].

Linoleic acid (LA), an n-6 PUFA with 18 carbon atoms and 2 double bonds, is the parent PUFA in the omega-6 family. The first double bond is between carbon atoms 6 and 7 from the methyl end, and thus omega 6. The body can convert it to arachidonic acid (ARA), which has 20 carbon atoms and 4 double bonds [50, 54]. ARA is an important part of cell structures, including the brain [56] and can be converted to various physiologically hormone-like molecules that affect many organs and tissues. Certain metabolic products are pro-inflammatory and can cause inflammation [55] and others help in the resolution of the inflammation [56].

Health benefits. EPA and DHA have been shown to have anti-inflammatory properties and can benefit some people with rheumatoid arthritis [50, 53]. They can also help lower fasting hypertriglyceridemia and contribute to normal blood triglyceride level maintenance thereby reducing risk for cardiovascular disease [50, 57]. DHA's contribution to normal brain function and vision is supported by evidence [58, 59]. A different analysis, however, showed that the favorable association with cognitive ability measures is inconsistent and needs further study [50]. Because the n-6 to n-3 ratio has received conflicting perceptions and "anti-inflammatory diets" seem to have evolved from it, it is worth discussing here. Experts have noted that the ratio of n-6 (linoleic) to n-3 (alpha-linolenic) is important because excessive n-6 can interfere with the conversion of ALA to EPA and DHA. The imbalance can not only reduce the EPA and DHA formed but also increase the proinflammatory substances in an over reactive "arachidonic cascade". The excessive n-6 hormones can cause inflammation, cardiovascular diseases, thrombosis and a host of other disorders. Increased EPA and DHA can moderate this cascade [54, 55]. The Western diet's ratio of linoleic/alpha-linolenic, which is between 10:1 and 20:1, is too high for good health and should be reduced to 2:1 or 1:1 [54].

The adequate intakes (AIs) for LA for men, aged 19 to 50 years and 51 to >70, are 17 g/day and 14 g/day, respectively. For women in the same age groups, the AIs are 12 g/day and 11 g/day, respectively. Regarding the ALA, the AIs for men and women, aged 19 to >70 years, are 1.6 g/day and 1.1 g/day, respectively [13]. A lower n-6/n-3 ratio can be anti-inflammatory. However, other experts noted no rationale for a specific ratio as long as the LA and ALA intakes are within the recommended amount [60]. It is important to note also that cardiovascular and other chronic diseases have multifactorial etiology and not this ratio or lipids alone. In the context of a balanced diet, people can eat less omega-6-rich oils like corn, sunflower, safflower, cottonseed, and soybean and more omega-3-rich oils like canola, flax seed, perilla and chia [54]. Walnuts, dried chia seeds, and ground flax seeds are also good sources [61]. Because the conversion of ALA to EPA and DHA is low, consuming at least two servings (1 serving = 3.5 ounces) of fatty fish each week is recommended. Individuals should be aware of the fish advisory regarding mercury. Children and pregnant women are advised to avoid shark, swordfish, king mackerel, or tile fish because these contain high levels of mercury [62].

Now, what do we do? Synthesizing a practical guide from the complex nutrition science of n-3 and n-6 PUFAs, the Academy of Nutrition and Dietetics included the following principle in its position statement [50]. "It is the position of the Academy of Nutrition and Dietetics (the Academy) that dietary fat for the healthy adult population should provide 20–35% of energy, with an increased consumption of n-3 polyunsaturated fatty acids and limited intake of saturated and trans fats. The Academy recommends a food-based approach through a diet that includes regular consumption of fatty fish, nuts and seeds, lean meats and poultry, low-fat dairy products, vegetables, fruits, whole grains, and legumes". The World Health Organization [60] concluded similarly after analyzing the data on lipids.

13.3.5 Fluid

It is widely recognized that people can live longer without food than they can without water. Maintaining fluid and electrolyte balance is critical to health.

Functions. Water maintains cell volume, participates in chemical reactions, acts as a solvent, transports nutrients and other substances in the circulation, excretes waste products of metabolism, regulates body temperature, and maintains normal fluid and electrolyte balance [63]. In addition, it aids in maintaining normal blood pressure and cardiac and renal function [64]. The body has mechanisms involving hormones, organs, and the central nervous system that precisely control fluid balance [11]. However, age-related changes and dementia-related factors affect these mechanisms in older adults with intellectual disability, increasing their susceptibility to dehydration [65]. Low fluid intake and dehydration are common among residents in long-term care facilities [65, 66].

Recommended intake. The recommended intakes (AIs) of total water per day for men and women (aged 19 to >70 years) are 3.7 L and 2.7 L, respectively. This includes all fluid from beverages and foods [67]. To prevent dehydration, 1500 ml or more of fluid daily should be provided [65]. Fluid intake varies from day to day and many factors, such as heat, physical activity, diet composition, diarrhea and vomiting, incontinence and some medications affect fluid balance [67]. Renal insufficiency and congestive heart failure, may need fluid restriction to help alleviate fluid retention. It is helpful to remember that fluid volume and electrolyte concentrations in the blood are interrelated [64].

Staff or caregivers should monitor the hydration status of an adult with intellectual disability as dehydration can be life-threatening. Dehydration disrupts cognitive and physical performance and causes fatigue and delirium [65]. Monitoring fluid intake and balance becomes much more important for older people and those with intellectual disability who cannot communicate their basic needs [65]. As noted before, fiber, with adequate fluid, can help relieve constipation which is prevalent in older adults [45, 46] and in people with intellectual disability [44]. At home, establishing a hydration schedule and flavoring water with orange or lime slices can enhance the appeal of plain water. Watery fruits and vegetables, milk, and fruit juices add not only fluid but also nutrients. Sugar-sweetened beverages should be avoided as they supply calories without the nutrients. Excessive sugar intake contributes to obesity [5].

13.4 Fat-Soluble Vitamins: Vitamins A, D, E, and K

13.4.1 Vitamin A

Vitamin A refers to retinoids, substances which have vitamin A (or all-trans-retinol) activity. These include retinol, retinal, retinoic acid, retinyl esters, and the synthetic forms [11]. In nature, retinol is stored in animal tissues as an ester (e.g., retinyl palmitate) which serves as a precursor for retinol. Retinol and its esters must be converted in the body to retinal and retinoic acid which are the main active forms of the vitamin. Retinol and its esters are the preformed vitamin A in animal-derived foods [68, 69].

In addition to the retinoids, provitamin A carotenoids, which are fat-soluble compounds in plants, also provide vitamin A. Carotenoids give plants the red, yellow, and orange pigments although chlorophyll in green vegetables mask them [11]. Beta-carotene is the most significant carotenoid as it yields the highest amount of vitamin A bioactivity. However, the conversion is not 1:1 ratio. One mcg of physiologically active retinol is equivalent to 12 mcg of beta-carotene [70]. Plant sources provide an alternative source of vitamin A to people who do not eat animal-derived foods. The absorption of carotenoids is variable. Fats (~10 g) are needed for the absorption of fat-soluble vitamins and carotenoids [70].

Functions. Sensory problems (including vision) are common among people with intellectual disability [7]. Vitamin A is essential to vision. Retinal and protein opsin are required to synthesize rhodopsin, a light-sensitive pigment in the rods of the eye, which enables people to see in dim light. Low supply can cause night blindness, an early sign of vitamin A deficiency. Vitamin A is also important in cellular differentiation that affects epithelial cells growth and for immunity or resistance to infection [71, 72]. Carotenoids have an antioxidant function, stopping the free radicals from damaging the cells and tissues. It may protect against cataract and age-related macular degeneration [11].

Recommended intake. The RDA for vitamin A is expressed as Retinol Activity Equivalent (RAE). The RDAs for men and women (19 to >70 years) are 900 mcg RAE/day and 700 mcg RAE/day, respectively. Excessive intake of vitamin A is toxic. Therefore a Tolerable Upper Intake Level (UL) of 3000 mcg RAE/day has been set for all adults [69]. Excessive intake can also cause birth malformations. Carotene, in contrast, is known not to cause birth malformation. Excessive carotene can cause orange discoloration of the skin which carotene supplement discontinuation can reverse [70]. Table 13.3 shows a summary of the minerals and vitamins, their major functions, deficiency effects, and key food sources.

Food sources. Beta-carotene is abundant in orange, yellow, and dark green plant foods. Sources include sweet potatoes, spinach, carrots, pumpkin, red sweet pepper, cantaloupe, broccoli, squash, mangoes and fortified cereals. Rich sources of pre-formed vitamin A include liver and some fish oils, fortified milk and other dairy products [70].

Primary deficiency is rare in the United States but can occur secondary to disorders causing fat malabsorption. In contrast, primary deficiency is prevalent in developing countries. According to the WHO [73], vitamin A deficiency is the leading preventable cause of blindness in children, it noted that "an estimated 250 000 to 500 000 vitamin A-deficient children become blind every year, half of them dying within 12 months of losing their sight." The World Health Organization has implemented a vitamin A supplementation program [73].

Table 13.3 Minerals and vitamins and their functions

Mineral	Function	Deficiencies can lead to	Sources
Minerals and their function in the human body			
[a]Calcium	Needed for muscle and neuron function; heart health; builds bone and supports synthesis and function of blood cells; nerve function	Osteoporosis, rickets, muscle spasms, impaired growth	Milk, yogurt, fish, green leafy vegetables, legumes
[a]Chlorine	Needed for production of hydrochloric acid (HCl) in the stomach and nerve function; osmotic balance	Muscle cramps, mood disturbances, reduced appetite	Table salt
Copper (trace amounts)	Required component of many redox enzymes, including cytochrome c oxidase; cofactor for hemoglobin synthesis	Copper deficiency is rare	Liver, oysters, cocoa, chocolate, sesame, nuts
Iodine	Required for the synthesis of thyroid hormones	Goiter	Seafood, iodized salt, dairy products

(continued)

Table 13.3 (continued)

Mineral	Function	Deficiencies can lead to	Sources
Iron	Required for many proteins and enzymes, notably hemoglobin, to prevent anemia	Anemia, which causes poor concentration, fatigue, and poor immune function	Red meat, leafy green vegetables, fish (tuna, salmon), eggs, dried fruits, beans, whole grains
[a]Magnesium	Required co-factor for ATP formation; bone formation; normal membrane functions; muscle function	Mood disturbances, muscle spasms	Whole grains, leafy green vegetables
Manganese (trace amounts)	A cofactor in enzyme functions; trace amounts are required	Manganese deficiency is rare	Common in most foods
Molybdenum (trace amounts)	Acts as a cofactor for three essential enzymes in humans: sulfite oxidase, xanthine oxidase, and aldehyde oxidase	Molybdenum deficiency is rare	
[a]Phosphorus	A component of bones and teeth; helps regulate acid-base balance; nucleotide synthesis	Weakness, bone abnormalities, calcium loss	Milk, hard cheese, whole grains, meats
[a]Potassium	Vital for muscles, heart, and nerve function	Cardiac rhythm disturbance, muscle weakness	Legumes, potato skin, tomatoes, bananas
Selenium (trace amounts)	A cofactor essential to activity of antioxidant enzymes like glutathione peroxidase; trace amounts are required	Selenium deficiency is rare	Common in most foods
[a]Sodium	Systemic electrolyte required for many functions; acid-base balance; water balance; nerve function	Muscle cramps, fatigue, reduced appetite	Table salt
Zinc (trace amounts)	Required for several enzymes such as carboxypeptidase, liver alcohol dehydrogenase, and carbonic anhydrase	Anemia, poor wound healing, can lead to short stature	Common in most foods
Water-soluble essential vitamins			
Vitamin B$_1$ (Thiamine)	Needed by the body to process lipids, proteins, and carbohydrates coenzyme removes CO_2 from organic compounds	Muscle weakness, beriberi: reduced heart function, CNS problems	Milk, meat, dried beans, whole grains

Table 13.3 (continued)

Mineral	Function	Deficiencies can lead to	Sources
Vitamin B$_2$ (Riboflavin)	Takes an active role in metabolism, aiding in the conversion of food to energy (FAD and FMN)	Cracks or sores on the outer surface of the lips cheilosis); inflammation and redness of the tongue; moist, scaly skin inflammation (seborrheic dermatitis)	Meat, eggs, enriched grains, vegetables
Vitamin B$_3$ Niacin)	Used by the body to release energy from carbohydrates and to process alcohol; required for the synthesis of sex hormones; component of coenzyme NAD$^+$ and NADP$^+$	Pellagra, which can result in dermatitis, diarrhea, dementia, and death	Meat, eggs, grains, nuts, potatoes
Vitamin B$_5$ (Pantothenic acid)	Assists in producing energy from foods (lipids, in particular); component of coenzyme A	Fatigue, poor coordination, retarded growth, numbness, tingling of hands and feet	Meat, whole grains, milk, fruits, vegetables
Vitamin B$_6$ (Pyridoxine)	The principal vitamin for processing amino acids and lipids; also helps convert nutrients into energy	Irritability, depression, confusion, mouth sores or ulcers, anemia, muscular twitching	Meat, dairy products, whole grains, orange juice
Vitamin B$_7$ (Biotin)	Used in energy and amino acid metabolism, fat synthesis, and fat breakdown; helps the body use blood sugar	Hair loss, dermatitis, depression, numbness and tingling in the extremities; neuromuscular disorders	Meat, eggs, legumes and other vegetables
Vitamin B$_9$ (Folic acid)	Assists the normal development of cells, especially during fetal development; helps metabolize nucleic and amino acids	Deficiency during pregnancy is associated with birth defects, such as neural tube defects and anemia	Leafy green vegetables, whole wheat, fruits, nuts, legumes
Vitamin B$_{12}$ (Cobalamin)	Maintains healthy nervous system and assists with blood cell formation; coenzyme in nucleic acid metabolism	Anemia, neurological disorders, numbness, loss of balance	Meat, eggs, animal products
Vitamin C (Ascorbic acid)	Helps maintain connective tissue: bone, cartilage, and dentin; boosts the immune system	Scurvy, which results in bleeding, hair and tooth loss; joint pain and swelling; delayed wound healing	Citrus fruits, broccoli, tomatoes, red sweet bell peppers

(continued)

Table 13.3 (continued)

Mineral	Function	Deficiencies can lead to	Sources
Fat-soluble essential vitamins			
Vitamin A (Retinol)	Critical to the development of bones, teeth, and skin; helps maintain eyesight, enhances the immune system, fetal development, gene expression	Night-blindness, skin disorders, impaired immunity	Dark green leafy vegetables, yellow-orange vegetables fruits, milk, butter
Vitamin D	Critical for calcium absorption for bone development and strength; maintains a stable nervous system; maintains a normal and strong heartbeat; helps in blood clotting	Rickets, osteomalacia, immunity	Cod liver oil, milk, egg yolk
Vitamin E (Tocopherol)	Lessens oxidative damage of cells,and prevents lung damage from pollutants; vital to the immune system	Deficiency is rare; anemia, nervous system degeneration	Wheat germ oil, unrefined vegetable oils, nuts, seeds, grains
Vitamin K (Phylloquinone)	Essential to blood clotting	Bleeding and easy bruising	Leafy green vegetables, tea

Source: https://cnx.org/contents/GFy_h8cu@11.1:cXkGrzS-@5/Nutrition-and-Energy-Productio
Licensed under a Creative Commons Attribution 4.0 License
[a]Greater than 200 mg/day required

13.4.2 Vitamin D

Vitamin D is a group of fat-soluble vitamins that includes both vitamin D2 and vitamin D3 [74]. It is available naturally in foods, as a supplement or added to foods [75]. It is called a hormone [76] and a member of the steroid hormone family [77]. Vitamin D is synthesized in the skin from a precursor (7-dehydrocholesterol) during exposure to solar ultraviolet light band B (UVB). The precursor is converted to previtamin D3 which is quickly transformed to vitamin D3 or cholecalciferol [76–78]. Vitamin D3 then goes to the liver where it is hydroxylated to form 25-hydroxyvitamin D, or 25(OH)D or calcidiol. This is the form that is measured to assess vitamin D status. Calcidiol then circulates to the kidneys for another hydroxylation to form 1,25-dihydoxyvitamin D or 1,25(OH)$_2$D, or calcitriol, the active form [77–79]. Vitamin D2 (ergocalciferol) is derived from the irradiation of plant ergosterol and is the form often used for food fortification [79]. It is clear that skin exposure to sunlight and healthy liver and kidneys are critical to the transformation of inactive vitamin D to its active form and that organ abnormalities will adversely affect vitamin D metabolism, calcium and phosphorus utilization, and bone health. In adults with intellectual disability, age-related changes in the skin, liver, kidneys and absorption can affect vitamin D and calcium utilization [80].

Vitamin D has two main types of functions, namely endocrine and autocrine [78]. The classic role of vitamin D is in bone formation and maintenance. Based on its thorough assessment of more than 1000 studies and reports and testimonials, a review committee of the Institute of Medicine [74] concluded that strong evidence supports the benefits of vitamin D (and calcium) for bone health but not for other conditions that have been reported (diabetes mellitus, multiple sclerosis, rheumatoid arthritis, and several others).

Functions The main endocrine function of vitamin D (calcitriol) is to help build and maintain the bones. It does this by promoting the intestinal absorption of calcium and phosphorus and maintaining their homeostasis for bone mineralization [77–79]. The function of vitamin D is a well-coordinated endocrine system, involving other hormones (parathyroid hormone) and the target organs (intestine, bones, and kidneys). One primary goal is to maintain blood calcium balance. For example, hypocalcemia triggers physiological responses to restore normocalcemia. Normocalcemia is important because calcium in body fluids has critical functions in nerve impulses transmission, muscle contraction, functions of enzymes and cell metabolism [74].

Vitamin D deficiency causes rickets in children and osteomalacia in adults. Osteoporosis is a multifactorial disease and vitamin D and calcium deficiency contributes to its etiology. A public health problem, it can cause bone fractures and disability [75, 81].

Recommended intake. The RDAs for adults aged 19–70 years and for those older than 70 are 600 IU (15 mcg of cholecalciferol)/day and 800 IU (20 mcg)/day, respectively. This amount is for people with inadequate exposure to sunlight. The conversion for International Unit is 40 IU = 1 mcg of cholecalciferol. Since long-term excessive use of vitamin D is toxic, the IOM [74] set the UL at 4000 IU (100 mcg) as the maximum daily intake. Holick [82] noted that vitamin D toxicity is rare although some conditions may cause hypercalcemia. The prevalence of osteopenia and osteoporosis, including their risk factors, in adults with intellectual disability is well documented [83, 84]. Timely screening and risk assessment for osteoporosis can identify the disorder early for further assessment and intervention [84]. Osteoporosis is preventable and treatable [81].

Food sources. Very few foods are naturally high in vitamin D. The best sources include cod liver oil and fatty fish (e.g., salmon, tuna, and mackerel). Beef liver, cheese and egg yolk contain small amounts. Additional food sources include some varieties of mushrooms, fortified foods such as milk and milk substitute beverages, cereals, orange juice, and some brands of yogurt [75]. The sun is the most dependable source; however individuals should also observe sun safety. Information on vitamin D food sources is available at https://health.gov/dietaryguidelines/2015/guidelines/appendix-12/.

13.4.3 Vitamin E

Vitamin E is a general name for a family of fat-soluble compounds that share certain similar characteristics and possess antioxidant properties. The biologic activities of the compounds vary and only the alpha-tocopherol has biologic activity. The synthetic form used in fortified foods and in supplements is not as biologically active as the naturally occurring form [11, 85].

Functions. Vitamin E has other functions outside of its anti-oxidant properties. As an antioxidant, vitamin E stops the propagation of the reactive oxygen species which can damage the cells causing cellular death and tissue injury. The damage can initiate a disease process. Biochemical processes in the body yield free radicals; in addition, the environment exposes people to free radicals. An antioxidant system, which includes vitamin E, can stop the formation of free radicals or can intercept the free radicals preventing their chain reaction that will damage the polyunsaturated lipids, DNA, and protein. The damage has been implicated in the development of chronic diseases such as CVD and cancer [11, 85]. The RDA for vitamin E for persons 14 years and older is 15 mg/day of alpha-tocopherol. Excessive vitamin E can have a hemorrhagic effect especially for adults with intellectual disability taking anticoagulant or have low vitamin K status. Therefore, a UL is set at 1000 mg/day for any form of alpha-tocopherol supplementation [86].

Food sources include nuts, seeds, vegetable oils, and wheat germ oil. Significant amounts are available in green leafy vegetables and fortified cereals [85, 86].

13.4.4 Vitamin K

Vitamin K is a family of compounds consisting of vitamin K1 (phylloquinone) and vitamin K2 (a family of menaquinone). Phylloquinones are synthesized in plants and menaquinones are mostly synthesized by the intestinal bacteria. The body recycles vitamin K repeatedly using the small amount available to it [87].

Functions. Vitamin K functions primarily to promote blood clotting. It is a cofactor for enzymes that synthesize coagulation factors, (e.g. prothrombin) and anticoagulation proteins (e.g., protein C) thus it prevents bleeding or hemorrhage. Additionally, it aids in the synthesis of other proteins that may help with bone processes and maintenance. Warfarin or Coumadin, an oral anticoagulant used to prevent clot formation, antagonizes vitamin K and thins the blood. Adults with intellectual diasbility who are Coumadin users should keep their vitamin K intake consistent because vitamin K can change the effect of the drug [11, 87, 88]. Other proteins that require vitamin K for their synthesis are the matrix Gla protein and osteocalcin. The matrix Gla protein in the smooth blood vessels, bones, and connective tissue may help reduce abnormal calcification of these tissues. Osteocalcin may aid in bone mineralization [11, 88].

Recommended intake. The Adequate Intakes for adult men and women are 120 mcg/day and 90 mcg/day, respectively [69]. Primary deficiency is rare. Deficiency may develop secondary to disorders that cause chronic fat malabsorption. Exclusively breastfed newborn infants are at risk for bleeding because their liver store of vitamin K is very low, their vitamin K cycle is not fully functional yet, and milk is low in vitamin K. They are given prophylactic dose of vitamin K to prevent a rare but serious disorder called vitamin K deficiency bleeding, As previously noted, Coumadin makes vitamin K functionally deficient [87].

Signs of Vitamin K deficiency, if present, include long prothrombin time, a measure for blood clotting time [87, 88], easy bruising and bleeding such as nosebleeds and bleeding gums. In infants, vitamin K deficiency may result in intracranial hemorrhage [87].

Food sources. Vitamin K is present mostly as phylloquinones in plant foods like green leafy vegetables and oils. Menaquinones are found in fermented foods; fermented soybeans (Natto) are the richest source. Bacterial synthesis of menadione and the body's recycling of vitamin K add to the dietary sources [87].

13.5   Water-Soluble Vitamins: Vitamin C, Folate/Folic acid and Vitamin B-12

13.5.1   Vitamin C

Vitamin C, also known as L-ascorbic acid or ascorbate, is a water-soluble vitamin that is structurally related to glucose. However, humans do not have the enzyme to synthesize vitamin C from glucose. Therefore, they must get the vitamin in the diet [11].

Functions. Vitamin C functions in reactions that generally involve the formation of substances essential to the body's regulatory processes and structures. For example, the synthesis of collagen, L-carnitine, neurotransmitters such as epinephrine and serotonin, and some hormones requires vitamin C as a cofactor. In addition, vitamin C acts as an antioxidant, enhances the absorption of iron and activates folate which are needed for red blood cell formation [11]. Collagen is required for the normal development and maintenance of the bones, tendons, cartilage, blood vessels, and skin and for wound healing. L-Carnitine transports the long-chain fatty acids from the cell cytoplasm into the mitochondria where they are oxidized to release energy (ATP) needed by many cellular reactions. Neonatal brain appears to be sensitive to vitamin C deficiency; the beginning event might affect early brain development and function later [89].

The classic vitamin C-deficiency disease is scurvy. It is rare in most countries, but it still occurs and can affect people with chronic vitamin C-deficient intake. The four Hs is a mnemonic for these scurvy signs: Hemorrhagic signs, hyperkeratosis of the hair follicles, hypochondriasis (psychological manifestations), and hematologic abnormalities [11]. The typical signs of scurvy, including poor wound healing, are related to the defective collagen synthesis in collagen-containing tissues. Collagen is needed as an organic matrix of the bones where minerals are deposited. Hemorrhage which can happen in any organ is a distinctive feature of scurvy. The skin becomes rough and dry and shows purpura due to easy bruising. Bleeding and poor iron absorption can lead to anemia [89].

Recommended intake. The RDAs for vitamin C for adults are 90 mg/day and 75 mg/day for men and women, respectively. It is recommended that smokers add 35 mg daily [86].

Food Sources. Fresh fruits and vegetables in general are excellent sources of vitamin C. Examples are citrus fruits, kiwi, strawberries, red pepper, green pepper, broccoli, Brussel and many others. Vitamin C is sensitive to air, light, and heat and is destroyed in improper storage and food preparation [11, 90]. Vegetables should be cooked as quickly as possible and in a small amount of water to conserve the water-soluble vitamins (microwaving vegetables is effective in retaining vitamin value). They should be stored properly and protected from air, heat, and sunlight.

13.5.2 Vitamin B-12

Functions. Vitamin B-12 (Cobalamin), a water-soluble vitamin, is important for DNA and red blood cell synthesis and neurological function. It works synergistically with folate in converting homocysteine to methionine thereby preventing elevated homocysteine and also providing a universal methyl donor, S-adenosyl methionine (SAM), through this methionine cycle. DNA and RNA methylation, myelin maintenance and neural function use SAM in methylation reactions. Elevated plasma homocysteine is considered a risk factor for CVD [91], which increases risks for vascular dementia [11, 28].

As summarized by the Office of Dietary Supplements (ODS) [92], "symptoms of vitamin B-12 deficiency include megaloblastic anemia, fatigue, weakness, constipation, loss of appetite, and weight loss. Neurological changes, such as numbness and tingling in the hands and feet, can also occur. Additional symptoms of vitamin B12 deficiency include difficulty maintaining balance, depression, confusion, dementia, poor memory, and soreness of the mouth or tongue."

Age-related changes in the digestive system can reduce the absorption of food-bound vitamin B-12. Atrophic gastritis, which affects 10–30% of older adults, can reduce gastric secretion of hydrochloric acid needed to free the food-bound vitamin B-12 during digestion. The free vitamin B-12 can then bind with intrinsic factor (also secreted by the stomach) for absorption in the ileum. Lack of intrinsic factor, gastric surgery and disorders [92] and *H. pylori* infection can also reduce vitamin B-12 absorption. Fayaz et al. [93] reported that out of their 75 study participants with intellectual disability and Down syndrome, 41 (54.7%) tested positive for *H. pylori* infection.

Most of older adults can absorb the synthetic vitamin B-12 in fortified foods and dietary supplements [92]. The Institute of Medicine (IOM) [94] therefore recommends that adults older than 50 years obtain most of their vitamin B-12 from vitamin supplements or fortified foods.

Recommended intake. The RDA for adults (aged 19 to >70 years) is 2.4 mcg/day [94]. Naturally occurring vitamin B-12 is present only in animal-derived foods (beef liver, clams, fish, meat, poultry, eggs, milk and milk products). Thus people with intellectual disability especially as they age should be aware of foods rich in or fortified with vitamin B-12. Vegans are advised similarly [92]. Information on vitamin B-12 food sources is available at http://www.ars.usda.gov/nutrientdata and https://oldwayspt.org/programs/oldways-vegetarian-network/oldways-vegetarian-network-resources/vegetarian-vitamin-b12-food [95].

13.5.3 Folate

Folate is a water-soluble vitamin which has been well established as a prophylactic against neural tube defects (NTD), spina bifida and anencephaly. The incidence of NTD has declined since folic acid fortification of foods in 1998 [91, 96].

Functions. Folate functions as a coenzyme or co-substrate in single carbon transfer involved in the formation of nucleic acids for DNA and RNA synthesis and in amino acid metabolism. It transfers several single carbon units; however, this section focuses only on the methyl group as an example. Its role in the homocysteine-methionine cycle, a vitamin B12-dependent process, is already described in the vitamin B-12 section. Impairment in the step for DNA formation can cause megaloblastic anemia because the red blood cells continue to grow in size but fail to mature and divide. DNA is critical to cell division and growth [11, 91].

Vitamin B-12 deficiency will impair folate's function in transferring the methyl group. Vitamin B-12 is needed as a methyl acceptor to complete the transfer in the methionine cycle. In addition, by releasing the methyl group, folate is re-activated and can resume its normal function. Otherwise, it is held non-functional in a "methyl trap" [11]. Either vitamin B-12 or folate deficiency causes megaloblastic anemia. Treatment with folate can correct the anemia but not the neurologic damage due to vitamin B-12 deficiency [91]. This means that folate is "masking" the effects of vitamin B-12 deficiency. Excessive intake of folic acid from fortified foods has raised this concern [91, 96]. The IOM [94] has set a UL for the synthetic form (folic acid in fortified foods and dietary supplements) because of the metabolic interactions between folate and vitamin B-12 [96].

Recommended intake. The RDA for folate (which includes both the folate in foods and folic acid added to supplements and food) for adults (>19 years) is 400 mcg dietary folate equivalent (DFE)/day. The UL is 1000 mcg/day from supplements and fortified foods, but excluding the folate in foods. The RDA for pregnancy is 600 mcg DFE /day [94]. It is important to note that genetic polymorphism in the sequence for the gene encoding for the enzyme methylenetetrahydrofolate reductase can raise folate requirements and has disease implications. Additionally, certain medications (methotrexate, phenytoin, and sulfasalazine) have anti-folate activity [97].

Food sources. In general, green leafy vegetables, legumes and some fruits have high folate content whereas fortified grains and grain products are high in folic acid. Spinach, liver, yeast, asparagus, and Brussels sprouts are among the foods with the highest levels of folate [96]. Information on folate, folic acid, and total folate content is available at http://www.ars.usda.gov/nutrientdata.

13.6 Minerals: Calcium, Iron, and Iodine

13.6.1 Calcium

Calcium is the most abundant mineral in the body where approximately 99% is stored as calcium hydroxyapatite in the bones and teeth and 1% is in the body fluids. Calcium in the bones, along with other minerals such as phosphorus, maintain bone structure and strength. The bone serves as a reservoir for calcium, releasing calcium into the blood in response to hypocalcemia to maintain normal blood calcium level [74].

Functions. Calcium in body fluids, muscles, and other tissues function in vascular contraction and vasodilation, nerve transmission, and many cellular reactions. Serum calcium balance is tightly regulated by the endocrine system including the hormonal form of vitamin D, bones, intestine, and kidneys. The role of vitamin D in calcium absorption and balance and results of deficiency are already described in the vitamin D section. Factors that impair vitamin D functions negatively affect calcium metabolism and balance and thus bone health. Factors that affect bone health include genetics, age-related physiological changes, lifestyle factors (diet and physical activity/mechanical loading), hormones, disorders that affect absorption, and medications [74, 81, 98].

Bone remodeling occurs throughout life where bone resorption is coupled with new bone formation. Women with intellectual disability need to pay special attention to bone builders. In menopausal and post-menopausal women, due to lack of estrogen, bone breakdown exceeds bone formation. Calcium is released from the bones reducing bone density. Overtime, the bones become fragile and susceptible to fracture [74]. Physical activity or mechanical loading of the bones (weight-bearing exercise such as walking, running, or jumping) promotes bone formation from younger to later years [74].

Recommended intake. The RDAs for men, aged 19–70 years, and older than 70, are 1000 mg/day and 1200 mg/day, respectively. The RDA for women, aged 19–50 years, is 1000 mg/day; it is 1200 mg/day for older women [74].

Food sources. Calcium-rich foods include milk products, some vegetables and fish (eaten with their soft bones). Calcium-fortified products such as orange juice, soy and almond beverages, rice drink, and ready-to-eat cereals; tofu; and certain vegetables (e.g., kale and turnip greens) offer choices for vegetarian and lactose-restricted diets. Vegetables, however, contain inhibitors that bind with calcium and reduce its absorption [5, 98]. Information on food sources of calcium is available at https://health.gov/dietaryguidelines/2015/guidelines/appendix-11/ and http://www.ars.usda.gov/nutrientdata.

13.6.2 Iron

Iron is so important to health that the WHO has included it among its priorities as iron-deficiency anemia (IDA) is interlinked with its other nutrition targets, namely stunting, low birth weight, childhood obesity, exclusive breastfeeding, and wasting. "The control of anemia is essential to prevent low birth weight and prenatal and maternal mortality as well as the prevalence of diseases later..." [99]. Iron deficiency is the most common cause of anemia worldwide although other nutritional deficiencies (folate, vitamin B-12 and vitamin C) are contributors as well.

Functions. Iron is a part of hemoglobin which transfers oxygen from the lungs to the tissues. It promotes growth and development and normal cellular functioning and also aids in the synthesis of some hormones and connective tissues [11, 100].

Dietary iron exists in two major forms: heme and non-heme. Meats, seafood and poultry contain heme and non-heme, while plants and fortified foods contain only non-heme. Heme is more absorbable than non-heme [100]. This difference in absorbability may have implications for individuals who eat mostly plant foods although mixing plant foods and eating a variety of them can reduce the potentially negative effect of certain foods.

Recommended intake. The RDAs for iron show sex-related differences. Adult women in their reproductive stage (aged 19–50 years) need more iron (18 mg/day) than men (8 mg/day) because women lose iron through their monthly menstruation. The RDA for older women (51 to >70 years) is 8 mg/day, which is the same as the RDA for men. The RDAs for women (19–50 years old) for pregnancy and lactation are 27 mg/day and 9 mg/day, respectively [69].

Food sources. The richest sources of heme iron include lean meats and seafoods; non-heme iron is found in nuts, beans, vegetables, and fortified grain products. As noted before, non-heme is less bioavailable than non-heme. However, vitamin C, can improve its absorbability [100]. In recipes, vitamin C-rich foods (e.g., tomatoes), when combined with non-heme iron-containing foods (e g. spinach), can increase the absorption of non-heme iron.

13.6.3 Iodine

"Iodine deficiency is the world's most prevalent, yet easily preventable, cause of brain damage. Iodine deficiency is one of the main causes of impaired cognitive development in children. It is a public health problem…It can cause congenital abnormalities such as cretinism, a grave irreversible form of [intellectual disability]" [101].

Functions. The above statement emphasizes the urgency of iodine nutrition to the health of the children starting with their mothers, in their fetal development and through adulthood. The impact of this public health problem on human lives is profound. Iodine is a trace element that, along with the amino acid tyrosine, is needed to synthesize the thyroid hormones, thyroxine (T4) and triodothyronine (T3). Insufficient production of these hormones adversely affects many biochemical reactions, physiological systems, and vital organs, including the developing brain. The resulting disorders are collectively called iodine deficiency disorders [101, 102].

In iodine-deficient geographic areas, endemic cretinism is prevalent. Cretinism is a severe form of the disorder caused by severe iodine deficiency during fetal, neonatal, and childhood stages of development. Signs include severe and reversible intellectual disability, short stature, deaf-mutism, and spastic dyplegia, and squints [102]. Goiter, enlargement of the thyroid gland, is an early clinical sign of iodine deficiency [102, 103].

Iodine is present in the soil and plants grown in iodine-rich soil can be good dietary sources of iodine. However, soil erosion, flooding, and deforestation have depleted the soil content. Plants grown on coastal areas originally thought to provide iodine may not be good sources anymore [102]. Certain vegetables contain goitrogens that interfere with thyroxine synthesis. Foods high in goitrogens include soy and cassava, cabbage, broccoli, cauliflower, and other cruciferous vegetables.

More than 70 countries, including the United States and Canada have salt iodization programs [103] and the program has achieved progress; however 54 countries are still iodine-deficient. The program uses salt because this item is widely used and inexpensive, costing only US $0.05 per person [101, 104].

Recommended intake. The RDAs are 150 mcg/day for adults, and 220 mcg/day and 290 mcg/day for pregnancy and lactation, respectively [69]. Major food sources include seaweed (the richest source), fish, dairy products, grains, and iodized salt [103]. Excessive intake can have adverse health effects, thus a UL (900–1100 mcg/day for adolescents, adults, and pregnant and lactating women) has been set [69].

13.7 Food-Based Dietary Guidelines and Healthy Eating Patterns

This section applies the background information on the nutrients and the recommended intakes to meal planning, selecting a combination of foods in the proper amount to meet the estimated calorie levels. *The Dietary Reference Intakes* connect with the food and the eating pattern. The Food Guide is used to ensure that each of the five food groups is represented in the days' menu. The Dietary Guidelines for Americans are used only as an example, fully recognizing that other countries have their own Food-Based Dietary Guidelines (FBDG). This section also includes other eating patterns, the Mediterranean Diet (Fig. 13.3) and the Vegetarian Diet (Fig. 13.4). They reinforce the principle that eating patterns can be modified to meet the person's personal and cultural preferences and health goals. Many resources are available to consumers regarding these topics. However, the overwhelming volume of information, many of which are often contradictory, can be confusing. Health professionals can help people with intellectual disability and their families separate sound information from hype and make well-informed decisions.

FBDG. The fact that the Food and Agricultural Organization (FAO) of the United Nations has been assisting other countries develop their FBDG illustrates the importance of such guidelines. With FAO's assistance, more than 100 countries have developed or are developing their FBDG. These guidelines affect the countries' food and nutrition, health, agriculture and nutrition education policies and programs. They can also be used as a teaching tool at various education points [105]. http://www.fao.org/nutrition/education/food-dietary-guidelines/background/en/. The FBDGs of the different countries are available at http://www.fao.org/nutrition/education/food-dietary-guidelines/regions/en/. Dietary guidelines from around the world are available at https://www.nal.usda.gov/fnic/dietary-guidelines-around-world. Ethnic cultural food guide pyramids are available at https://www.nal.usda.gov/fnic/ethniccultural-food-pyramids.

Graphics. The key messages of the Dietary Guidelines for Americans are communicated to the consumers through a colorful graphic ChooseMyPlate (Fig. 13.1). MyPlate visually represents the variety of foods in a meal majority of which are from plants. Half of the plate beams the fruits and vegetables, about ¼ the grains, and the remaining small space has the protein foods. Milk is on the side of the place setting. People who do not want milk can use a calcium-rich

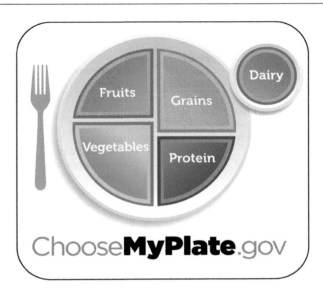

Fig. 13.1 Choose MyPlate. https://www.choosemyplate.gov/myplate-graphic-resources

substitute. Liberal amounts of water are available. At least half of the day's grain selections are whole grain, protein foods are lean and oils or fats are unsaturated. Regular physical activity is part of a healthy lifestyle (e.g., ChooseMyPlate.gov; [29]) (Table 13.4).

Some of the key messages in Fig. 13.2 include:

- All foods and beverages matter; focus on amount, variety and nutrition.
- Choose nutrient-dense foods. These foods contain vitamins, minerals, fiber, and other healthful nutrients or components at an appropriate calorie level.
- Include vegetables, fruits, whole grains, seafood, eggs, beans and peas, unsalted nuts and seeds, fat-free and low-fat dairy products, and lean meats and poultry and foods with little or no saturated fats, sodium, and added sugars.
- Choose an eating style that is low in saturated fat, sodium and added sugar. (https://www.choosemyplate.gov/translating-dietary-guidelines-consumer-messages [106]).

Food-based guidelines are recommended as teaching tools for nutrition education of the consumers or the public [5]. The MyPlate method is simple and practical for teaching meal planning to different groups of consumers, including older adults and people with low literacy and cognitive difficulties [107, 108]. The USDA Food Patterns have a plan for different calorie levels (1000–3200 calories) with the recommended amount of foods from each food group. The USDA Healthy Mediterranean Style and Vegetarian Style Eating Patterns are also available (https://health.gov/dietaryguidelines/2015/guidelines/appendix-3/). Practical nutritional guidelines and other helpful resource for children and adults with intellectual disability are available in the report published by Caroline Walker Trust ([109]; https://www.cwt.org.uk/wp-content/uploads/2015/02/EWLDGuidelines.pdf).

Table 13.4 Portions of food from each food group with selected examples

Food groups	Fruits (selected examples)	What counts as a cup of fruit	Other amounts (count as 1/2 cup of fruit unless noted
Fruits In general, 1 cup of fruit or 100% fruit juice, or ½ cup of dried fruit can be considered as 1 cup from the Fruit Group. Whole fruit is preferable to fruit juice. The fruits listed are selected examples. Detailed information is available at https://www.choosemyplate. gov/fruit	Apple	½ large (3¼″ diameter) 1 small (2¼″ diameter) 1 cup, sliced or chopped, raw or cooked	½ cup, sliced or chopped, raw or cooked
	Grapes	1 cup, whole or cut-up 32 seedless grapes	16 seedless grapes
	Orange	1 large (3 1/16″ diameter) 1 cup, sections	1 small (2 3/8″ diameter)
	Plum	1 cup, sliced raw or cooked 3 medium or 2 large plum	1 large plum
	Dried fruit (raisins, prunes, apricots, etc.)	½ cup dried fruit	¼ cup dried fruit or 1 small box raisins (1½ oz)
Vegetables	**Vegetables (selected examples)**	**Amount that counts as 1 cup of vegetable**	**Amount that counts as 1/2 cup of vegetable**
Any vegetable or 100% vegetable juice counts as a member of the Vegetable Group. Vegetables may be raw or cooked; fresh, frozen, canned, or dried/dehydrated; and may be whole, cut-up, or mashed. Based on their nutrient content, vegetables are organized into five subgroups: dark-green vegetables, starchy vegetables, red and orange vegetables, beans and peas, and other vegetables. The vegetables listed are selected examples. Detailed information is available at https://www.choosemyplate.gov/ vegetables Dark Green	Broccoli Spinach	1 cup, chopped or florets 3 spears 5″ long raw or cooked 2 cups, Raw 1 Cup Cooked	1 Cup, Raw

Table 13.4 (continued)

Food groups	Fruits (selected examples)	What counts as a cup of fruit	Other amounts (count as 1/2 cup of fruit unless noted
Red and Orange Vegetables	Carrots	1 cup, strips, slices, or chopped, raw or cooked 2 medium 1 cup baby carrots (about 12)	1 medium carrot about 6 baby carrots
	Red Peppers	1 cup, chopped, raw, or cooked 1 large pepper (3″ diameter, 3 3/4″ long)	1 Small Pepper
	Dry beans and peas (such as black, garbanzo, kidney, pinto, or soy beans, or black-eyed peas or split peas)	1 cup, whole or mashed, cooked	
Starchy Vegetables	Green Peas	1 cup, Cooked	
	White Potatoes	1 cup, diced, mashed 1 medium boiled or baked potato (2½″ to 3″ diameter)	
Other Vegetables	Cabbage, Green	1 cup, chopped or shredded raw or cooked	
Grains	**Grains (selected examples)**	**Amount that counts as 1 ounce-equivalent of grains**	**Common portions and ounce-equivalents**
Any food made from wheat, rice, oats, cornmeal, barley or another cereal grain is a grain product. Bread, pasta, oatmeal, breakfast cereals, tortillas, and grits are examples of grain products. Choose whole grains. **At least half of all the grains eaten should be whole grains.** Detailed information is available at https://www.choosemyplate.gov/grains	Bagel WG[a]: whole wheat RG[a]: plain, egg	1″ mini bagel	1 large (3″ diameter) = 2 ounce-equivalents

(continued)

Table 13.4 (continued)

Food groups	Fruits (selected examples)	What counts as a cup of fruit	Other amounts (count as 1/2 cup of fruit unless noted
	Biscuit baking powder/ buttermilk—RG[a])	1 small (2″ diameter)	Regular slices = 2 ounce-equivalents
	Bread WG[a]: 100% whole wheat RG[a]: white, wheat, French, sourdough	1 regular slice 1 small slice, French 4 snack-size slices rye bread	
	WG[a]: 100% whole wheat, rye RG[a]: saltines, snack cracker	5 whole wheat crackers 2 rye crisp breads 7 square or round crackers	
	Ready-to eat breakfast cereal WG[a]: toasted oat, whole wheat flakes RG[a]: corn flakes, puffed rice	1 cup, Flakes or Rounds 1 1/4 cups, Puffed	
	Rice	½ cup cooked 1 ounce, dry	1 cup, cooked = 2 ounce-equivalents

[a]WG = whole grains, RG = refined grains. This is shown when products are available both in whole grain and refined grain forms.

Protein foods	Protein foods (selected examples)	Amount that counts as 1 ounce-equivalent in the Protein Foods Group	Common portions and ounce-equivalents
All foods made from meat, poultry, seafood, beans and peas, eggs, processed soy products, nuts, and seeds are considered part of the Protein Foods Group. Beans and peas are also part of the Vegetable Group. For more information on beans and peas, see Beans and Peas are Unique Foods	Meats	1 ounce cooked lean beef 1 ounce cooked lean pork or ham	1 small steak (eye of round, filet) = 3½ to 4 ounce-equivalents 1 small lean hamburger = 2 to 3 ounce-equivalents

Table 13.4 (continued)

Food groups	Fruits (selected examples)	What counts as a cup of fruit	Other amounts (count as 1/2 cup of fruit unless noted
	Poultry	1 ounce cooked chicken or turkey, without skin 1 sandwich slice of turkey (4½″ × 2½″ × 1/8″)	1 small chicken breast half = 3 ounce-equivalents ½ Cornish game hen = 4 ounce-equivalents
	Seafood	1 oz. cooked fish or shellfish	1 can of tuna, drained = 3 to 4 ounce-equivalents 1 salmon steak = 4 to 6 ounce-equivalents 1 small trout = 3 ounce-equivalents
	Eggs	1 egg	3 egg whites = 2 ounce-equivalents 3 egg yolks = 1 ounce-equivalent

Additional information, including nuts and seeds, beans and peas, and cooking tips, is available at https://www.choosemyplate.gov/protein-foods

Dairy Group

What counts as a cup in the dairy group?

In general, 1 cup of milk, yogurt, or soymilk (soy beverage), 1½ ounces of natural cheese, or 2 ounces of processed cheese can be considered as 1 cup from the Dairy Group. Additional information is available at https://www.choosemyplate.gov/dairy

Oils: What are "oils"?

Oils are fats that are liquid at room temperature, like the vegetable oils used in cooking. Oils come from many different plants and from fish. Oils are NOT a food group, but they provide essential nutrients. Therefore, oils are included in USDA food patterns.

Some **commonly eaten oils** include: canola oil, corn oil, cottonseed oil, olive oil, safflower oil, soybean oil, and sunflower oil. Some oils are used mainly as **flavorings**, such as walnut oil and sesame oil. A number of foods are naturally high in oils, like nuts, olives, some fish, and avocados.

Additional information is available at https://www.choosemyplate.gov/oils

Source: My Plate https://www.choosemyplate.gov/MyPlate

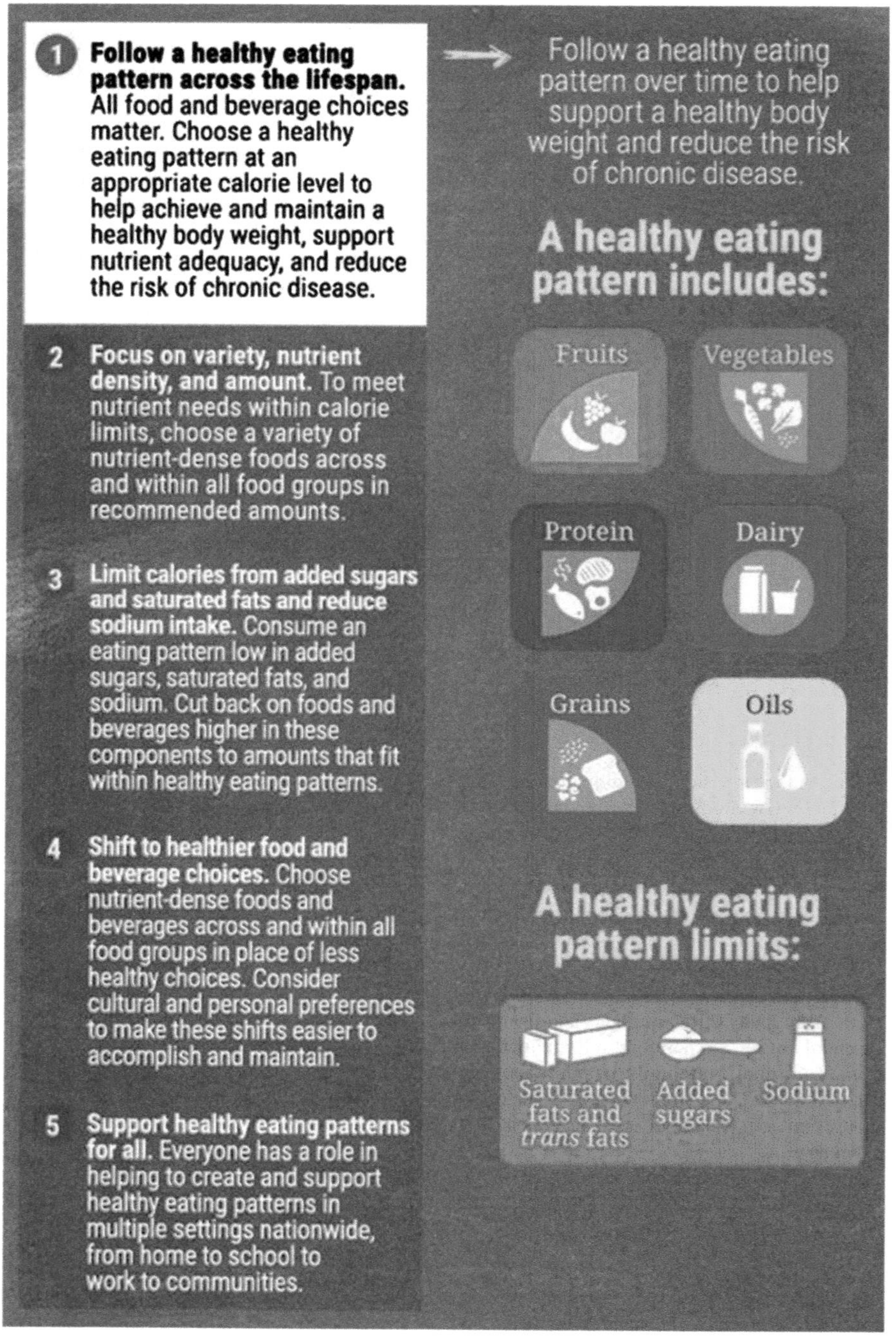

1. **Follow a healthy eating pattern across the lifespan.** All food and beverage choices matter. Choose a healthy eating pattern at an appropriate calorie level to help achieve and maintain a healthy body weight, support nutrient adequacy, and reduce the risk of chronic disease.

2. **Focus on variety, nutrient density, and amount.** To meet nutrient needs within calorie limits, choose a variety of nutrient-dense foods across and within all food groups in recommended amounts.

3. **Limit calories from added sugars and saturated fats and reduce sodium intake.** Consume an eating pattern low in added sugars, saturated fats, and sodium. Cut back on foods and beverages higher in these components to amounts that fit within healthy eating patterns.

4. **Shift to healthier food and beverage choices.** Choose nutrient-dense foods and beverages across and within all food groups in place of less healthy choices. Consider cultural and personal preferences to make these shifts easier to accomplish and maintain.

5. **Support healthy eating patterns for all.** Everyone has a role in helping to create and support healthy eating patterns in multiple settings nationwide, from home to school to work to communities.

Follow a healthy eating pattern over time to help support a healthy body weight and reduce the risk of chronic disease.

A healthy eating pattern includes:

Fruits   Vegetables

Protein   Dairy

Grains   Oils

A healthy eating pattern limits:

Saturated fats and *trans* fats   Added sugars   Sodium

Fig. 13.2 Snapshot of the 2015–2020 Dietary Guidelines for Americans

Table 13.5 Sample 1800- and 2000-calorie meal plans for 1 day

Food groups	1800 kcal Amount of foods	2000 Kcal Amount of foods
Vegetables	2½ c—equivalent 2 cups Fresh Greens (Equivalent to 1 cup) 1 cup Cooked Carrots ½ cup Mashed Potatoes	2½ c—equivalent The same amount of vegetables
Fruits	1½ c—equivalent 1 Orange, Large 1 Apple, Small	2 c—equivalent I Orange, Large 1 Apple, Large
Grains See the list for "What Counts as 1 oz.— equivalent of grains"	6 oz –equivalent 2 Slices, 100% Whole Grain Bread 1/2 cup Cooked Oatmeal, Plain ½ cup, Cooked Brown Rice or White, Enriched ½ cup Cooked Pasta, Whole Grain 1 small Whole Grain Muffin (2½″ diameter)	6 oz—equivalent The same amount
Dairy Choose fat-free or low-fat products. Low-fat or reduced-fat cheeses	3 c—equivalent 1 cup Milk 1½ ounces hard cheese (cheddar, mozzarella, Swiss, Parmesan) 1 Cup Yogurt	3 c—equivalent The same amount
Protein Foods See the list for examples of other protein foods. Choose lean protein foods.	5 oz—equivalent 2 oz. Chicken or Turkey Cooked, Without Skin, White Meat, or 2 oz. Cooked Fish 2 oz. Beef, Very Lean, Cooked 1 Egg, Cooked Note: Dried beans and legumes are protein foods.	5 ½ oz c—equivalent 3 oz. Chicken or Turkey Cooked, Without Skin. White Meat 2½ oz. Beef, Very Lean, Cooked
Oils Vegetable oils (such as canola, corn, cottonseed, olive, peanut, safflower, soybean, and sunflower) Vegetable oils (such as canola, corn, cottonseed, olive, peanut, safflower, soybean, and sunflower) See the list for other items in this group.	24 g 2½ tsp./11 g, Soft Margarine 3 tsp. Vegetable Oil/14 g	27 g For practical purposes, use the same amount of oils. Some foods have invisible fat.
Limit on Calories for Other Uses. Calories (% of calories)[a]	170 kcal (9%) Choose extra healthy items to use the calories wisely.	270 kcal (14%) Choose extra healthy items to use the calories wisely.

https://health.gov/dietaryguidelines/2015/guidelines/appendix-3/
Source: https://www.choosemyplate.gov/MyPlate
[a]All foods are assumed to be in nutrient-dense forms, lean or low-fat and prepared without added fats, sugars, refined starches, or salt. If all food choices to meet food group recommendations are in nutrient-dense forms, a small number of calories remain within the overall calorie limit of the pattern (i.e., limit on calories for other uses). The number of these calories depends on the overall calorie limit in the pattern and the amounts of food from each food group required to meet nutritional goals

Table 13.5 illustrating the 1800-calorie and 2000-calorie levels for the U.S.-Style Eating Pattern is shown below. Table 13.4 shows how to count a portion of food in each of the five food groups (Figs. 13.3 and 13.4).

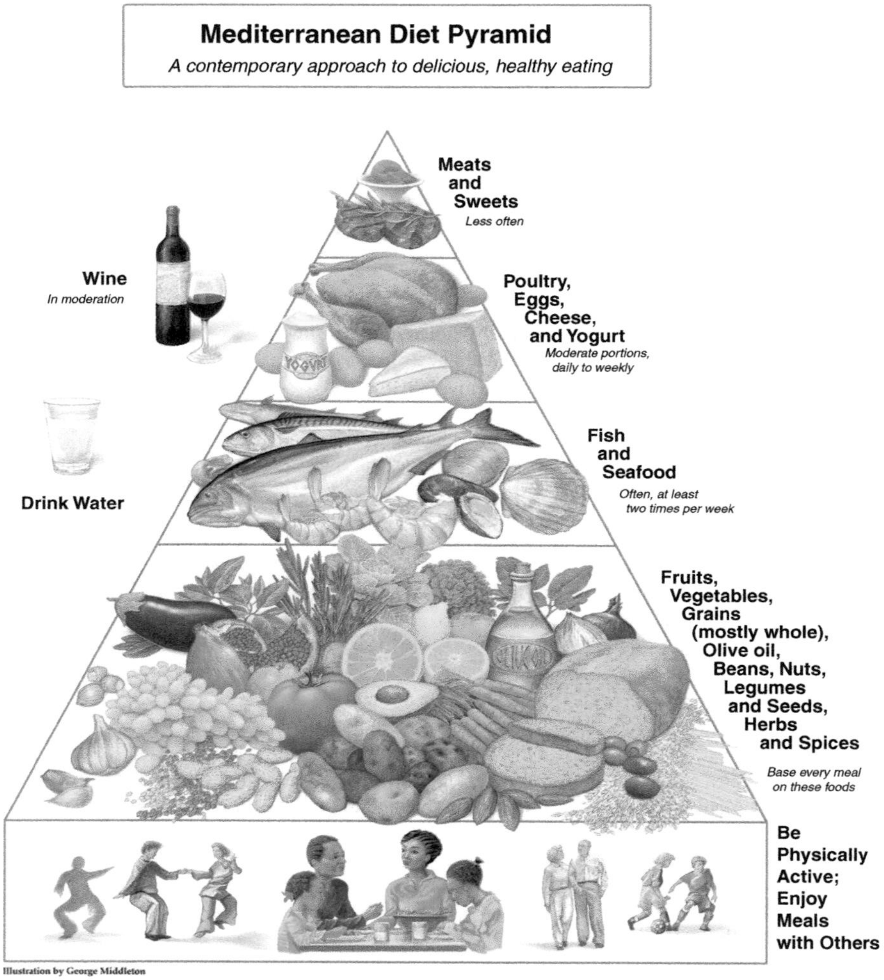

Fig. 13.3 Mediterranean DIET PYRAMID. © 2009 Oldways Preservation and Exchange Trust, www.oldwayspt.org

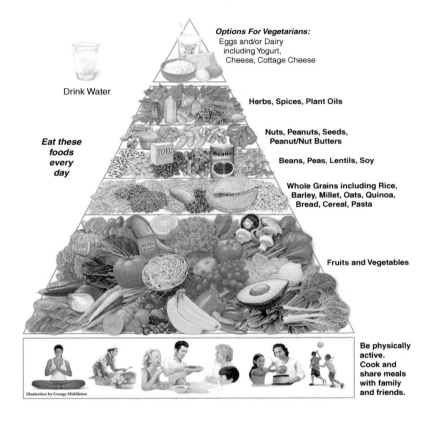

Fig. 13.4 Vegetarian and vegan diet pyramid. © 2013 Oldways Preservation and Exchange Trust, www.oldwayspt.org

13.8   Conclusion

This section "pulls" the pieces together by applying them to different eating patterns. There are other eating plans that this chapter did not discuss. For example, the
DASH style diet (Dietary Approaches to Stop Hypertension) and the Mediterranean-
DASH Intervention for Neurodegenerative Delay diet (MIND) offer similar principles. The diverse eating patterns re-inforce the principle that eating patterns can be
modified to fit the person's social and cultural preferences. Depending on their level
of functioning, persons with intellectual disability can participate in menu planning
and food preparation to practice their culinary skills and knowledge of foods.
MyPlate is a simple meal planning guide. Some eating patterns explicitly emphasize
the sense of community gained from preparing and eating foods with friends and
family. They also emphasize minimally processed foods, eco-friendliness and preservation of the environment (such as the Mediterranean diet [110]). Socialization
should be part of good nutrition care.

The key in all eating patterns is to eat a variety of foods in the proportion and
amount that are appropriate for nutrient and energy needs. General eating pattern recommendations are for healthy people and are not intended as therapeutic diets. They
are not applicable to children under 2 years of age [5]. Many people with intellectual
disability have special nutrition-related needs that should have timely assessment and
intervention by qualified health professionals. Optimal care requires interdisciplinary
collaboration among health team, effective partnerships with the persons with intellectual disability and their families, community support, and education of all people
involved. Diet and nutrition are determinants of health; however, the social context
affects their effectiveness in achieving person-centered health outcomes.

References

 1. Slawson DL, Fitzgerald N, Morgan KT. Position of the academy of nutrition and dietetics:
    the role of nutrition in health promotion and chronic disease prevention. J Acad Nutr Diet.
    2013;113:972–9. https://doi.org/10.1016/j.jand.2013.05.005.
 2. Freeland-Graves JH, Nitzke S. Position of the academy of nutrition and dietetics: Total diet
    approach to healthy eating. J Acad Nutr Diet. 2013;113:307–17.
 3. Davis R, Campbell R, Hildon Z, Hobbs L, Michie S. Theories of behaviour and behaviour
    change across the social and behavioural sciences: a scoping review. Health Psychol Rev.
    2015;9:323–44. https://doi.org/10.1080/17437199.2014.941722.
 4. Glanz K. Social and behavioral theories. Office of Behavioral and Social Sciences Research.
    OBSSR e-Source online resource for Behavioral and Social Sciences. e-Source Book; n.d.,
    p. 1–32. Accessed from http://www.esourceresearch.org/tabid/724/default.aspx
 5. U.S. Department of Health and Human Services (DHHS) and U.S. Department of Agriculture
    (USDA). 2015–2020 dietary guidelines for Americans. 8th ed; 2015 Accessed from: https://
    health.gov/dietaryguidelines/2015/guidelines/.
 6. Ptomey LT, Wittenbrook W. Position of the academy of nutrition and dietetics for individuals
    with intellectual and developmental disabilities and special health care needs. J Acad Nutr
    Diet. 2015;115:593–608. https://doi.org/10.1016/j.jand.2015.02.002.
 7. Davis R, Proulx R, van Schrojenstein Lantman-De Valk H. Health issues for people with
    intellectual disabilities: the evidence base. In: Taggart L, Cousins W, editors. Health promo-

tion for people with intellectual and developmental disabilities. London: Open University Press; 2014. p. 7–16. https://www.mheducation.co.uk/openup/chapters/9780335246946.pdf.

8. Haveman M, Perry J, Salvador-Carulla L, Walsh PN, Kerr M, Van Schrojenstein Lantman-De Valk H, Weber G. Ageing and health status in adults with intellectual disabilities: results of the European POMONA II study. J Intellect Dev Disabil. 2011;36:49–60. https://doi.org/10.3109/13668250.2010.549464.

9. Coppus AM. People with intellectual disability: what do we know about adulthood and life expectancy? Dev Disabil Res Rev. 2013;18:6–16.

10. Matthews DE. Proteins and amino acids. In: Ross CA, Caballero B, Cousias R, Tucker KL, Ziegler TR, editors. Modern nutrition in health and disease. 11th ed. Philadelphia: Lipincott, Williams and Wilkins; 2014. p. 4–36.

11. Gropper SAS, Smith JL, Groff JL. Advanced nutrition and human metabolism. Belmont: Wadsworth/Cengage Learning; 2009.

12. National Institutes of Health (NIH). National Institute of General Medical Sciences. (2011). Structures of life. Chapter 1. Proteins. Accessed from https://publications.nigms.nih.gov/structlife/chapter1.html

13. Institute of Medicine (IOM)/Food and Nutrition Board. Dietary reference intakes for energy, carbohydrate, fiber, fat, fatty acids, cholesterol, protein, and amino acids. Washington, DC: National Academies Press; 2005.

14. Dorner B, Friedrich EK. Position of the academy of nutrition and dietetics: individualized nutrition approaches for older adults: long-term care, post-acute care, and other settings. J Acad Nutr Diet. 2018;118:724–35.

15. Chernoff R. Protein and older adults. J Am Coll Nutr. 2004;23(6 Suppl):627s–30s.

16. Morley JE, Argiles JM, Evans WJ, Bhasin S, Cella D, Deutz NEP, The Society for Sarcopenia, Cachexia, and Wasting Disease. Nutritional recommendations for the management of sarcopenia. J Am Med Dir Assoc. 2010;11:391–6. https://doi.org/10.1016/j.jamda.2010.04.014.

17. Nowson C, O'Connell S. Protein requirements and recommendations for older people: a review. Nutrients. 2015;7:6874–99. https://doi.org/10.3390/nu7085311.

18. Morley JE, Cao L. Rapid screening for sarcopenia. J Cachexia Sarcopenia Muscle. 2015;6:312–4. https://doi.org/10.1002/jcsm.12079.

19. International Working Group on Sarcopenia. Sarcopenia: an undiagnosed condition in older adults. Current consensus definition: prevalence, etiology, and consequences. J Am Med Dir Assoc. 2011;12:249–56. https://doi.org/10.1016/j.jamda.2011.01.003.

20. von Haehling S, Morley JE, Anker SD. An overview of sarcopenia: facts and numbers on prevalence and clinical impact. J Cachexia Sarcopenia Muscle. 2010;1(2):129–33. https://doi.org/10.1007/s13539-010-0014-2.

21. Bastiaanse LP, Hilgenkamp TI, Echteld MA, Evenhuis HM. Prevalence and associated factors of sarcopenia in older adults with intellectual disabilities. Res Dev Disabil. 2012;33:2004–12.

22. Anker SD, Morley JE, von Haehling S. Welcome to the ICD-10 code for sarcopenia. J Cachexia Sarcopenia Muscle. 2016;7:512–4. https://doi.org/10.1002/jcsm.12147.

23. Melina V, Craig W, Levin S. Position of the academy of nutrition and dietetics: vegetarian diets. J Acad Nutr Diet. 2016;116:1970–80.

24. Slavin J, Carlson J. Carbohydrates. Adv Nutr. 2014;5(6):760–1. https://doi.org/10.3945/an.114.006163.

25. Kein ML, Levin RJ, Havel PJ. Carbohydrates. In: Ross CA, Caballero B, Cousias R, Tucker KL, Ziegler TR, editors. Modern nutrition in health and disease. 11th ed. Philadelphia: Lipincott, Williams and Wilkins; 2014. p. 36–57.

26. Taggart L, Coates V, Truesdale-Kennedy M. Management and quality indicators of diabetes mellitus in people with intellectual disabilities. J Intellect Disabil Res. 2013;57:1152–63. https://doi.org/10.1111/j.1365-2788.2012.

27. American Diabetes Association. Standards of medical care in diabetes—2018 abridged for primary care providers clinical diabetes. Diabetes Care. 2018;41(Suppl 1):S1–S159. Accessed from: http://clinical.diabetesjournals.org/content/diaclin/early/2017/12/07/cd17-0119.full.pdf

28. Alzheimer's Association. Alzheimer's disease facts and figures; 2018. Accessed from: https://www.alz.org/documents_custom/2018-facts-and-figures.pdf
29. US Department of Agriculture (USDA). ChooseMy Plate; n.d.. Accessed from: http://www.choosemyplate.gov/.
30. Clemens R, Kranz S, Mobley RA, Nicklas TA, Raimondi MP, Rodriguez JC, Slavin JL, Warshaw H. Filling America's fiber intake gap: summary of a roundtable to probe realistic solutions with a focus on grain-based foods. J Nutr. 2012;142:1390S–401S. https://doi.org/10.3945/jn.112.160176.
31. Jones JM. CODEX-aligned dietary fiber definitions help to bridge the "fiber gap". Nutr J. 2014;13:34. https://doi.org/10.1186/1475-2891-13-3.
32. Thompson HJ, Brick MA. Perspective: closing the dietary fiber gap: an ancient solution for a 21st century problem. Adv Nutr. 2016;7:623–6. https://doi.org/10.3945/an.115.009696.
33. Adolfsson P, Sydner YM, Fjellström C, Lewin B, Andersson A. Observed dietary intake in adults with intellectual disability living in the community. Food Nutr Res. 2008;52 https://doi.org/10.3402/fnr.v52i0.1857.
34. McRorie JW. Evidence-based approach to fiber supplements and clinically meaningful health benefits. Part 1: What to look for and how to recommend an effective fiber therapy. Nutr Today. 2015;50:82–9. https://doi.org/10.1097/NT.0000000000000082.
35. Dahl WJ, Stewart ML. Position of the academy of nutrition and dietetics: health implications of dietary fiber. J Acad Nutr Diet. 2015;115:1861–70.
36. Drake VJ. Fiber. Linus Pauling Institute, Oregon State University; 2012. http://lpi.oregonstate.edu/mic/other-nutrients/fiber.
37. Khan K, Jovanovski E, Ho HVT, Marques ACR, Zurbau A, Mejia SB, Sievenpiper JL, Vuksan V. The effect of viscous soluble fiber on blood pressure: a systematic review and meta-analysis of randomized controlled trials. Nutr Metab Cardiovasc Dis. 2018;28:3e13. https://www.nmcd-journal.com/article/S0939-4753(17)30222-3/pdf
38. Lambeau KV, McRorie JW. Fiber supplements and clinically proven health benefits: how to recognize and recommend an effective fiber therapy. J Am Assoc Nurse Pract. 2017;29:216–23. Published online 02 Mar 2017. https://doi.org/10.1002/2327-6924.12447.
39. McRorie JW, McKeown NM. Understanding the physics of functional fibers in the gastrointestinal tract: an evidence-based approach to resolving enduring misconceptions about insoluble and soluble fiber. J Acad Nutr Diet. 2017;117:251–64.
40. Perry JR, Ying W. A review of physiological effects of soluble and insoluble dietary fibers. J Nutr Food Sci. 2016;6:476. https://doi.org/10.4172/2155-9600.1000476.
41. Slavin J. Fiber and prebiotics: mechanisms and health benefits. Nutrients. 2013;5(4):1417–35. https://doi.org/10.3390/nu504141.
42. Sharon V, Thompson BA, Hannon RA, Holscher HD. Effects of isolated soluble fiber supplementation on body weight, glycemia, and insulinemia in adults with overweight and obesity: a systematic review and meta-analysis of randomized controlled trials. Am J Clin Nutr. 2017;106:1514–28. https://doi.org/10.3945/ajcn.117.163246.
43. Connor M, Hunt C, Lindley A. Using abdominal massage in bowel management. Nurs Stand. 2014;28(45):37–42. https://doi.org/10.7748/ns.28.45.37.e8661.
44. Robertson J, Baines S, Emerson E, Hatton C. Prevalence of constipation in people with intellectual disability: a systematic review. J Intellect Dev Disabil. Published online: 25 May 2017. 2017; https://doi.org/10.3109/13668250.2017.1310829.
45. Mounsey A, Raleigh M, Wilson A. Management of constipation in older adults. Am Fam Physician. 2015;92:500–4.
46. Schuster BG, Kosar L, Kamrul R. Constipation in older adults: stepwise approach to keep things moving. Can Fam Physician. 2015;61:152–8.
47. Quagliani D, Felt-Gunderson P. Closing America's fiber intake gap: communication strategies from a food and fiber summit. Am J Lifestyle Med. 2015;11:80–5.
48. Institute of Shortening and Edible Oils. Food fats and oils. 10th ed. Washington, DC: Author; 2016. Accessed from: http://www.iseo.org/httpdocs/FoodFatsOils2016.pdf

49. European Food and Information Council (EUFIC). Facts on fats: dietary fats and health; 2015. Accessed from: http://www.eufic.org/en/whats-in-food/article/facts-on-fats-dietary-fats-and-health.
50. Vannice G, Rasmussen H. Position of the academy of nutrition and dietetics: dietary fatty acids for healthy adults. J Acad Nutr Diet. 2014;114:136–53. https://doi.org/10.1016/j.jand.2013.11.001.
51. Liu AG, Ford NA, Hu FB, Zelman KM, Mozaffarian D, Kris-Etherton PM. A healthy approach to dietary fats: understanding the science and taking action to reduce consumer confusion. Nutr J. 2017;16(1):53. https://doi.org/10.1186/s12937-017-0271-4.
52. International Food Information Council (IFIC). 2017 food and health survey: "A healthy perspective: Understanding American food values"; 2017. Accessed from: https://www.foodinsight.org/2017-food-and-health-survey
53. Jones PJH, Rideout T. Lipids, sterols and their metabolites. In: Ross CA, Caballero B, Cousias R, Tucker KL, Ziegler TR, editors. Modern nutrition in health and disease. 11th ed. Philadelphia: Lipincott, Williams and Wilkins; 2014. p. 65–87.
54. Simolopoulos AP. The omega-6/omega-3 fatty acid ratio: health implications. Oilseeds Fats Crops Lipids. 2010;17(5):267–75. https://doi.org/10.1051/ocl.2010.0325. Accessed from: https://www.ocl-journal.org/articles/ocl/abs/2010/05/ocl2010175p267/ocl2010175p267.html
55. Lands B. Dietary omega-3 and omega-6 fatty acids compete in producing tissue compositions and tissue responses. Mil Med. 2014;179(Suppl 11):76–81. https://doi.org/10.7205/MILMED-D-14-00149.
56. Tallima H, El Ridi R. Arachidonic acid: physiological roles and potential health benefits – a review. J Adv Res. 2018;11:33–41. https://doi.org/10.1016/j.jare.2017.11.004.
57. European Food Safety Authority (EFSA). Scientific opinion the substantiation of a health claim related to docosahexaenoic acid (DHA) and maintenance of normal (fasting) blood concentrations of triglycerides (ID 533, 691, 3150). EFSA J. 2010;8:1734. https://doi.org/10.2903/j.efsa.2010.1734.
58. Dyall SC. Long-chain omega-3 fatty acids and the brain: a review of the independent and shared effects of EPA, DPA and DHA. Front Aging Neurosci. 2015;7:52. https://doi.org/10.3389/fnagi.2015.00052.
59. European Food Safety Authority (EFSA). Scientific opinion on the substantiation of a health claim related to alpha linolenic acid and contribution to brain and nerve tissue development pursuant to Article 14 of Regulation (EC) No 1924/2006. EFSA J. 2011;9:2130. https://doi.org/10.2903/j.efsa.2011.2130.
60. World Health Organization (WHO). Fats and fatty acids in human nutrition. Report of an expert consultation; 2010. Accessed from: http://www.who.int/nutrition/publications/nutrientrequirements/fatsandfattyacids_humannutrition/en/
61. Angelo G. Essential fatty acids. Corvallis, OR: Linus Pauling Institute, Oregon State University; 2014.
62. American Heart Association. Fish and omega-3 fatty acids; 2016. Accessed from: http://www.heart.org/HEARTORG/HealthyLiving/HealthyEating/HealthyDietGoals/Fish-and-Omega-3-Fatty-Acids_UCM_303248_Article.jsp#.WxPtKO4vx0w
63. Armstrong L. Rationale for renewed emphasis on dietary water intake. Nutr Today. 2010;45(6):S4–6. https://doi.org/10.1097/NT.0b013e3181fe1597.
64. Roumelioti ME, Glew RH, Khitan ZJ, Rondon-Berrios H, Argyropoulos CP, Malhotra D, Tzamaloukas AH. Fluid balance concepts in medicine: principles and practice. World J Nephrol. 2018;7:1–28. https://doi.org/10.5527/wjn.v7.i1.1. https://health.gov/dietaryguidelines/2015/27/wjn.v7.i1.1
65. Archibald C. Promoting hydration in patients with dementia in healthcare settings. Nurs Stand. 2006;20:49–52. https://www.ncbi.nlm.nih.gov/pubmed/16872119
66. Keller H, Carrier N, Duizer L, Lengyel C, Slaughter S, Steele C. Making the most of mealtimes (M3): grounding mealtime interventions with a conceptual model. J Am Med Dir Assoc. 2014;15:158–61. https://doi.org/10.1016/j.jamda.2013.12.001.

67. Institute of Medicine (IOM)/Food and Nutrition Board. Dietary reference intakes for water, potassium, sodium, chloride, and sulfate. Washington, DC: National Academies Press; 2005.
68. Delage B. Vitamin A. Linus Pauling Institute, Oregon State University; 2015. http://lpi.oregonstate.edu/mic/vitamins/folate
69. Institute of Medicine (IOM)/Food and Nutrition Board. Dietary reference intakes for vitamin A, vitamin K, arsenic, boron, chromium, copper, iodine, iron, manganese, molybdenum, nickel, silicon, vanadium, and zinc. Washington, DC: The National Academies Press; 2001. https://doi.org/10.17226/10026
70. Office of Dietary Supplements (ODS)/National Institutes of Health. Vitamin A; 2018. Accessed from: https://ods.od.nih.gov/factsheets/VitaminA-HealthProfessional/
71. Conaway HH, Henning P, Lerner UH. Vitamin A metabolism, action, and role in skeletal homeostasis. Endocr Rev. 2013;34(6):766–97. https://doi.org/10.1210/er.2012-1071.
72. Ross AC. Vitamin A. In: Ross AC, et al., editors. Modern nutrition in health and disease. 11th ed. Philadelphia: Lippincott, Williams, and Wilkins; 2014.
73. World Health Organization (WHO). Micronutrient deficiencies: vitamin A deficiency; 2018. Accessed from: http://www.who.int/nutrition/topics/vad/en/
74. Institute of Medicine (IOM)/Food and Nutrition Board. Dietary reference intakes for calcium and vitamin D. Washington, DC: National Academies Press; 2011. Accessed from http://books.nap.edu/openbook.php?record_id_13050
75. Office of Dietary Supplements (ODS)/National Institutes of Health. Vitamin D; 2018. Accessed from: https://ods.od.nih.gov/factsheets/VitaminD-HealthProfessional/
76. Holick MF, Chen TC, Lu Z, Sauer E. Vitamin D and skin physiology: a D-lightful story. J Bone Miner Res. 2007;22(Suppl 2):V28–33. https://doi.org/10.1359/JBMR.07S211. https://www.foodinsight.org/2017-food-and-health-survey
77. Wang H, Chen W, Li D, Yin X, Zhang X, Olsen N, Zheng SG. Vitamin D and chronic diseases. Aging Dis. 2017;8(3):346–53. https://doi.org/10.14336/AD.2016.1021.
78. Lappe JM. Role of vitamin D in health: a paradigm shift. J Evid Based Complementary Altern Med. 2010;16:58–72.
79. Zhang R, Naughton DP. Vitamin D in health and disease: current perspectives. Nutr J. 2010;9:65. https://doi.org/10.1186/1475-2891-9-65. (on-line)
80. Gallagher JC. Vitamin D and aging. Endocrinol Metab Clin N Am. 2013;42:319–32. https://doi.org/10.1016/j.ecl.2013.02.004.
81. Cosman F, de Beur FJ, Leboff MS, Lewiecki EM, Tanner B, Randall S, Lindsay R. Clinician's guide to prevention and treatment of osteoporosis. Osteoporos Int. 2014;25:2359–81. https://doi.org/10.1007/s00198-014-2794-2.
82. Holick M. Vitamin D is not as toxic as was once thought: a historical and an up-to-date perspective. Mayo Clin Proc. 2015;90:561–4.
83. Jasien J, Daimon CM, Maudsley S, Shapiro BK, Martin B. Aging and bone health in individuals with developmental disabilities. Int J Endocrinol. 2012;2012:469235. https://doi.org/10.1155/2012/469235.
84. Srikanth R, Cassidy IG, Joiner C, Teeluckdharry S. Osteoporosis in people with intellectual disabilities: a review and a brief study of risk factors for osteoporosis in a community sample of people with intellectual disabilities. J Intellect Disabil Res. 2011;55:53–62.
85. Office of Dietary Supplements (ODS)/National Institutes of Health. Vitamin E; 2018. Accessed from: https://ods.od.nih.gov/factsheets/VitaminE-HealthProfessional/
86. Institute of Medicine (IOM)/Food and Nutrition Board. Dietary reference intakes for vitamin C, vitamin E, selenium, and carotenoids. Washington, DC: National Academy Press; 2000.
87. Delage B. Vitamin K. Linus Pauling Institute, Oregon State University; 2014. http://lpi.oregonstate.edu/mic/vitamins/vitamin-K
88. Office of Dietary Supplements (ODS)/National Institutes of Health. Vitamin K; 2018. Accessed from: https://ods.od.nih.gov/factsheets/VitaminK-HealthProfessional/
89. Goebel L, Mose M. Scurvy. Medscape; 2017. https://emedicine.medscape.com/article/125350-overview#a6

90. Office of Dietary Supplements (ODS)/National Institutes of Health. Vitamin C; 2018. Accessed from: https://ods.od.nih.gov/factsheets/VitaminC-HealthProfessional/

91. Coffey-Vega K, Gentili A, Vohra M, Chen K-HD. Folic acid deficiency. Medscape, July 19, 2017. https://emedicine.medscape.com/article/200184-overview.

92. Office of Dietary Supplements (ODS)/National Institutes of Health. Vitamin B-12; 2018. Accessed from: https://ods.od.nih.gov/factsheets/VitaminB12-HealthProfessional/

93. Fayaz F, Gachkar L, Rahmati Roodsari S, Pourkaveh B. Prevalence of Helicobacter pylori infection in patients with Down syndrome and mental retardation. Arch Clin Infect Dis. 2014;9:e22064. https://doi.org/10.5812/archcid.22064.

94. Institute of Medicine (IOM)/Food and Nutrition Board. Dietary reference intakes: thiamin, riboflavin, niacin, vitamin B6, folate, vitamin B12, pantothenic acid, biotin, and choline. Washington, DC: National Academies Press; 1998. Accessed from www.ncbi.nlm.nih.gov/pubmed/23193625

95. Oldways. Vegetarian and vegan diet; n.d.-b Accessed from: https://oldwayspt.org/traditional-diets/vegetarian-vegan-diet

96. Office of Dietary Supplements (ODS)/National Institutes of Health. Folate; 2018. Accessed from: https://ods.od.nih.gov/factsheets/Folate-HealthProfessional/

97. Delage B. Folate. Linus Pauling Institute, Oregon State University; 2014. http://lpi.oregonstate.edu/mic/vitamins/folate.

98. Office of Dietary Supplements (ODS)/National Institutes of Health. Calcium; 2017. Accessed from: https://ods.od.nih.gov/factsheets/Calcium-HealthProfession

99. WHO. Anemia; n.d.. http://www.who.int/topics/anaemia/en/

100. Office of Dietary Supplements (ODS)/National Institutes of Health. Iron; 2018. Accessed from: https://ods.od.nih.gov/factsheets/Iron-HealthProfessional/

101. World Health Organization (WHO). Nutrition. Micronutrient deficiencies: iodine deficiency disorder, 2018. Accessed from: http://www.who.int/nutrition/topics/idd/en/

102. Kapil U. Health consequences of iodine deficiency. Sultan Qaboos Univ Med J. 2007;7(3):267–72.

103. Office of Dietary Supplements (ODS)/National Institutes of Health. Iodine; 2018. Accessed from: https://ods.od.nih.gov/factsheets/Iodine-HealthProfessional/

104. World Health Organization (WHO). Goitre as a determinant of the prevalence and severity of iodine deficiency disorders in populations. In: Vitamin and mineral nutrition information system. Geneva: World Health Organization; 2014. Accessed from: http://www.who.int/vmnis/indicators/goitre_idd/en/.

105. Food and Agricultural Organization of the United Nations. Food-based dietary guidelines; 2010. Accessed from: http://www.fao.org/nutrition/education/food-dietary-guidelines/background/en/.

106. US Department of Agriculture (USDA). Translating the dietary guidelines into consumer messages; 2018. Accessed from: https://www.choosemyplate.gov/translating-dietary-guidelines-consumer-messages.

107. University of Idaho Extension. Planning meals by photo; 2009. Accessed from: https://www.extension.uidaho.edu/diabetesplate/planning/index.html

108. Wright I, Safaii S, Raidl M, Buck JH, Spencer MR, Deringer N. Effectiveness of the healthy diabetes plate and social media project. J Nutr Health. 2015;1(2):1–6. Accessed from: http://www.avensonline.org/wp-content/uploads/JNH-2469-4185-01-0007.pdf

109. Caroline Walker Trust. Eating well: children and adults with learning disabilities – nutritional and practical guidelines. Abbots Langley (Herts): Author; 2007. Accessed from https://www.cwt.org.uk/wp-content/uploads/2015/02/EWLDGuidelines.pdf

110. Oldways. Mediterranean diet; n.d.-a Accessed from: https://oldwayspt.org/traditional-diets/mediterranean-diet

111. American Diabetes Association. Create your plate; 2016. Accessed from: http://www.diabetes.org/food-and-fitness/food/planning-meals/create-your-plate/?referrer=https://search.yahoo.com/

112. Haveman MJ, Heller T, Lee L, Maaskant M, Shooshtari S, Strydom A. Major health risks in aging persons with intellectual disabilities: an overview of recent studies. J Policy Pract Intellect Disabil. 2010;7:59–69.
113. Jones JM. Dietary fiber future directions: integrating new definitions and findings to inform nutrition research and communication. Adv Nutr. 2013;4:8–15. https://doi.org/10.3945/an.112.002907.
114. Raidl M, Safaii S. The healthy diabetes plate website teaches meal planning skills. J Diabetes Metab. 2013;4:284. https://doi.org/10.4172/2155-6156.1000284. Accessed from: https://www.omicsonline.org/the-healthy-diabetes-plate-website-teaches-meal-planning-skills-2155-6156.1000284.php?aid=16627
115. Strydom A, Lee LA, Jokinen N, Shooshtari S, Raykar V, Torr J, Tsiouris JA, Courtenay K, Bass N, Sinnema M, Maaskant MA. Report on the state of science on dementia in people with intellectual disabilities. IASSID Special Interest Research Group on ageing and intellectual disabilities; 2009. Accessed from: https://www.iassidd.org/content/aging-and-intellectual-disability-documents-and-publications

Improving Lives Through Alleviating Malnutrition

14

Sunil J. Wimalawansa

14.1 Introduction

Approximately 4.6 million individuals resident in the USA have an intellectual disability [1], while others reported increasing incidences and the prevalence of, up to 15% of the population in some countires [2]. Varying prevalence of intellectual disability has been reported in other countries [3–5]. The Centers for Disease Control and Prevention reported a gradual increase of the prevalence of intellectual and developmental disabilities in children resident in the United States, currently up to 7% [6] and 6% in United Kingdom [7]. IT is important to note that virtually, any syndrome associated with intellectual disability is aggravated by concomitant presence of nutritional deficiencies. These worsen their behavior and the underlying health conditions and the overall health [8].

Severe malnutrition is deleterious at any stage of the life. Malnutrition during the fetal life or infancy in animals and humans, decreases brain size and reduces the number of brain and kidney cells. These are known to results in both, behavioral and physiological abnormalities. However, this is complicated by underlying genetic abnormalities, birth defects, epigenetic factors, and socio-economic and other factors that are common in adults with intellectual disability [9].

Whilst body mass index (BMI) could be normal, many adults with intellectual disability have visceral (abdominal) obesity. Since intra-abdominal fat produce a host of inflammatory agents [10, 11] it leads to insidious metabolic derangements, and thus, negatively alter metabolism [12]. Thus, in addition to taking care of controlling caloric intake and energy consumption, attention should be given to healthful lifestyle, associated conditions, and micronutrient requirements. These would minimize the associated comorbidities [13]. Data suggests that timely, and appropriate nutritional interventions could reverse not only the nutritional deficiencies, but also

S. J. Wimalawansa (✉)
Department of Medicine, Cardio Metabolic Institute (hon.),
North Brunswick, NJ, USA

© Springer Nature Switzerland AG 2019
V. P. Prasher, M. P. Janicki (eds.), *Physical Health of Adults with Intellectual and Developmental Disabilities*, https://doi.org/10.1007/978-3-319-90083-4_14

complications from illnesses that commonly present in those with intellectual disability by modifying and stabilizing the internal milieu including the gut microbiota [14]. These include but not limited to, protein-energy malnutrition, iodine, iron, antioxidants and vitamin deficiencies [8, 15].

14.2   Fundamental Issues Related to Nutrition Issues in Adults with Intellectual Disability

Chronic diseases demand both general treatment and targeted, disease modifiers and replacement therapies. In addition, whether it is primary, secondary or tertiary prevention, putting efforts on root-cause alliviation for disease prevention is equally important. Many adults with intellectual disability have behavioural issues. However, purely focusing on behaviour modification to achieve consistent and sustainable healthy eating and physical activity is untenable. Considering this, none of the currently published, *evidence-based* clinical practice guidelines are applicable in general, to persons with intellectual disability. Direct implementation of such is inappropriate for those with intellectual disabilities, in defining the standard of care for healthy eating or management, and prevention of nutritional, metabolic and other disorders.

Nutritional education and evidence-based behavioral modifications that considered standard for those community-dwelling ambulatory persons, do not apply to adults with intellectual disability. The latter group and caregivers alike, face many unique obstacles that preclude following the standard guidelines published for ambulatory people. In fact, many of those are irrelevant, and unpractical in most situations in adults with intellectual disability. Trying to emulate the guidelines and counselling, published for general health nutrition education, such as medical nutrition therapy for diabetes mellitus and nutrition for chronic kidney disease, thus, should not be directly imposed on those with intellectual disability.

14.3   What Makes Adults with Intellectual Disability Different?

Most common medical diseases, such as overweight and obesity, dyslipidaemia, hypertension, thyroid diseases, prediabetes and type 2 diabetes (T2D), polycystic ovarian syndrome, osteopenia and osteoporosis, chronic obstructive airways diseases, gastro-oesophageal/reflux diseases, chronic kidney disease (CKD), eating disorders, malnutrition, also affect adults with intellectual disability. However, presentation of these disease may be different in those with intellectual disability. In addition, there are a host of other diseases, particularly conditions with genetic ailments are inherent in some adult with intellectual disability; this further complicate the situation.

While the above is a simplified statement, many obstacles exist to implementing healthy eating strategies in adults with intellectual disability. These includes, appetite, non-corporations, oesophageal abnormalities and reflux (swallowing difficulty) diseases, and digestion difficulties, and so forth. Moreover, there is no standardized protocol that can be easily used or adapted for the variety of conditions that adults with intellectual disability. In addition, the cultural habits, believes, and resources vary much in different countries, making any global recommendations impractical. Given the importance and the emphasize on disease prevention, health promotion and wellness care, focus should shift to improving the quality of life, early identification of root-causes, and thus, preventing complications.

In addition, targeting and providing, low cost, palatable, nutritious food, designed for easy ingestion and digestion for adults with challenging eating conditions is virtually non-existent. Market should explore the provision of such food at an affordable cost to the public. Another complicated area is the variability of nutrigenomics and nutrigenetics (i.e., nutrient-gene interactions), epigenetics, ethnic, cultural, religious, social, and economic factors that are associated with individual food preferences, affordability, and availability.

14.4   Common Nutritional Deficiencies Among Adults with Intellectual Disability

Nutrients, such as trace minerals requirements that requires less than 100 mg/day/person, are considered as micronutrients, as opposed to macronutrients (carbohydrate, protein, fat, fibre, etc.) and macro-minerals (calcium, magnesium, etc.), which are required in larger quantities. Single micronutrient deficiency states are easier to recognized than multiple deficiencies [16, 17]. Micronutrients are essential throughout the life; these are need in small quantities, and are necessary for a range of physiological functions and maintaining good health. Moreover, except for some B-vitamins and vitamin D, micronutrients are not produced within the body and thus, must be taken from the diet [16].

14.5   Macronutrient Deficiencies

The broader groups of nutritional components include, macronutrients, micronutrients, fibre, and water. These must be incorporated into chosen foods and beverages these are also need to be palatable to the recipients and affordable. Macronutrients provide the opportunity for calorie-control. Generally, this goes 'hand-in-hand' with healthy lifestyle, such as regular physical activity (e.g., 150 min or more per week recommended for ambulatory people), ways to avoid a sedentary lifestyle, appropriate sleep time (7 to 9 h, each night) and age- and sex-appropriate recreational activities. Nevertheless, these may not necessarily practical or applicable to those with intellectual disability. Especially for those with intellectual disability who have multiply-physical and cognitive impairments.

General meal plans should provide 45–65% of ingested energy, through carbohydrates. This is an area that can be easily modify and adapt to each person. Whether the person consumes the recommended 5–7 servings (a serving is considered as equivalent of 15 g of carbohydrate), containing high fiber and whole-grain products, fruits (e.g., any type of berries) and vegetables (≥4.5 cups per day), will increase the fiber content, while simplifing caloric control.

Reduced fat dairy products (3–4 ounces per day) facilitate balance in the protein to calorie ratio and add certain micronutrients. Nevertheless, a higher proportion of adults with intellectual disability are intolerant or allergic to dairy products, especially, lactose. Instead of animal proteins that may cause subsidiary issues in some plant protein such as pulses, beans, lentils, and some nuts, together with vegetables like broccoli and spinach, can be substituted in the meal plan.

Fat supposed to provide approximately 25–35% of daily calories (or less). Consumption of poly- and mono-unsaturated fats (e.g., liquid, seeds, nuts, and fish oils, including omega-3 fatty acids), should mostly replace high saturated fatty foods (butter, margarine, and animal fats).

14.6   Micronutrients Deficiencies

Micronutrient deficiencies in adults with intellectual disability are much higher than in the typical ambulatory populations. These include vitamins, (micro) minerals, and antioxidants deficiencies. Diets provided in congregate care settings, such as nursing homes and disability residential care centres, generally provide adequate amounts of vitamin A, B, and E, and (macro)minerals like calcium, magnesium, iron, etc. However, others such as vitamin D and C, micro-minerals and antioxidants that are necessary as co-factors and for enzymatic functions, and the fiber contents are generally low. Combination of such are known to affect intellectual functions, including memory, behaviour, neuro-muscular coordination, and fine motor functions [18].

Since gastrointestinal abnormalities such as intestinal malabsorption (e.g., celiac disease, inflammatory bowel disease, exocrine pancreatic insufficiency, pernicious anaemia, bariatric surgery, short bowel syndrome, chronic kidney and chronic liver diseases) are common in adults with intellectual disability, fractional absorption of many of these micronutrients are less than that of ambulatory healthy people. Thus, such adults are likely to require higher intake of micronutrients, compared to adults without these conditions [19, 20].

Other micro-nutritional areas that require attention include vitamin B12 (especially among vegans and adults on metformin therapy), folate, and micro-minerals (also a part of antioxidants), like selenium and zinc [21]. In the case of vitamin D deficiency, it can be only confirmed by the measurement of 25-hydroxyvitamin D [25(OH)D] concentration [22]. In some residential care facilities, it has been reported that the incidence of vitamin D deficiency reaches 90% [23, 24].

While, many adults with intellectual disability do not get exposed to adequate amounts of sunlight. In addition, those with pigmented or damaged skin, elderly, or who are over-covered with clothing and use sunscreens are more prown to develop hypovitaminosis D [24–26]. Average amount of vitamin D obtained from a

Western diet is between 200–500 IU/day, while in general, the requirements in adults are more than 2,000 IU/day. Thus, in the absence of sun expose and regular eating of fatty fish, such as salmon or mackerel, or sun-exposed mushrooms, virtually all adults with intellectual disability need vitamin D supplementation of between 2000 and 4000 international units (IU) per day.

14.7 Avoiding Saturated Fats, Processed Food, Trans-Fat (barbecued meat), and Pastry Products

Reducing the intake of saturated fat intake lowers the LDL-cholesterol. The Dietary Guidelines Advisory Committee stated that, "there is strong evidence to support that increased saturated fat intake, intensifies CVD via increasing non-HDL-cholesterol and insulin resistance." On the other hand, replacing 5% of energy with mono unsaturated fat (MUFAs) or poly unsaturated fat (PUFAs), instead of saturated fat can reduce the risk of CVD and T2D in healthy adults. These incidences can also decrease by reducing the intake of red meat and processed food [27] and increase the intake of fruit and vegetables [28].

Large randomized control clinical trials (RCTs), such as Oslo Diet Heart, Finnish Mental Hospital, and Veteran Affairs, and others have demonstrated consistently, that there is a reduced risk of mortality following decrease intake of saturated fat and increasing PUFA intake [29]. Many RCTs have shown that replacing saturated fat with PUFA tangibly decreases LDL-cholesterol, and reduces risk for cardiovascular mortality [30, 31]. The current recommendation is to replace saturated fats with increased intake of unsaturated fats.

Communities that consume diets that consistently have high refined grains (less bran/fiber), have increased risk for cardiovascular diseases, cancer, and all-cause mortality [32]. In addition, high intake of refined grains (also have high glycemic index), independently associated with raised plasma plasminogen activator inhibitor type 1 (PAI-1), a marker of chronic inflammation [33] and C-reactive proteins. Thus, it is best to consume the whole grain products than refined ones.

14.8 Malnutrition

Both under-nutrition and over-nutrition are common among adults with intellectual disability. Extremes of nutrition, *kwashiorkor* and *marasmus*, and overweightness and obesity, have significant negative consequences and have increased comorbidities and reduce life expectancy. Because of relative inactivity in adults with intellectual disability, these conditions are common in this group. However, one should not simply rely on the use of BMI to diagnose this; in adults with intellectual disability, the measurement of abdominal girth is much more informative than the calculated BMI [34].

Obesity should be considered as a chronic inflammatory disease that can aggravate other metabolic conditions [34–36]. The goal here is to reduce the intra-abdominal fat content, not the BMI. There is no established weight-reduction goal for adults with intellectual disability. This is due to marked individual variations, intra-abdominal fat does not reflect linearly the total body weight, and the unreliability of the use of BMI. A combined approach of using a low-calorie diet, increased physical activity, a psychological and behaviour therapy (but not through pharmacotherapy) is more cost-effective. In rare cases, such as severe insulin resistance syndrome, bariatric surgery can be considered as the last resort to improve quality of life and metabolic risk reduction.

14.9 Undernutrition

Key manifestations of severe under-nutrition caused by macronutrient malnutrition are marasmus (stunting, wasting, and underweight) and kwashiorkor (severe protein malnutrition). However, numerous other nutritional disorders exist secondary to different micronutrient insufficiency. Since it is cost-prohibitive to correct these individual deficiencies based on personal biochemical diagnosis, food fortification has become a practical and a cost-effective approach to solve this problem. The costs of the adding ingredients, such as vitamins and minerals to food, for fortification are estimated between 0.5% and 2.0% of the cost of a typical staple food [37]. Thus, it is an efficient and affrodable way to provide micronutrients to a given community.

Underlying causes for micronutrient deficiencies vary from underlying diseases to economic reasons, such as lack of access to nutritious food and food affordability, transportation and storage issues, processing and cooking issues, and cultural and eating habits. Understanding the causes would facilitate designing cost-effective solutions to an individual, as well as for a given community. Micronutrient deficiencies are associated morbidities, thus, treatment costs and loss of productivity. These could be overcome cost-effectively by proactively preventing nutritional disorders.

14.10 Dietary, Lifestyle, and Medical Choices in Promoting Health

To achieve the best health status, one need to follow (a) balanced diet, (b) regular weight-bearing exercise, (c) avoid bad lifestyle habits, and (d) relaxation of the mind and the body. These would in turn, shift the negative spiral of mental and physical imbalance and stresses, to a positive cycle leading to an optimum health and happiness. Lifestyle changes are always useful, if these can be implemented effectively. Achieving and maintaining a healthy body weight, and age-, sex- and height/weight appropriate abdominal girth, will also facilitate normalization of serum lipids, blood pressure, reduce insulin resistance, and the overall metabolism. In general, trying to manipulate solely, sodium and sugar intake (if they are used to higher amounts) may not be sufficient.

In constructing diets, staff and caregivers should strive to eliminate processed food and limit red meat intake to fewer less than 2 servings per week. Also, useful is the substitution of refined grain products (e.g., white flour products) with whole grain products as much as possible, striving for at least one-half of daily servings of grains to be from whole-grains would be beneficial.

Many adults with intellectual disability have low bone mineral density (BMD) and co-existing vitamin D-deficiency related osteomalacia [38]. To decrease osteoporosis and associated fracture risks (which are at least ten-fold higher in some adults with intellectual disability [39, 40], it is recommended to have the total elemental calcium intake of 1,000 mg/day for men and premenopausal women, and 1200 mg/day for post-menopausal women, together with 2,000 IU of vitamin D. Considering the sedentary lifestyles of many adults with intellectual disability, exceeding elemental calcium intake beyond 1,500 mg/day may cause hypercalciuria and increase the risk of renal stones.

14.11 Addressing Healthy Eating

Many adults with intellectual disability have many barriers to overcome, including nutritional adequacy and balance. Nutritional barriers are not limited to the access, affordability, and the availability of nutritious food, but also the need for one-on-one attention or supervision on direct feeding, when self-feeding is not adequate. Meanwhile the associate comorbidities such as depression, airways and gastrointestinal diseases, oral hygiene and dental problems, chewing or swallowing problems, sexual desires and other personal needs, social isolation, and rectifying underlying diseases needs appropriate concomitant treatment.

Healthy eating benefits from being presented with likable and palatable proper meals, that provide adequate amounts of macro- and micronutrients to sustain normal physiology and avoid nutritional deficiencies. In addition to healthy eating, physical activity, adequate sleep and healthy sleep patterns, all contribute to wellness.

A healthy lifestyle benefits general health as well as cardiovascular health. In addition, overcoming obesity and having reasonable physical activity, reduces the incidence of most common cancers, such as breast, lung, and colorectal cancer. Moreover, the increase consumption of fruits and vegetables, and whole grain food products that contain vitamins, minerals, and antioxidants, also reduce the risks of cancers.

The daily ingestion of at least eight servings of fresh fruits and vegetables should be recommended for most adults with intellectual disability. Many potentially anti-carcinogenic and antioxidant agents are present in fish, fruits, vegetables, fibre, and plant compounds (e.g., flavonoids, phenols, protease inhibitors, sterols, allium compounds, and limonene) [41]. Healthy eating, such as the Mediterranean diets and their adaptions, contributes significantly to human health maintenance and disease prevention.

At the clinical level, micronutrient status can be assessed or measured for an individual, and potentially appropriate intake levels and/or supplements can be supplied. However, in population strategies, all complicating factors must be considered.

Special fortified foods for the elderly and those with disabilities were proposed to provide to fulfil the estimated requirements for micronutrients, which may otherwise not be met by their reduced energy diets [42]. Chronic low-grade inflammation is common in elderly persons and among persons who live in unsanitary conditions; this can lead to less efficient intestinal absorption through hepcidin regulation [43].

In industrialized countries, medical drug prescriptions and intakes are increasing, especially in aging populations, often inappropriately. Elderly adults and those adults with disability on average are taking six medications. Some of these medications either enhance or reduce availability of other medications and micronutrients (i.e., drug-drug or drug-food interactions). Especially with new medications; while, many of such interactions with micronutrients are known, few have been properly investigated. For example, the regular intake of aspirin, commonly used for prevention of cardiovascular diseases, is associated with lower serum ferritin [43] and taking iron tablets can increase the susceptibility to infections.

Although many diseases can lead to changes in micronutrient absorption and the requirements, these are not well defined. As a recent review of micronutrients and cancer stated, "the optimal age for intervention, optimum dose in a given individual, and the duration needed to test nutritional agents for cardiovascular diseases or cancer prevention are largely unknown" [44]. Alterations in micronutrient status in diseases such as, diabetes mellitus and obesity are documented. Clinical trials have shown benefits from both single nutrients and in combinations; the latter being more cost-effective. However, one need to select subjects who are deficient in a particular nutrient, to demonstrate a positive outcomes from a nutritional intervention. The recommended intakes for prevention of prediabetes while important, except for vitamin D, such are not defined yet [45].

14.12 Specific Interactions of Drugs with Food

Calcium supplements and calcium rich foods and iron supplements interfere the absorption of thyroxine; thus, thyroid supplements should be taken 2-h or more after oral dosing of thyroid hormone. In persons with osteoporosis, the intestinal bioavailability (absorption) of bisphosphonates are markedly reduced in the presence of calcium, milk, orange juice, mineralized water, etc. When taken simultaneously, these food items containing calcium in particular, chelat with bisphosphonates and thus, prevent their gastrointestinal absorption. Therefore, oral bisphosphonates agents should be taken on empty stomach with glass of unmineralized water, at least 60 min before taking anything other than water. However, chelating mechanisms have beneficial effects. For example, excess divalent cations such as calcium and magnesium present in the intestine, avidly binds to toxins, heavy metals, and pesticides (if any ingested) in the gastrointestinal tract and making insoluble complexes, thus preventing their absorption.

Most anti-epileptic (anticonvulsants) agent, particularly phenytoin and phenobarbital frequently used by adults with intellectual disability [46], deplete the storage form and increased catabolism of vitmain D, thus, markedly reducing the serum

25(OH)D concentrations [47]. Thus, in the long term, these drugs can cause hypovitaminosis-associated muscle weakness (e.g., shoulder-girdel myopathy), lethargy, osteomalacia, and increase oxidative stress. In part, this is due to enhancement of hepatic cytochrome enzymes [hydroxylation at C-24 by a 24-hydroxylase; CYP24A1] that increases the catabolism of 25(OH)D. Whereas, most atypical antipsychotic agents use by those with intellectual disability causes abdominal obesity, weight gain, and precipitate diabetes [48, 49].

14.13 Conclusions

Impaired nutrition is a frequently occurring element in persons with intellectual and developmental disabilities. Consequently, malnutrition augments many common diseases affecting this community. While macronutrient deficiencies lead to conditions such as marasmus and kwashiorkor are uncommon, micronutrient, vitamin, mineral, and anti-oxidant deficiencies are common in adults with intellectual disability. However, most of these deficiencies and associated morbidities go undiagnosed [50, 51].

These deficiencies can insidiously affect the well-being and the quality of life. Associations and correlations have been reported with micronutrients, vitamin and antioxidant deficiencies, such as selenium, zinc, vitamins C and D, and skeletal and extra-skeletal diseases and conditions. While the negative outcomes can be dramatic in children, adults with intellectual disability are not immune from multiple nutritional deficiencies and associated conditions related to malnutrition. Underlying disease status and genetic abnormalities worsen these situations.

Most adequately powered, RCTs, ecological, and epidemiological studies have reported favorable outcomes with sufficient doses of nutrients in vulnerable groups. Nevertheless, the RCTs in adults with intellectual disability are few, under-powered, and the number of participants and study duration are too little to make meaningful conclusions [52]. Stratergic planning and implementation of policies to scale-up resources for alleviation of micro- and nano-nutrient deficiencies, healthy food intake and composition data, making nutritious food available and affordable, educating about and encouraging healthful lifestyles, and disseminating the information on the importance of balanced diet and good nutrition, would greatly facilitate overcoming micronutrient deficiencies not only among the healthy ambulatory population but also among the vulnerable groups.

References

1. Maulik PK, Mascarenhas MN, Mathers CD, Dua T, Saxena S. Prevelance of interllectual disabilitiy: a meta-analysis of population-based studies. Res Dev Disabili. 2011;32(2):419–36.
2. Boyle CA, Boulet S, Schieve LA, Cohen RA, Blumberg SJ, Yeargin-Allsopp M, Visser S, Kogan MD. Trends in the prevalence of developmental disabilities in US Children, 1997–2008. Pediatrics. 2011;127:1034.
3. Chen J, Simeonsson RJ. Prevention of childhood disability in the People's Republic of China. Child Care Health Dev. 1993;19:71–88.

4. Deb S, Thomas M, Bright C. Mental disorder in adults with intellectual disability. 1: prevalence of functional psychiatric illness among a community-based population aged between 16 and 64 years. J Intellect Disabil Res. 2001;45:495–505.
5. Salvador-Carulla L, Garcia-Gutierrez JC, Ruiz Gutierrez-Colosia M, Artigas-Pallares J, Garcia Ibanez J, Gonzalez Perez J, Nadal Pla M, Aguilera Ines F, Isus S, Cereza JM, Poole JM, Portero Lazcano G, Monzon P, Leiva M, Parellada M, Garcia Nonell K, Hernandez L, Martinez A, Rigau E, Martinez-Leal R. Borderline intellectual functioning: consensus and good practice guidelines. Rev Psiquiatr Salud Ment. 2013;6:109–20.
6. Zablotsky B, Black LI, Blumber SJ. Stimulated prevalence of children with diagnosed developmental disabilities in the United States, 2014–2016. In NCHS Data Brief No. 291. CDC/National Center for Health Statistics, CDC; 2017.
7. Blackburn C, Read J, Spencer N. Children with neurodevelopmental disabilities. In: Annual report of the Chief Medical Officer, 2012; our children deserve better: prevention pays. UK: UK Government; 2013. Chapter 9; pages 1–13.
8. Humphries K, Traci MA, Seekins T. Nutrition and adut with interllectual or developmenetal disabilities: systematic literature reviw results. Intellect Dev Disabil. 2009;47(3):163–85.
9. Read MS. Malnutrition and behavior. Appl Res Ment Retard. 1982;3:279–91.
10. du Plessis J, van Pelt J, Korf H, Mathieu C, van der Schueren B, Lannoo M, Oyen T, Topal B, Fetter G, Nayler S, van der Merwe T, Windmolders P, Van Gaal L, Verrijken L, Hubens G, Gericke M, Cassiman D, Francque S, Nevens F, van der Merwe S. Association of adipose tissue inflammation with histologic severity of nonalcoholic fatty liver disease. Gastroenterology. 2015;149:635–48. e14
11. Wensveen FM, Valentic S, Sestan S, Wensveen T, Polic B. The "Big Bang" in obese fat: Events initiating obesity-induced adipose tissue inflammation. Eur J Immunol. 2015;45:2446–56.
12. Wimalawansa SJ. Associations of vitamin D with insulin resistance, obesity, type 2 diabetes, and metabolic syndrome. J Steroid Biochem Mol Biol. 2018;175:177–89.
13. Bronberg RA, Alfaro EL, Bejarano IF, Dipierri JE. Prevalence of malnutrition in institutionalized intellectually disabled patients. Medicina (B Aires). 2011;71:1–8.
14. Colombo M, de la Parra A, Lopez I. Intellectual and physical outcome of children undernourished in early life is influenced by later environmental conditions. Dev Med Child Neurol. 1992;34:611–22.
15. Grantham-McGregor SM, Fernald LC. Nutritional deficiencies and subsequent effects on mental and behavioral development in children. Southeast Asian J Trop Med Public Health. 1997;28(Suppl 2):50–68.
16. Shenkin A. Micronutrients in health and disease. Postgrad Med J. 2006;82:559–67.
17. Smith G, Wimalawansa SJ. Reconciling the irreconcilable: micronutrients in clinical nutrition and public health. Vitam Miner. 2015;4:1–4.
18. Christian P, Murray-Kolb LE, Khatry SK, Katz J, Schaefer BA, Cole PM, Leclerq SC, Tielsch JM. Prenatal micronutrient supplementation and intellectual and motor function in early school-aged children in Nepal. JAMA. 2010;304:2716–23.
19. Ashworth CJ, Antipatis C. Micronutrient programming of development throughout gestation. Reproduction. 2001;122:527–35.
20. Fenech MF. Dietary reference values of individual micronutrients and nutriomes for genome damage prevention: current status and a road map to the future. Am J Clin Nutr. 2010;91:1438S–54S.
21. Sobiecki JG, Appleby PN, Bradbury KD, Key TJ. High compliance with dietary recommendations in a cohort of meat eaters, fish eaters, vegetarians, and vegans: results from the European Prospective Investigation into Cancer and Nutrition-Oxford study. Nutr Res. 2016;36:464–77.
22. Wimalawansa SJ. Vitamin D in the new millennium. Curr Osteoporos Rep. 2012a;10:4–15.
23. Wimalawansa SJ. Vitamin D: An essential component for skeletal health. Ann N Y Acad Sci. 2012c;1240:90–8.
24. Wimalawansa SJ. Extra-skeletal benefits, endocrine functions, and toxicity of vitamin D. J Endocrinol Diabetes. 2016a;3:1–5.
25. Holick MF. The vitamin D deficiency pandemic: Approaches for diagnosis, treatment and prevention. Rev Endocr Metab Disord. 2017;18:153–65.

26. Wimalawansa SJ. Vitamin D: Everything You Need to Know. Homagama: Karunaratne & Sons; 2012b. ISBN: 978-955-9098-94-2
27. Sinha R, Cross AJ, Graubard BI, Leitzmann MF, Schatzkin A. Meat intake and mortality: a prospective study of over half a million people. Arch Intern Med. 2009;169:562–71.
28. Dauchet L, Amouyel P, Hercberg S, Dallongeville J. Fruit and vegetable consumption and risk of coronary heart disease: a meta-analysis of cohort studies. J Nutr. 2006;136:2588–93.
29. Skeaff CM, Miller AJ. Dietary fat and coronary heart disease: summary of evidence from prospective cohort and randomised controlled trials. Ann Nutr Metab. 2009;55:173–201.
30. National Heart, Lung, and Blood Institute. Third Report of the National Cholesterol Education Program (NCEP) Expert Panel on Detection, Evaluation, and Treatment of High Blood Cholesterol in Adults (Adult Treatment Panel III) final report. Circulation. 2002;106:3143–421.
31. Siri-Tarino PW, Sun Q, Hu FB, Krauss RM. Meta-analysis of prospective cohort studies evaluating the association of saturated fat with cardiovascular disease. Am J Clin Nutr. 2010;91:535–46.
32. Heidemann C, Schulze MB, Franco OH, van Dam RM, Mantzoros CS, Hu FB. Dietary patterns and risk of mortality from cardiovascular disease, cancer, and all causes in a prospective cohort of women. Circulation. 2008;118:230–7.
33. Masters RC, Liese AD, Haffner SM, Wagenknecht LD, Hanley AJ. Whole and refined grain intakes are related to inflammatory protein concentrations in human plasma. J Nutr. 2010;140:587–94.
34. Wimalawansa SJ. Visceral adiposity and cardio-metabolic risks: Epidemic of Abdominal Obesity in North America. Res Rep Endocr Disord. 2013b;3:17–30.
35. Egger G, Dixon J. Inflammatory effects of nutritional stimuli: further support for the need for a big picture approach to tackling obesity and chronic disease. Obes Rev. 2010;11:137–49.
36. Yang P, Xiao Y, Luo X, Zhao Y, Zhao L, Wang Y, Wu T, Wei L, Chen Y. Inflammatory stress promotes the development of obesity-related chronic kidney disease via CD36 in mice. J Lipid Res. 2017;58:1417–27.
37. Wimalawansa SJ. Food fortification programs to alleviate micronutrient deficiencies. J Food Process Technol. 2013a;4:257–67.
38. Cooper C, Javaid K, Westlake S, Harvey N, Dennison E. Developmental origins of osteoporotic fracture, the role of maternal vitamin D insufficiency. J Nutr. 2005;135:2728S–34S.
39. Buchele G, Becker C, Cameron ID, Auer R, Rothenbacher D, Konig HH, Rapp K. Fracture risk in people with developmental disabilities: results of a large claims data analysis. Osteoporos Int. 2017;28:369–75.
40. Burke EA, McCallion P, Carroll R, Walsh JB, McCarron M. An exploration of the bone health of older adults with an intellectual disability in Ireland. J Intellect Disabil Res. 2017;61:99–114.
41. Steinmetz KA, Potter JD. Vegetables, fruit, and cancer. II. Mechanisms. Cancer Causes Control. 1991;2:427–42.
42. Tsikritzi R, Moynihan PJ, Gosney MA, Allen VJ, Methven L. The effect of macro- and micronutrient fortification of biscuits on their sensory properties and on hedonic liking of older people. J Sci Food Agric. 2014;94:2040–8.
43. Fairweather-Tait SJ, Wawer AA, Gillings R, Jennings A, Myint PK. Iron status in the elderly. Mech Ageing Dev. 2014;136-137:22–8.
44. Mayne ST, Ferrucci LM, Cartmel B. Lessons learned from randomized clinical trials of micronutrient supplementation for cancer prevention. Annu Rev Nutr. 2012;32:369–90.
45. Kaur B, Henry J. Micronutrient status in type 2 diabetes: a review. Adv Food Nutr Res. 2014;71:55–100.
46. Faridi MM, Aggarwal A. Phenytoin induced vitamin D deficiency presenting as proximal muscle weakness. Indian Pediatr. 2010;47:624–5.
47. Mikati M, Wakim RH, Fayad M. Symptomatic antiepileptic drug associated vitamin D deficiency in noninstitutionalized patients: an under-diagnosed disorder. J Med Liban. 2003;51:71–3.
48. Almandil NB, Liu Y, Murray ML, Besag FM, Aitchison KJ, Wong IC. Weight gain and other metabolic adverse effects associated with atypical antipsychotic treatmentof children and adolescents: a systematic review and meta-analysis. Paediatr Drugs. 2013;15:13–50.

49. Lord CC, Wyler SC, Wan R, Castorena CM, Ahmed N, Mathew D, Lee S, Liu C, Elmquist JK. The atypical antipsychotic olanzapine causes weight gain by targeting serotonin receptor 2C. J Clin Investig. 2017;127:3402–6.
50. Black MM. Micronutrient Deficiencies and Cognitive Functioning. J Nutr. 2003;133: 3927S–31S.
51. Gladstone M, Mallewa M, Jalloh AA, Voskuijl W, Postels D, Groce N, Kerac M, Molyneux E. Assessment of neurodisability and malnutrition in children in Africa. Semin Pediatr Neurol. 2014;21:50–7.
52. Wimalawansa SJ. Vitamin D adequacy and improvements of comorbidities in persons with intellectual developmental disabilities. J Child Dev Disord. 2016b;2:22–33.

Aging and Physical Health

15

Meindert Haveman

15.1   Introduction

Aging is affecting all of us, but in an individual way with many layers. "Aging" is a complex concept with many facets (see Table 15.1). Age can be measured by past time (*chronological age*), and is documented in this sense in administrations, statistics, and science (*administrative age*). Rights, privileges and duties are regulated in age-transition points by law (*legal age*) (see Table 15.1).

Chronological age does not feel the same for people. There are individuals who are still feeling young at 70 years old, when others feel old at 50 years of age and may no longer celebrate their birthday (*psychological age*). The position of people according to age is also determined by culture and social group. Societal roles and norms regarding chronological age differ between cultures and countries, but also within one's own culture the same person who feels old in his or her family, feels young living with elderly adults in a senior home (*social age*). Age-appropriate moral values of responsible conduct because of ethical awareness are changing in time regarding, e.g. independence and sexuality (*ethical age*). Age and cognitive change are related to young and old age (*mental age*). Also, the concept of mental age has been used, and often abused, to label persons as "mentally retarded" or "intellectually disabled". Each individual has a unique relationship with the period of time they live in with their surroundings, her or his personal history. Severity of intellectual disability can be influenced by living in periods of war, hunger, poverty, and institutionalization *(historical age)*. Age can also have a religious dimension. So can the experience of end-of-life be influenced by religious faith and spiritual lifestyle derived in earlier phases of life (*religious age*).

M. Haveman (✉)
Department of Rehabilitation Sciences, University of Dortmund, Dortmund, Germany
e-mail: meindert.haveman@uni-dortmund.de

© Springer Nature Switzerland AG 2019
V. P. Prasher, M. P. Janicki (eds.), *Physical Health of Adults with Intellectual and Developmental Disabilities*, https://doi.org/10.1007/978-3-319-90083-4_15

Table 15.1 Facets of aging

* Chronological aging (measured by past time)
* Administrative aging (by classification of individual in age-groups in administration, statistics and science: e.g. 65+)
* Legal aging (rights, priviliges and duties according to chronological age)
* Psychological aging (individual's relationship with its own lived time; feeling "old" or "young" and behave accordingly)
* Social aging (acquisition of and comparison withnormal age-specific roles and positions in society)
* Ethical aging (age-appropriate moral values of responsible conduct because of ethical awareness)
* Cognitive or mental aging (changes in mental capacity to learn, record and evaluate differences about himself, and his physical and social environment, as well as, as the ability to adjust appropriately)
* Historical aging (influenced by events, physical and social circumstances in a past period of personal life)
* Religious aging (influence of age-appropriate faith and spiritual lifestyle obtained in earlier phases of life)
* Biological aging (physical condition of people due to biological processes such as growth, maturation, degradation and decay)
* Functional aging (age-appropriate functionality, overall performance in social life)

Haveman and Stöppler [1]

Growth, maturation, and decay of our body show the biological side of age (*biological age*). Loosing hair and teeth are minor signs that we are getting older. Biological aging, however, is not an autonomous process; it can be influenced, for example, by a healthy lifestyle. It is possible that a person of 60 years of age can catch the bus whereas a young adult running for the same bus does not succeed because of lack of breath, stamina and muscle power (*functional age*). In this chapter, especially the last two aspects of aging for persons with intellectual disability will be addressed.

Age as well as disability are both important factors that could lead without emancipatory and political action to exclusion, neglect, and poverty. In this sense, aging people with intellectual disability are at risk for a double hazard and should have support and protection as formulated in the Convention of the Rights on Persons with Disabilities [2]: "Persons with disabilities include those who have long-term physical, mental, intellectual or sensory impairments which in interaction with various barriers may hinder their full and effective participation in society on an equal basis with others." (Article 1, CRPD, [2]). From a perspective of physical functioning, there are at least three groups of elderly people with disabilities in society: people with life-long or early-onset disability, with mid- to later-life onset of disability, and those whose health is affected leading to impairment at older age. People with intellectual disability are part of the first group, but as do other people also be affected by adverse health conditions in mid- and later-life.

15.2   Population Aging

Population aging is likely to affect all countries. The population will be slightly higher in 2060, while the age structure will be much older than it is now (see Fig. 15.1). Population aging has a profound impact on societies. It affects educational institutions, labour markets, social security, health care, long-term care, and relationships between generations. Life expectancy at birth is rising in all parts of the world. In a 45–50-year age band, it is expected that longevity will increase worldwide with 10%, with a maximum of 18% for parts of Africa and 6% for countries with development market economies [3].

Except for Japan, the world's 15 oldest countries are all in Europe. Japan has the highest older population; the next highest are Italy, Germany, and Greece. The U.S. population is relatively "young" by European standards, with less than 13% age 65 or older. The aging of the baby-boom generation in the United States will push the proportion of older Americans to 20% by 2030; however, it will still be lower than in most Western European countries.

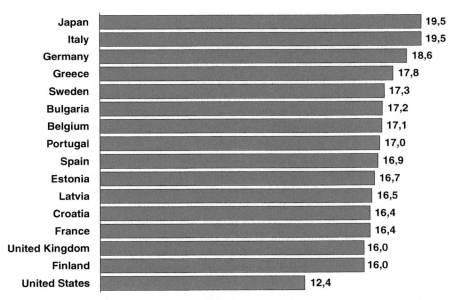

Sources: Haub 2006, World Population Data Sheet.

Fig. 15.1 The world's 15 'Oldest' countries and the U.S. Sources: [3], World Population Data Sheet

15.3   Aging and Health Disparities

Risk factors and preventive health practices for adults with intellectual disability have received increased attention over the past 20 years, as evidenced by several overview and review publications [4, 5]. General conclusion from these reviews is that most persons with intellectual disability experience a lower level of health age compared with peers in the general population. The likelihood of illness increases with age for all people, but many of those reaching old age with intellectual disability can expect a greater burden of illness than people without intellectual disability [6, 7]. This health differential may be considered in two ways: health inequalities and health disparities. *Health inequality* refers to differences caused or facilitated by social or access issues, and *health disparity* refers to differences due to underlying health pathologies.

Whitehead [8] identified seven main determinants of health differentials which were closely linked to poor outcome across a range of health measures—not least mortality:

> natural biological variation, health-damaging behaviour if freely chosen (e.g. participation in certain sports and behaviours), transient advantage to one group when they are first to adopt a health promoting behaviour, health damaging behaviour where the degree of choice of lifestyles is greatly restricted, exposure to unhealthy stressful living and working conditions, inadequate access to essential health and other public services, and natural selection or health-related social mobility involving the tendency for sick people to drift down the social ladder with long-lasting disease or disability. Regarding people with lifelong severe disabilities the category of comorbidities with specific syndromes could be added (or specified within the determinants of natural biological variation).

The observed poorer health status of many persons with intellectual disability can be explained in most countries by both concepts, health disparities and health inequalities. Higher incidence and prevalence rates reflect a combination of factors, including genetic predispositions to certain health conditions, less favourable social circumstances typically experienced by people with intellectual disability (or social and economic deprivation), reluctance or inability to utilise generic and special health services, poor nutrition and conditioning, omission from public health awareness campaigns, and residential circumstances that foster inactivity and poor lifestyle choices. Some of these health inequalities are linked to poor quality primary and special health care provided to people with intellectual disability [9, 10].

There is almost a total lack of information about the aging process and its consequences for persons with intellectual disability in low- and middle-income countries [11]. In this respect, the information and evidence in this chapter comes from and may be biased to the situation of North American, European, and industrialized Asian-Pacific countries.

15.4   Aging and Life Expectancy

Life expectancy at birth is rising in all parts of the world. In a 45–50-year period it is expected that longevity will increase worldwide 10%, with a maximum of 18% for parts of Africa and 6% for more economically developed countries [3]. Also people with mild intellectual disability can now expect to live as long as their age peers in the general population [12, 13]. The increase in life expectancy has been particularly marked for people with Down syndrome, from 12 in 1949 to nearly 60 in 2004 [14]. Reasons for this dramatic shift include reduced childhood mortality and better knowledge, healthcare, advocacy, and services. Despite this positive trend, life expectancy for persons with moderate and severe intellectual disability is still significantly below that of the general population. With an average age of death of 65 years for men with intellectual disability and 63 years for women, life expectancy for persons with intellectual disability in England was 16 years less than for the general population,. Mortality rates for people with intellectual disability are approximately twice that of the general population in England [15].

Mortality increases sharply after the age of 40 years [16, 17]. Pneumonia was reported as the primary cause of death in 40% of people with Down syndrome aged 40 years and older [18]. As pneumonia is a major cause of death associated with dementia [19] and given the high rates of dementia in older people with Down syndrome, dementia of the Alzheimer type (DAT) is expected to be an important secondary cause of death. Coppus et al. [20] examined risk factors for mortality according to morbidity at baseline in a prospective longitudinal study of almost 500 people with Down syndrome in the Netherlands, followed up on average over 4.5 years. A two- to threefold higher risk of dying was found for adults affected by epilepsy, vision impairment, mobility restriction, and dementia during follow-up.

15.5   Aging and Life-Course-Development

In gerontology, the process of aging and the phase of old age is seen as part of the life course in which the cornerstones of active ageing and health are already laid in early phases of life [21]. Although there might be more disruptive events in old age (like death of relatives and the onset of dementia), biographical trajectories through childhood, adolescence and adulthood shape the "third" and "fourth" phase in life. As lifespans of persons with intellectual disability have increased substantially, more individuals often experience health issues associated with aging at an early age and at higher rates than the general population. These health issues include: gait and mobility limitations, changes in bone health, over- or undernutrition, dental problems, decreases in vision/hearing, cardiovascular health risks, hypertension, type II diabetes, dementia, and depression [11, 22, 23]. This higher risk of developing conditions at younger ages than other adults is due to the confluence of biological factors related to syndromes and associated comorbidities or developmental impairments, access to adequate health care, and lifestyle and environmental issues. Hence, these risks are associated with potentially avoidable factors, including increased rates of exposure to social determinants of health (e.g., poverty, social exclusion) and discrimination in the implementation of health care systems [24] throughout the life course. Many of these conditions could be prevented and or improved with programs targeting lifestyle behaviors and increasing health care access [25].

15.6   Lifestyle Health Risks

The most common illness-related lifestyle health risks in industrialized nations include smoking and exposure to second hand smoke, maintaining excessive weight, and low physical activity levels. These risk factors also apply for adults with intellectual disability [26]. The European POMONA data (see Fig. 15.2) show some age-related trends with regard of some of the lifestyle risk factors in samples from 14 EU-member states [27].

Age	19–34 y (n = 436)	35–54 y (n = 516)	55–64 y (n = 198)	65+ y (n = 103)	Total (N = 1253)
Smoking					
No	91.5	90.0	90.4	85.1	90.1
Now and then	3.7	4.3	3.0	4.0	3.9
Daily	4.8	5.7	6.6	10.9	6.0
Alcohol use					
Never	71.2	61.5	60.5	60.0	64.6
Less than twice a month	23.0	26.1	29.1	27.0	25.6
1–2 days a week	4.0	8.5	4.1	10.0	6.3
3–6 days a week	0.7	1.8	2.6	3.0	1.6
Every day	1.2	2.2	3.6	0.0	1.9
Physical activity					
Sedentary	52.4	49.0	53.3	60.9	51.8
Light activities 4 hours a week	36.8	45.4	42.8	37.0	41.4
Gardening, jogging, recreational sports 4 hours a week	9.0	5.0	2.8	1.1	5.7
Hard training, competitive sports more than once a week	1.8	0.6	1.1	1.1	1.1

Haveman et al., 2011

Fig. 15.2 Lifestyle risk factors in adults with ID according to age (%). Haveman et al. [27]

15.6.1 Tobacco Use and Exposure

While tobacco use is generally a low frequency behavior among adults with severe to moderate intellectual disability community-dwelling adults, those with mild or marginal intellectual disability, do show higher rates of use [28, 29]. They are at-risk by exposure to second-hand smoke, as other people, when adults live or work in settings where staff or visitors are permitted to smoke. Steinberg et al. [29] found for community-dwelling adults with intellectual disability in the US that they are three times more likely to live in poverty, are more affected by the financial expense of tobacco use, and that their use of tobacco use may decrease the effectiveness of the medications they take. Tobacco addiction may have begun when older adults were institutional residents and tobacco use was "normalized" when dispensed as a "reward". The European Pomona II study found that elderly adults with intellectual disability (65+ years) had the highest proportion of smokers [27]. When adults with intellectual disability were offered access to smoking cessation programs, they often may fail as they may have difficulty understanding the health information presented to them. With this in mind, some efforts to provide stop-smoking education information adapted for adults with intellectual disability have emerged (see [30]). Problematic also are high BMIs and coincident smoking or exposure to second-hand smoke, which have been linked to higher rates of asthma [28]. As these studies show, the health risks associated with tobacco use or exposure are of concern.

15.6.2 Overweight and Obesity

People with intellectual disability are at-risk of obesity at an earlier age than the general population and are consequently experience obesity-related health problems at earlier in life [31]. Overweight (BMI 25.5–30) and obesity (BMI > 30; [32]) increases the risk of cardiovascular, pulmonary, metabolic, and neoplastic diseases, osteoarthritis, impaired fertility and complications of pregnancy, anesthetics, and surgery [33]. Health behaviors, such as consuming high-fat foods and participating in low levels of physical activity, play a role in the development of obesity in adults with intellectual disability living in community settings. Draheim et al. [34] found that individuals with intellectual disability who are overweight or have abdominal obesity are 3–10 times more likely to have elevated biological risk factors, such as hypertension, hypertriglyceridemia, hyperinsulinemia, and low high-density lipo-protein (good) cholesterol levels than those who are not overweight or who do not have abdominal obesity.

Prolonged obesity can lead to serious medical problems, such as diabetes mellitus, hypertension, and cardio-vascular disease (CVD). The rates of overweight and obesity are higher in adults with intellectual disability in many industrialized countries [11], but there is a wide range in the estimates. Stanish and Draheim [35], for example, reported that almost 80% of adults with mild to moderate intellectual disability who resided in community settings in the U.S. tended to be overweight or obese (including 45% obese and 8% morbidly obese). Also, in the Netherlands overweight and obesity were highly prevalent in older people with intellectual disability, with more obesity (26%) than in the general Dutch older population (10%) as measured by BMI, and 46–48% obesity as measured by waist circumference and waist-hip ratio respectively [36]. Women, adults with Down syndrome, higher age, less severe intellectual disability, autism, not being able to eat independently or prepare meals and shopping for groceries, being physically inactive, and use atypical antipsychotics were significantly more at risk of being overweight or obese. Bhaumik et al. [37], however, reported that the differences in BMI between the intellectual disability and general populations in England were not found with regard to obesity, but were found in the underweight category.

Genetic disorders, such as Prader-Willi syndrome, carry a high risk of severe obesity and it has been estimated that 24–48% of adults with Down syndrome are classified as obese. Use of psychotropic medication in adults with intellectual disability is considered to be a major cause of weight gain in this particular group. Eating practices, such as consuming high-fat foods and not eating sufficient fresh fruits and vegetables likely play a role in the development of excessive weight and obesity and elevated risk for cardio-vascular diseases and diabetes among adults with intellectual disability [38, 39]. Being low-income and poorly informed about sound nutritional practices, as reported for the majority of adults with intellectual disability [40, 41], may limit access to healthy food and sound food choices. Nutritional practices among adults with intellectual disability living independently may be less than ideal and this finding may apply also to those adults living in congregate care. For example, studies of adults with intellectual disability in the U.S. who resided in group homes indicated that they consume a diet that is high in carbohydrates and fat, and low in fruits and vegetables [38, 39], much like the diet of the homes' staff.

15.6.3 Interventions and Recommendations Regarding Lifestyle Risk Factors

Evidence exists that physical activity reduces mortality and morbidity not only in coronary heart disease and hypertension [42], but also on obesity, type 2 diabetes, constipation, and osteoporosis for people with and without intellectual disability. Increasing levels of physical activity is the most effective single intervention to improve the health status of a population of adults with intellectual disability [43]. Studies examining exercise practices and reports show that a lack of regular physical activity (along with unhealthy eating habits), a factor associated with obesity in the general population, is also a growing problem among persons with intellectual disability [38, 44]. Physical activity and exercise levels among adults with intellectual disability are generally considered to be low and are noted to be even lower among the older adults [43, 44].

Key barriers to participation in exercise for this population include cognitive and social emotional barriers (e.g., lack of motivation, lack of self-efficacy, poor outcome expectations), issues of accessibility (e.g., transportation, accessibility of equipment, money), and lack of staff/family motivation to promote and support physical activity [25]. Bodde and Seo [45] highlight the difficulties for people with intellectual disability to overcome social and environmental barriers and to engage in physical activity. The key barriers outlined are lack of money, transportation, access and support from family and caregivers. It has to be highlighted that parents and caregivers need to change their perception of individuals with intellectual disability as being too fragile to participate in exercise and especially in vigorous physical activity, and provide encouragement rather than negative support. For this group of persons, physical activity and exercise should be stimulated wherever and whenever possible. As a preventative health measure, the standard recommendation is accruing 30 min of moderate intensity physical activity on most, preferably all, days of the week [32].

Hamilton et al. [46] reviewed interventions for weight loss amongst adults with intellectual disability and obesity. They noted four key interventional approaches: (a) focused on dietary intake, (b) physical approaches looking at increasing energy expenditure, (c) health promotion and health education approaches, and (d) multifaceted approaches incorporating more than one of the above interventions. Each of the above approaches has demonstrated some effectiveness at producing weight loss in the short term in people with intellectual disability and obesity.

In reviewing eight studies on physical activity of adults with intellectual disability in the U.S., Stanish et al. [47] concluded that less than one-third of this population engage in sufficiently robust physical activity to accrue health benefits using the criterion of 30 min of moderate to vigorous activity at all or most days of the week or 10,000 steps per day. Others have reported similar findings using the criterion of at least 12 bouts of 20 min of moderate-to-vigorous activity occurring over 4 weeks [43, 44]. The proportion of participants meeting this criterion ranged from 4% to 20% [47]. Extensive physical activity and exercise may, however, remain very limited in non-ambulatory adults (e.g. blind, cerebral palsy) and who are permanently reliant on using wheelchairs.

Most of the exercise studies addressed younger adults with intellectual disability and demonstrated fitness benefits from exercise. Podgorsky et al. [48] showed that it was possible to introduce physical activity to a group of older adults with intellectual disability with relatively severe cognitive and physical functional disabilities. The findings indicated that 92% of the participants experienced improvement in at least one domain of physical functioning.

15.7 Deterioration and Diseases More Prevalent with Age

15.7.1 Diseases Affecting Vision and Hearing

Older people often experience increasing *problems with seeing*, such as: presbyopia (age related long-sightedness), difficulties with light/dark adaptation, age related macular degeneration (damage to the macular which is the part of the retina responsible for central vision), cataracts (clouding of the lens), and glaucoma (caused by raised pressure in the eye). See Chap. 7.

Compared to the general population eye problems are more common among older adults with intellectual disability. People with intellectual disability have high rates of life-long, early-onset, and midlife onset of eye pathologies such as refraction errors, strabismus, cataract and keratoconus. The prevalence of eye problems is especially very high in persons with severe and profound intellectual disability [49]. These eye conditions get more pronounced with aging and new cases are added at old age [50, 51]. Even at old age many of the eye problems are unknown and under-diagnosed. Persons who are daily in contact with adults with intellectual disability, family members or staff persons, are often not sensitive, experienced, or informed enough to deal effectively with significant regression of vision function in their clients. In the UK, nursing caregivers assessed vision as "perfectly normal" for 49% of their clients although less than 1% were assessed as having normal vision on ophthalmological testing [52].

Older persons with intellectual disability with lifelong vision impairment are in many cases not well prepared by educational measures, attitudes from others, rehabilitative efforts or changes in the physical environment to cope well with their vision problem. Responding to the high rates of formerly undetected cases of visual impairment in their study, Van Splunder et al. [53] advised that all persons with severe and profound intellectual disability, and all older adults with Down syndrome, should be considered as visually impaired until proven otherwise.

The prevalence of *hearing impairment* in the population of persons with intellectual disability is considerably higher than in the general population [54] and advances with age. There is a high prevalence for conductive hearing loss caused by chronic middle ear infections and ear wax blocking the canal, and a moderate prevalence for sensorineural and mixed hearing loss. Again, and similar to vision problems, the age-related hearing loss of persons with Down syndrome considerably exceeds the age-related hearing loss in other persons with intellectual disability, and reaches almost 100% after the age of 60 years [55]. See Chap. 8.

The proportion of undetected hearing impairment is large, even among people with mild and moderate intellectual disability. Reversible changes in hearing function are often neglected by staff members who are in direct contact with adults with intellectual disability. In a British study, nursing staff reported that 74% of the persons with intellectual disability had imperfect hearing. Formal assessment indicated only 11% to have normal hearing, with 61% having mild hearing loss, 15% having moderate to severe loss, and 13% having profound loss. For many, but certainly not for all, removal of ear wax, was a solution to the problem [52]. This significant lack in detection of bad hearing by laymen and support staff was also found in the Netherlands [56]. High risk groups for hearing impairment are persons with Down syndrome and the older adults (age 60 + yrs). Routine screening for age-related hearing loss for all adults with intellectual disability at age 45 and every 5 years thereafter has been recommended [57]. If possible, this should be done by an audiologist. Screening of the hearing function of adults with Down syndrome is recommended every 3 years throughout life [4].

15.7.2 Epilepsy

The International League Against Epilepsy [58] states that epilepsy is a disease of the brain defined by any of the following conditions: (a) at least two unprovoked (or reflex) seizures occurring greater than 24 h apart; (b) one unprovoked (or reflex) seizure and a probability of further seizures similar to the general recurrence risk (at least 60%) after two unprovoked seizures, occurring over the next 10 years; and (c) diagnosis of an epilepsy syndrome. In the adult general population epilepsy is the second commonest serious chronic neurological disorder after stroke. Prasher and Kerr [59] suggest that the existence of the combination of the conditions epilepsy and intellectual disability in an individual can pose unique challenges to the individual and his social environment. See Chap. 9.

The diagnosis of epilepsy in older adults with intellectual disability is quite common in general practice, as well as in outpatient and institutional settings. The prevalence rate of epilepsy amongst people with intellectual disability has been reported as at least 20 times higher than for the general population, with seizures commonly multiple and resistant to drug treatment [60, 61]. This is especially true in severe and profound intellectual disability.

Uncontrolled epilepsy can have serious negative consequences on both quality of life and mortality [62]. Consequences of epilepsy include sudden unexpected death, trauma caused by falls leading to fracture and soft tissue injury, hospital admission, the impact on learning and development, and social life [63, 64]. Loss of consciousness in fits can lead to burns and drowning. It is also apparent that epilepsy adds to caregiver strain and burden [65]. As is pointed out by van Schrojenstein Lantman-de Valk [66] inadequate dosage of anticonvulsants may diminish alertness. Long-term use of anticonvulsants may cause osteoporosis—an additional risk for fractures [67, 68]. Seizures may develop in people with Down syndrome as they age as a precursor or as a consequence to the manifestation of dementia [69].

15.7.3 Dementia

Dementia is the syndrome of progressive memory loss, other cognitive loss (from a stable baseline), epilepsy, and behavioral change that occurs with pathological deterioration of the brain. However, in advanced stages primary body functions are also affected, such as loss of vision and speech, mobility, and continence. Generally it was considered an older person's disorder, but it now seen as potentially affecting some middle-age persons as well (e.g., early-onset dementia). Amongst the population with intellectual disability, however, some genetic syndromes are associated with extremely early dementia —e.g., Rett Syndrome, Angelman Syndrome. It is well established that people with Down syndrome develop dementia of the Alzheimer type (DAT) at a younger age than the general population [70–72]. There is also evidence for increased prevalence of dementia in community populations of people with intellectual disability over the age of 65 years without Down syndrome, compared with the general population (possibly because of the extenuating earlier life conditions [73, 74].

It is important to diagnose dementia early, especially in adults with Down syndrome who are at increased risk. Alertness to dementia symptoms might be missed because changes in emotion and social behavior, or loss of motivation can be gradual and subtle. A baseline of functioning against which to measure changes is needed. Differentiating dementia from depression and delirium can be especially challenging. It is important for patients at risk of dementia, to assess or refer for psychological testing and to establish a baseline of cognitive, adaptive, and communicative functioning [71]. Family and other care providers should be educated about early signs of dementia. When symptoms are present, potential reversible causes (e.g., depression, vascular dementia) other than Alzheimer's disease should be investigated. Referral to an appropriate specialist (i.e., psychiatrist, neurologist, neuropsychologist) should be considered if it is unclear whether symptoms and behavior are due to emotional disturbance, psychiatric disorder, or a neurocognitive disorder (such as dementia) [75, 76].

15.7.4   Hypertension

The existing data on rates of hypertension in adults with intellectual disability are somewhat conflicting. Adults with intellectual disability may have more risk factors for the development of hypertension, such as obesity and inactivity [37]. Some studies noted lower rates of hypertension, but similar death rates from cardiovascular disease in adults with intellectual disability compared with the general population [50, 77, 78]. Some have noted higher rates of hypertension as adults with intellectual disability age [79]; others [80], noted similar rates of hypertension as the general population. There are indications that adults with Down syndrome have, compared with other adults with intellectual disability, significantly lower rates of hypertension [81].

15.7.5   Heart Disease

As in the general population, cardiovascular disease is also the primary cause of death in people with intellectual disability in most western countries. The mortality rates in various vary considerably as a result of factors related to patient selection, sample size, and quality and reliability of datasets. Only one study is country-wide population centered [82]. This Finnish study is based on a 35 year follow-up of a nation-wide population of 2313 persons with intellectual disability aged between 2 and 97 years. Of these persons 46% died within this long period. Vascular diseases constituted the largest group of primary causes of death at 36%. This percentage was lower than in the sex- and age-matched general population. The relative risk for vascular mortality was lower for men with intellectual disability in all age-groups and for most women except those with mild or moderate intellectual disability aged between 20 and 39 years. Mean age at death as a result of cardiovascular disease was 63.2 years. Of those who died at an older age, vascular disease was noted less frequently than in the general Finnish population. The findings from the Finnish study with regard to causes of death in persons with intellectual disability are similar to those found in the USA [83–85]. The three most common causes of death in those studies were cardiovascular diseases, respiratory diseases and cancer.

The behavioral risk factors for cardiovascular disease for adults with intellectual disability are similar to those for the general population, and they include smoking [86], poor nutritional intake [39] and deficient exercise or physical activity levels [35, 47, 87]. In a Dutch study [88], hypertension (53%), diabetes (14%), and metabolic syndrome (45%) were present similarly as in the general Dutch population. Hypercholesterolemia was present less often (23%). Fifty percent of the people with hypertension had not been previously diagnosed with this condition.

15.7.6 Diabetes

Diabetes is more common in persons with intellectual disability in the US compared to the general population [50, 77], but their proportion is smaller in older age groups. There is a significant chance that type 2 diabetes is systematically underestimated for older adults with intellectual disability [50, 51]. It is notable that the percentage of adults with known cardiovascular disease risk factors, such as type 2 diabetes, hyperlipidemia, BMI more than 27, lack of weekly exercise, and hypertension, decreases with intellectual disability severity [51]. It is postulated that underdiagnoses may be occurring, or that nutritional intake and non-smoking may be affecting health outcomes. See Chap. 10.

15.7.7 Gastrointestinal Problems

Gastrointestinal and eating problems are common among adults with intellectual disability. These are often different than in the general population and might include changes in behavior or weight. In some countries, many older adults with intellectual disability were, or are, residents of institutional settings and therefore at higher risk for hepatitis B, tuberculosis and Helicobacter pylori infections.

Adults with intellectual disability might have an increased risk of *helicobacter pylori (HP) infection* due to exposure to pathogens having lived in a group home or institution, rumination, or exposure to saliva or feces due to personal behavior or environmental contamination. Numerous studies have verified high prevalence rates for HP infection in participants with intellectual disability who had been formerly institutionalized [89, 90] and higher rates for those who had lived longer in institutional care [91] and for those with lower IQ [92]. One study conducted in Canada [89] examined prevalence rates for HP and discovered that 80% of participants who had been formerly institutionalized suffered from the infection. This was 3–4 times higher than adults who never lived in an institution. Similar high prevalence rates of HP were found for persons with intellectual disability in other studies [90–92]. Clarke et al. [93] showed that 22% of the persons who stayed shorter than 4 years had a positive antibody test compared to 84% of those who stayed longer than 4 years. Treatment led to eradication of HP infection in 11 of the 12 people who were able to cooperate with testing.

The high occurrence rate of HP among persons with intellectual disability is troubling. Many persons with intellectual disability are infected, and some of them can develop serious consequent conditions, including peptic ulcers and gastric cancer [94]. Duff et al. [95] reviewed deaths from cancer in the Stoke Park Group of hospitals in England, and found that stomach cancer accounted for 48% of all deaths from cancer, with additional residents dying from perforated stomach ulcers. They hypothesized that HP infections might be a factor. HP is recognized as the most important cause of chronic active gastritis, and HP colonization of the stomach is almost inevitably followed by histological signs of chronic inflammation. Chronic gastritis is now believed to predispose to metaplasia (cell abnormalities) and stomach cancer.

Although effective treatment of HP infections is available, recurrence rates are quite high. Wallace et al. [96] re-tested 28 adults with intellectual disability 36 months after successful eradication therapy and found a recurrence rate for HP infection of 21% (7% per year). *Gastro-esophageal reflux disease* (GERD), a disorder affecting 5–7% of the general population [97], is a major clinical problem in people with intellectual disability. It may be overlooked and underestimated [98–100] in both institutionalized and community-dwelling people with intellectual disability [101]. GERD is a disorder characterized by frequent backflow of gastric content into the esophagus.

Common GERD symptoms in the general population are heartburn, regurgitation, dysphagia, angina-like pain, and bronchospasm. The prevalence of GERD and reflux esophagitis in people living in institutions is very high. In a population of Dutch residential facilities, approximately one third of individuals with intellectual disability were diagnosed as having reflux esophagitis [98], though other studies have found even higher prevalence rates (40–50%) ([99]; Tracy & Wallace, 2001). Possible predisposing factors include non-ambulancy, scoliosis, cerebral palsy, use of anticonvulsant drugs, benzodiazepines, and IQ less than 35. Symptoms in this population indicative of reflux are: vomiting, hematemesis, regurgitation, food refusal, recurrent pneumonia, rumination, and behavior problems (such as self-injurious behavior, aggression, fear, screaming episodes, restlessness, and depression).

In the Canadian Consensus guidelines [76] recommendations for management of GERD problems among adults with intellectual disability can be found: "a. Screen annually for manifestations of GERD and manage accordingly. If introducing medications that can aggravate GERD, monitor more frequently for related symptoms; b. If there are unexplained gastrointestinal findings or changes in behavior or weight, investigate for constipation, GERD, peptic ulcer disease, and pica; c. Screen for H pylori infection in symptomatic adults with intellectual disability or asymptomatic ones who have lived in institutions or group homes. Consider retesting at regular intervals (e.g., 3–5 years); and d. Consider urea breath testing, fecal antigen testing, or serologic testing depending on the indication, availability, and tolerability of the test" (p. 544).

15.7.8   Skeletal Disorders

In the general population it has been established that there is a relationship between aerobic fitness and bone mineral density (BMD) [102], with the association suggesting that in those individuals who undertake regular exercise there are higher BMD scores; and a decrease in the value is associated with decreased levels of loading on the musculoskeletal system [103].

Osteoporosis and associated fractures are more prevalent among the population with intellectual disability compared to the general population [104]. Factors associated with osteoporosis are small body size, hypogonadism, and Down syndrome [105], and combinations of these factors [106]. A lower peak BMD and lower muscle tone have been suggested among the predisposing factors [107, 108].

Fragility fractures occur 1.7–3.5 times more frequently among adults with intellectual disability [104, 109]. Fracture detection is often delayed in people with intellectual disability due to profound cognitive and skeletal disabilities and lack of communication skills, in spite of the presence of pain [110].

Musculoskeletal diseases are frequently found in persons with intellectual disability. A Dutch study showed a prevalence rate of congenital musculoskeletal diseases (CMD) of 6%, with a higher prevalence in persons with severe/profound intellectual disability. The prevalence of acquired musculoskeletal diseases (AMD) was 20%, with a lower prevalence among persons with Down syndrome. The risk of having CMD, and AMD in general was not related to age. However, older adults (age 50+) were more at risk of having arthrosis [111].

15.7.9   Immune System Pathology in People with Down Syndrome as They Age

It has been established that both the innate and the acquired immune systems in adults with Down syndrome undergo precocious aging with subsequent similar immune deficiency manifestations as in the general population [112, 113]. It has been noted that thyroiditis, coeliac disease, and diabetes mellitus occur more frequently in adults with Down syndrome than in the general population [114–116] and that this group has altered T-cell activity and tumor marker levels [117, 118]. The incidence rates of leukemia in adults with Down syndrome are significantly higher than for the general population [119, 120].

With respect to these conditions, the Canadian guidelines for primary care [76] recommend that for persons with Down syndrome: "a. monitor thyroid function regularly; and consider testing for thyroid disease in patients with symptoms (including changes in behavior and adaptive functioning) and at regular intervals (e.g., 1–5 years) in patients with elevated risk of thyroid disease (e.g., Down syndrome)=; and b. establish a thyroid baseline and test annually for patients taking lithium or atypical or second-generation antipsychotic drugs" (p. 546).

15.7.10 Cancer

One in ten persons with intellectual disability dies of cancer [121]. This disease is becoming more common as a consequence of the increasing life expectancy of persons with intellectual disability [122, 123]. The increase of the increasing occurrence of cancer with age is at about the same frequency and rate as in the general population. However, the cancer profile for people with intellectual disability is slightly different from the general population, with a higher than average incidence of gastrointestinal cancers [122]. Adults with Down syndrome have a significantly increased risk of leukemia and a lower risk of many solid tumors, including a lower risk of breast cancer [124].

Cancer screening is an essential aspect of preventive care. However, adults with intellectual disability are less likely than those in the general population to be included in preventive screening programs, such as cervical screening, breast examination, mammography, and digital rectal examination. They are also less likely to do self-examination or to report abnormalities.

The Canadian guidelines for primary care suggest the following with respect to cancer screening among adults with intellectual disability [76]:

"a. perform regular cervical screening for all women who have been sexually active;
b. perform annual breast screening, including mammography, for women with intellectual disability aged 50–69 years;
c. perform an annual testicular examination for all men with intellectual disability;
d. screen for prostate cancer annually using digital rectal examination from age 45 years for all men with intellectual disability; and e. screen for colon cancer regularly in all adults with intellectual disability older than 50 years."(p. 547).

With respect to terminal cancer care, adults with intellectual disability will require special pain and symptom control in palliative care. Other palliative care needs of people with intellectual disability are, in essence, the same as those of the general population. Due to unique issues, challenges and circumstances, adults with intellectual disability affected by cancer may pose some difficulties in meeting their needs; these may include communication impediments which affect all aspects of palliative care provision, as well as problems with insight and the ability to participate in decision-making. They may also present with unconventional ways of expressing signs and symptoms of ill health and distress, multiple co-morbidities, and higher levels of behavioral or psychiatric problems.

The European Association for Palliative Care published a White Paper [125] targeting best practices in supporting people with intellectual disability at the end of life, setting out 13 important areas of practice and service delivery that are relevant in a wide range of settings, including the family home, independent living arrangements, residential care settings, nursing homes, hospitals and specialist palliative care settings. The International Summit on Dementia and Intellectual Disability

[126] also resulted in set of guidelines on terminal care when dementia is present, which can also apply to providing palliative care in complex situations. Both of these are useful documents which contain aspirational norms, as well as best practice examples and links to useful resources.

15.8 Multimorbidity and Polypharmacy in Older Age

Multimorbidity can be defined as two or more conditions which occur together in individuals [127]. Multimorbity is more the rule than the exception and is increases with older age [128–130]. In a Canadian study [128] the prevalence of having two or more chronic medical conditions between age 45 and 64, and 65 and older was, respectively, 95% and 99% among women, and 89% and 97% for men. Similar high percentages of multi-morbidity in the general population were found by Britt et al. [131] in Australia and Marengoni et al. [132] in Sweden. In the Swedish study, cardiovascular and mental diseases were the most common chronic disorders. Advanced age, female sex, and lower education were independently associated with a more than 50% increased risk of multi-morbidity. See Chap. 15.

As in the general population, multi-morbidity is reported high in older adults with intellectual disability. Prevalence, associated factors and clusters of multi-morbidity have been studied by Hermans and Evenhuis [133] in older adults with intellectual disability in Dutch residential homes (≥50 years; N = 1047). Multi-morbidity was prevalent in 80% and associated with age and severe/profound intellectual disability. Four or more conditions were prevalent in 47% and associated with age, severe/profound intellectual disability, and Down syndrome.

A possible explanation for the differences in multi-morbidity prevalence rates and patterns between persons with intellectual disability and the general population may be the earlier onset of some diseases and comorbidities, such as epilepsy, mental health problems, and gastrointestinal conditions. There are indications that older people with intellectual disability seem to be more likely to have psychiatric diagnoses in inpatient or outpatient specialist care than their peers in the general population [134]. If this is an effect of different disorder prevalence, diagnostic difficulties, or differences in health care availability is still not known. The complexity of the multi-morbidity pattern and appropriate surveillance of medical care with two or more chronic conditions is further complicated in persons with intellectual disability by the diversity of syndrome specific aging issues. Older adults with Down syndrome, for example, experience a phenomenon of accelerated aging, characterized by increased rates of cataracts, hearing loss, hypothyroidism, osteoporosis, epilepsy, sleep apnea, and a genetically elevated risk of developing Alzheimer's disease. Older adults with cerebral palsy (some of whom have intellectual disability) are at greater risk of accelerated musculoskeletal system aging, often leading to loss of mobility, osteoporosis, chronic fatigue, and chronic pain. Aging related issues have also been identified in persons with Prader-Willi syndrome, Williams syndrome, and fragile X syndrome [135].

Measuring and comparing multi-morbidity in older adults with intellectual disability and the general Irish population was also one of the aims of a longitudinal IDS-Tilda study in Ireland (Intellectual Disability Supplement—The Irish Longitudinal Study on Aging") [136]. Data on 753 adults with intellectual disability over the age of 40 years were reviewed, corresponding to about 9% of the Irish population with intellectual disability in this age range. Information on the presence of 12 chronic diseases was analyzed using a standardized protocol applied in face-to-face interviews with people with intellectual disability and/or their caregivers. The eight highest disease categories in order of prevalence were: eye disease (51%), psychiatric conditions (48%), neurological disease (36%; of which 31% was epilepsy), gastrointestinal disease (27%), endocrine disease (22%), joint disease (21%), hypertension (15%), and heart disease (12%). The highest rate of chronic conditions experienced by an individual was seven, with a median of two conditions. Multi-morbidity, defined in this study as two or more chronic health conditions, was observed in 71% of the sample, with women at higher risk. Eye diseases and mental illnesses were more often associated with a second health problem, and the pattern of most prevalent multi-morbidity was mental/neurological pathology. Multi-morbidity increased from 63% in those aged 40–49 years, to 72% in those aged 50–65 years, and to 86% in those aged 65 years and older. Prevalence of eye disease, psychiatric conditions, endocrine disease, joint disease, hypertension, cancer, and stroke were all significantly associated with age [136, 137].

Type and prevalence of disorders can differ between people with mild-moderate and severe-profound intellectual disability. In this respect, a Dutch study [138] undertook an analysis of the multi-morbidity of persons with severe and profound intellectual disability. The most common combination of two physical health problems comprise the most prevalent physical health problems, which included visual impairment, constipation, epilepsy, spasticity, and scoliosis. These five issues occurred as a multi-morbidity combination in 37% of the participants. In 56% of the participants a multi-morbidity combination of four health problems emerged, namely constipation, visual impairment, epilepsy, and spasticity.

Polypharmacy is associated with multi-morbidity and chronic conditions. Very few studies have investigated associations between specific multi-morbidity and multi-drug therapy [139]; this is also the case for older adults with intellectual disability. The combination of mental health, neurological, and physical health conditions increases the likelihood of polypharmacy in people with intellectual disability [140]. Increasing emphasis on deinstitutionalization and community integration also means that different specialists are contacted and more primary care services are used. This trend can lead to fragmentation in the individuals' medication and reduction of specialist knowledge of the unique issues for people with intellectual disability as they age.

Information about polypharmacy related to older persons with intellectual disability is scarce [11, 141]. In an Irish study (IDS-TILDA), 90% of the participants reported use of medications. Polypharmacy (5–9 medicines) was observed in 31% of participants and excessive polypharmacy (10+ medicines) in 20% [142].

   The frequency of prescribed medications corresponded to the frequency of reported chronic conditions. Six of the most frequently reported medication groups were drugs for psychiatric conditions and epilepsy. Almost two-thirds (65%) of the excessive polypharmacy group and over half (55%) of those with polypharmacy reported one or more antipsychotics, compared with 26% with no polypharmacy. Antiepileptics were the second most frequently reported class (39%) and represented 63% of the excessive polypharmacy, 54% of the polypharmacy, but only 17% of the no polypharmacy groups. The increase in use of a drug class across the groups was greatest for anxiolytics with 16 times as many users in the excessive polypharmacy group compared with the no polypharmacy group. This contrasted with only 2.5 times as many reporting using an antipsychotic, emphasizing the high usage across all groups and the reported prevalence of mental ill health. Antipsychotic medications, however, increase risk of metabolic syndrome and can have other serious side effects (e.g., akathisia, cardiac conduction problems, swallowing difficulties, bowel dysfunction). The Canadian guidelines recommended ([76], p. 548)

– to not use antipsychotic medication as a first-line treatment of problem behaviors without a confirmed robust diagnosis of schizophrenia or other psychotic disorder;
– to monitor use of antipsychotic medications for side effects, including metabolic syndrome.
– to educate patients and caregivers to incorporate a healthy diet and regular exercise into their lifestyle;
– to reassess the need for ongoing antipsychotic medications at regular intervals and to consider dose reduction or discontinuation when appropriate.

   Laxatives (75%) and drugs for peptic ulcer disease (PUD)/gastro-esophageal reflux disease (GORD) (49%) were frequently reported by the excessive polypharmacy group, but were reported by only 12% and 9%, respectively, of the no polypharmacy group. Proton pump inhibitors were the principal drugs in this group reported by 22% of all participants and 44% of those in the excessive polypharmacy group. Of the sample, 43% reported that constipation was a problem, and almost one-fifth reported a doctor's diagnosis of chronic constipation [142]. Lipid modifying agents (25%) were the most frequently reported cardiovascular agents with a notably lower reported use of other cardiovascular agents: antithrombotics (11%) and agents acting on the renin–angiotensin system (6%). Thyroid disease and drugs were frequently reported and varied little across the groups and were around threefold greater than the number reporting diabetes and receiving antidiabetic drugs.
   The TILDA study showed that living in a residential institution, and having a psychiatric, neurological, or endocrine condition or hypertension were each independently associated with polypharmacy and excessive polypharmacy exposure at both levels. Those with severe/profound intellectual disability were likely to be exposed to polypharmacy, but not excessive polypharmacy. Gastrointestinal disease

was significantly associated with excessive polypharmacy only. Sex, age, eye conditions, heart disease or joint disease were not significantly associated with polypharmacy or excessive polypharmacy [142].

It can be concluded that multi-morbidity and polypharmacy is much higher in older adults with intellectual disability when compared with younger people with intellectual disability and age peers in the general population [142–144]. This means that healthcare, including general practitioner (GP) visits and monitoring, and hospital and specialist services, are intensively used by this group of adults. For the planning of adequate assessments and treatment of health problems of older adults with intellectual disability it would be of practical interest to know how different co-morbid conditions and their medication are clustered together and how different providers coordinate their services. More information is needed about effective models of cooperation.

It is clear those older adults with need a comprehensive and developmental approach on multi-morbidity and polypharmacy, because many of them have life-long physical impairments, diseases, and mental health problems which complicate the assessment, treatment, and prognosis of other medical problems acquired during adulthood and old age [145]. Systematic review of appropriateness of medication use is essential, as polypharmacy places aging people with intellectual disability at risk of adverse effects. It is important to sort out medication use, capacity to follow the medication regime, and assistance required to support medication use compliance. The Canadian Consensus Guidelines for primary care for adults with intellectual disability [76] recommend: (a) "review the date of initiation, indications, dosages, and effectiveness of all medications regularly (e.g., every 3 months);

(a) determine patient adherence capacity and recommend dosettes, blister-packs, and other aids if necessary;
(b) watch for both typical and atypical signs of adverse effects and regularly monitor potentially toxic medications or interactions of medications (e.g., liver function tests or serum drug levels) at the recommended interval for each medication; and
(c) ensure that patient and staff or caregivers are educated about appropriate use of medications, including over-the-counter, alternative, and as-needed medications" (p. 544).

15.9   Health Service Delivery for Older Adults with Intellectual Disability

Health goals for adults with intellectual disability are similar to those that apply to the general population: to maintain or improve community participation, support a good quality of life (as defined by the individual and/or caregiver), promote wellness, and minimize acute care visits. Current knowledge provides no specific age range or cutoff that clearly defines the "geriatric" adult with intellectual disability. Defining elderly issues by functional age could be much more helpful than using "chronical age" as a concept of reference.

For older adults with intellectual disability marked disparities are found in health and access to health services caused by genetic predispositions to certain health conditions, less favourable social circumstances, reluctance or inability to utilise generic health services, omission from public health awareness campaigns, and residential circumstances that foster inactivity and poor lifestyle choices [5].

Actually, persons with intellectual disability are much more heterogenous as they age than persons in the general population. Certain conditions are strongly associated with adults with intellectual disability and are also more prevalent among older adults. For example, there is a higher incidence of dental disease, functional decline, mental illness, bowel obstruction, gastrointestinal cancer, and obesity. Additionally, hearing impairment and vision loss are common in older adults with intellectual disability because of pre-existing undiagnosed pathologies. Health promotion programs and attention to prevention for service providers can help address such health care needs of adults with intellectual disability.

Increased supports for older parents and brothers and sisters are necessary for helping adults with intellectual disability that are living at home. This task becomes more challenging over the individual's life span as aging-related changes impact both the person with intellectual disability and his or her supporting family. Key challenges that must be addressed by service providers, families, and adults aging with intellectual disability include (a) learning about the characteristics, health care needs, and common clinical issues in this aging population, (b) improving the health and function of these adults, (c) enhancing consumer-directed and family-based care, and (d) reducing barriers to health and community participation.

Also, regularly scheduled screening and assessments (yearly or every 6 months, if required) are recommended along with a multidisciplinary approach to health maintenance. With potentially major changes in their health, it is critical that greater efforts are made to increase preventive care and health promotion activities. Health checks in people with intellectual disability have been shown to increase detection of vision and hearing impairments in detecting women's health issues [146]. Moreover, health checks have been found to identify new health problems in 51% of those who received a health check [63] and a subsequent repeat health check identified similar level of new health needs in the same group of patients [147].

Although older people are living now in the community compared to decades ago, they generally see general practitioners (GP) less often in comparison with the general population. Several barriers contribute to this, such as:

- lack of GPs who are knowledgeable and experienced with this population (e.g., availability, distance);
- accessibility of GP practices (barriers of building, signage, and interior);
- psychological and behavioral issues that negatively impact individual's cooperation for tests, injections, consultations etc. (e.g., autism, stereotypical behavior, cramped posture, crying, shouting);
- communication issues that make interaction among the provider and patient difficult (e.g., type of language and sensitivity of GPs, language proficiency of patient);

- physical challenges for social interaction (e.g., blindness, deafness, cerebral palsy);
- physical environmental issues involving sensory challenges (e.g., lighting, sound, smells, temperature); and social environmental issues (e.g., full and busy GP practice, lack of time of support persons).

The model of care in many economically developed countries shows three models of services for older people with intellectual disability: (a) generic health services, (b) geriatric health service for persons older than 60 or 65 years, and (c) specialized (aging-related) service provision to adults with ID. As is pointed out by Strydom et al. [148], the complexity of multiple morbidities in aging adults with intellectual disability is an argument for engaging specialist physicians and providing for multidisciplinary teams in intellectual disability. In the absence of specialist adult physicians in intellectual disability, geriatricians are well-placed to assess and manage the complex mix of disorders presenting in older people with intellectual disability. However, geriatricians will have to take a larger role in addressing the special health care needs of older adults with intellectual disability, which requires additional target group attention and training.

References

1. Haveman MJ, Stöppler R. Altern mit geistiger Behinderung. Grundlagen und Perspektiven für Begleitung, Bildung und Rehabilitation. Stuttgart: Verlag W.Kohlhammer; 2010.
2. United Nations. Convention on the rights of persons with disabilities. New York, NY: United Nations; 2006. Available from: www.un.org/disabilities
3. Haub C. World population data sheet; 2006. ftp://eos.atmos.washington.edu/pub/breth/PCC/SI2006/readings/PopRefBureau_2006.pdf. 30 Jan 2018.
4. Evenhuis H, Henderson CM, Beange H, Lennox N, Chicoine B. Healthy ageing—adults with intellectual disabilities: physical health issues. Geneva, Switzerland: World Health Organization; 2001.
5. Haveman MJ, Heller T, Lee LA, Maaskant MA, Shooshtari S, Strydom A. Report on the state of science on health risks and ageing in people with intellectual disabilities. IASSID special interest research group on ageing and intellectual disabilities/faculty rehabilitation sciences, University of Dortmund; 2009. Available at: http://www.iassid.org.
6. Bowers B, Bigby C, Webber R. Intellectual disability and ageing. In: Nay R, Garratt S, editors. Interdisciplinary care of older people: issues and innovations. Sydney, Australia: Elsevier; 2009. p. 60–77.
7. Janicki MP, Dalton AJ, McCallion P, Baxley DD, Zendell A. Group home care for adults with intellectual disabilities and Alzheimer's disease. Dementia. 2005;4:361–85.
8. Whitehead M. The concepts and principles of equity and health. Int J Health Serv. 1990;22:429–45.
9. DOH. Valuing people: a new strategy for learning disability for the 21st century. London: HMSO; 2001.
10. Michael J. Healthcare for all: independent inquiry into access to healthcare for people with learning disabilities. London: HMSO; 2008.
11. Haveman M, Heller T, Lee L, et al. Major health risks in aging persons with intellectual disabilities: an overview of recent studies. J Policy Pract Intellect Disabil. 2010;7:59–69.
12. Fisher K, Kettl P. Aging with mental retardation: increasing population of older adults with MR require health interventions and prevention strategies. Geriatrics. 2005;60:26–9.

13. Ouellette-Kuntz H, Garcin N, Lewis S, Minnes P, Freeman C, Holden J. Addressing health disparities through promoting equity for individuals with intellectual disabilities. Can J Public Health. 2005;96(2):8–S22.
14. Bittles A, Glasson E. Clinical, social, and ethical implications of changing life expectancy in Down syndrome. Dev Med Child Neurol. 2004;46:282–6.
15. Heslop P, Glover G. Mortality of people with intellectual disabilities in England: a comparison of data from existing sources. J Appl Res Intellect Disabil. 2015;28:414–22.
16. Day SM, Strauss DJ, Shavelle RM, Reynolds RJ. Mortality and causes of death in persons with Down syndrome in California. Dev Med Child Neurol. 2005;47:171–6.
17. Strauss D, Shavelle R. Life expectancy of persons with chronic disabilities. J Insur Med. 1998;30:96–108.
18. Bittles AH, Bower C, Hussain R, Glasson EJ. The four ages of Down syndrome. Eur J Pub Health. 2007;17:221–5.
19. Keene J, Hope T, Fairburn CG, Jacoby R. Death and dementia. Int J Geriatr Psychiatry. 2001;16:969–74.
20. Coppus A, Evenhuis H, Verbene GJ, Visser F, Oostra BA, Eikelenboom P, Van Duijin C. Survival in elderly persons with Down syndrome. J Am Geriatr Soc. 2008;56:2311–6.
21. Elder GH, Giele JZ. The craft of life course research. New York: The Guilford Press; 2009.
22. Humphries K, Traci MA, Seekins T. Nutrition and adults with intellectual or developmental disabilities: systematic literature review results. Intellect Dev Disabil. 2009;47:163–85.
23. Willgoss TG, Yohannes AM, Mitchell D. Review of risk factors and preventative strategies for fall-related injuries in people with intellectual disabilities. J Clin Nurs. 2010;19:2100–9.
24. Emerson E, Hatton C. Contribution of socioeconomic position to health inequalities of British children and adolescents with intellectual disabilities. Am J Ment Retard. 2007;112:140–50.
25. Heller T, Sorensen A. Promoting healthy aging in adults with developmental disabilities. Dev Disabil Res Rev. 2013;18:22–30.
26. Wilkinson J, Culpepper L, Cerreto M. Screening tests for adults with intellectual disabilities. J Am Board Fam Med. 2007;20(4):399–407.
27. Haveman M, Perry J, Salvador-Carulla L, et al. Ageing and health status in adults with intellectual disabilities: results of the European POMONA II study. J Intellect Develop Disabil. 2011;36:49–60.
28. Gale L, Naqvi H, Russ L. Asthma, smoking and BMI in adults with intellectual disabilities: a community-based survey. J Intellect Disabil Res. 2009;53:787–96.
29. Steinberg ML, Heimlich L, Williams JM. Tobacco use among individuals with intellectual or developmental disabilities: a brief review. Intellect Dev Disabil. 2009;47:197–207.
30. North Dakota Disability Health Project. Tobacco cessation resource materials for people with intellectual disabilities; n.d.. http://www.ndcpd.org/health/files/publications/tob%20cess%20info%201-09.pdf. Retrieved 08 Nov 2009
31. Doody CM. Health promotion for people with intellectual disability and obesity. Br J Nurs. 2012;21(460):2–5.
32. World Health Organization (WHO). Global strategy on diet, physical activity and health. Geneva: Author; 2003.
33. Haslam D, Sattar N, Lean M. ABC of obesity.Obesity—time to wake up. Br Med J. 2006;333:640–2.
34. Draheim CC, Williams DP, McCubbin JA. Prevalence of physical inactivity and recommended physical activity in community-based adults with mental retardation. Ment Retard. 2002;40:436–44.
35. Stanish H, Draheim C. Physical activity assessment using pedometer and questionnaire in adults with mental retardation. Adapt Phys Act Q. 2005;22:136–45.
36. de Winter CF, Bastiaanse LP, Hilgenkamp TI, Evenhuis HM, Echteld MA. Overweight and obesity in older people with intellectual disability. Res Dev Disabil. 2012;33:398–405.
37. Bhaumik S, Watson J, Thorp C, Tyrer F, McGrother C. Body mass index in adults with intellectual disability: distribution, associations and service implications: a population-based prevalence study. J Intellect Disabil Res. 2008;52:287–98.

38. Braunschweig C, Gomez S, Sheean P, Tomey K, Rimmer J, Heller T. Nutritional status and risk factors for chronic disease in urban-dwelling adults with Down syndrome. Am J Ment Retard. 2004;109:186–93.
39. Draheim CC, Stanish HI, Williams DP, McCubbin JA. Dietary intake of adults with mental retardation who reside in community settings. Am J Ment Retard. 2007;112:392–400.
40. Fujiura GT, Yamaki K. Analysis of ethnic variations in developmental disability prevalence and household economic status. Ment Retard. 1997;35:268–94.
41. Yamaki K, Fujiura GT. Employment and oncome status of adults with developmental disabilities living in the community. Ment Retard. 2002;40:132–41.
42. Sutherland G, Couch MA, Iacono T. Health issues for adults with developmental disability. Res Dev Disabil. 2002;23:422–45.
43. Robertson J, Emerson E, Gregory N, Hatto C, Turner S, Kessissoglou S, et al. Lifestyle related risk factors for poor health in residential settings for people with intellectual disabilities. Res Dev Disabil. 2000;21:469–86.
44. Emerson E. Underweight, obesity and exercise among adults with intellectual disabilities in supported accommodation in Northern England. J Intellect Disabil Res. 2005;49:134–43.
45. Bodde AE, Seo D-C. A review of social and environmental barriers to physical activity for adults with intellectual disabilities. Disabil Health J. 2009;2:57–66.
46. Hamilton S, Hankey CR, Miller S, Boyle S, Melville CA. A review of weight loss interventions for adults with intellectual disabilities. Obes Rev. 2007;8(4):339–45.
47. Stanish H, Temple V, Frey G. Health-promoting physical activity of adults with mental retardation. Ment Retard Dev Disabil Res Rev. 2006;12:13–21.
48. Podgorsky C, Kessler K, Cacia B, Peterson D, Henderson M. Physical activity intervention for older adults with intellectual disability: report on a pilot project. Ment Retard. 2004;42:272–83.
49. van den Broek E, Janssen C, van Ramshorst T, Deen L. Visual impairments in people with severe and profound multiple disabilities: an inventory of visual functioning. J Intellect Disabil Res. 2006;50(6):470–5.
50. Janicki MP, Davidson PW, Henderson CM, McCallion P, Taets JD, Force LT, et al. Health characteristics and health services utilization in older adults with intellectual disability living in community residences. J Intellect Disabil Res. 2002;46:287–98.
51. Merrick J, Davidson PW, Morad M, Janicki MP, Wexler O, Henderson CM. Older adults with intellectual disability in residential care centers in Israel: health status and service utilization. Am J Ment Retard. 2004;109:413–20.
52. Kerr AM, McCulloch D, Oliver K, McLean B, Coleman E, Law T, et al. Medical needs of people with intellectual disability require regular assessment, and the provision of client- and carer-held reports. J Intellect Disabil Res. 2003;47:134–45.
53. van Splunder J, Stilma J, Bernsen R, Evenhuis H. Prevalence of visual impairment in adults with intellectual disabilities in the Netherlands: cross-sectional study. Eye. 2006;20(9):1004–10.
54. Evenhuis H, Theunissen M, Denkers I, Verschuure H, Kemme H. Prevalence of visual and hearing impairment in a Dutch institutionalized population with intellectual disability. J Intellect Disabil Res. 2001;45:457–64.
55. Meuwese-Jongejeugd A, Vink M, Van ZB, Verschuure H, Eichhorn E, Koopman D, et al. Prevalence of hearing loss in 1598 adults with an intellectual disability: crosssectional population based study. Int J Audiol. 2006;45:660–9.
56. Aerts-Neggers TMA, Schoonbrood-Lenssen AMJ, Maaskant MA. Gehoorverlies bij mensen met een verstandelijke handicap, resultaten van een screeningsonderzoek in drie activiteitencentra. Nederlands Tijdschrift voor de Zorg aan verstandelijk gehandicapten. 2003;29(4):238–50.
57. Evenhuis HM, Nagtzaam LMD, editors. Early identification of hearing and visual impairment in children and adults with an intellectual disability. IASSID International Consensus Statement. SIRG Health Issues; 1998.
58. Fisher RS, Acevedo C, Arzimanoglou A, Bogacz A, Cross JH, Elger CE, Engel J, Forsgren L, French JA, Glynn M, Hesdorffer DC. ILAE official report: a practical clinical definition of epilepsy. Epilepsia. 2014;55:475–82.

59. Prasher VP, Kerr MP. Epilepsy and intellectual disabilities. 2nd ed. New York: Springer; 2016.
60. Amiet C, Gourfinkel-An I, Bouzamondo A, Tordjman S, Baulac M, Lechat P, et al. Epilepsy in autism is associated with intellectual disability and gender: evidence from a meta-analysis. Biol Psychiatry. 2008;64:577–82.
61. Matthews T, Weston N, Baxter H, Felce D, Kerr M. A general practice-based prevalence study of epilepsy among adults with intellectual disabilities and of its association with psychiatric disorder, behaviour disturbance and carer stress. J Intellect Disabil Res. 2008;52:163–73.
62. Kerr M, Bowley C. Evidence-based prescribing in adults with learning disability and epilepsy. Epilepsia. 2001;42(Suppl 1):44–5.
63. Baxter H, Lowe K, Houston H, Jones G, Felce D, Kerr M. Previously unidentified morbidity in patients with intellectual disability. Br J Gen Pract. 2006;56:93–8.
64. McGrother C, Bhaumik S, Thorp C, Hauck A, Branford D, Watson J. Epilepsy in adults with intellectual disabilities: prevalence, associations and service implications. Seizure. 2006;15:376–86.
65. Wilson R. Carer burden in learning disability with coexistent epilipsy. Unpublished M.Sc. thesis. University of Wales College of Medicine, Cardiff; 1998.
66. van SchrojensteinLantman-de Valk HM. Health in people with intellectual disa-bilities: current knowledge and gaps in knowledge. J Appl Res Intellect Disabil. 2005;18:325–33.
67. Jancar J, Jancar MP. Age-related fractures in people with intellectual disability and epilepsy. J Intellect Disabil Res. 1998;42. (Pt 5:429–33.
68. Wagemans AM, Fiolet JF, van der Linde ES, Menheere PP. Osteoporosis and intellectual disability: is there any relation. J Intellect Disabil Res. 1998;42(5):370–4.
69. Collacott R. Epilepsy, dementia and adaptive behaviour in Down's syndrome. J Intellect Disabil Res. 1993;37(2):153–60.
70. Holland AJ, Hon J, Huppert FA, Stevens F. Incidence and course of dementia in people with Down's syndrome: findings from a population-based study. J Intellect Disabil Res. 2000;44:138–46.
71. Prasher VP. Alzheimer's disease and dementia in Down syndrome and Inteilectual disabilities. Oxon, UK: Radcliffe Publishing; 2005.
72. Zigman WB, Schupf N, Sersen E, Silverman W. Prevalence of dementia in adults with and without Down syndrome. Am J Ment Retard. 1996;100:403–12.
73. Cooper SA. Psychiatry of elderly compared to younger adults with intellectual disabilities. J Appl Res Intellect Disabil. 1997;10:303–11.
74. Strydom A, Livingston G, King M, et al. Prevalence of dementia in intellectual disability using different diagnostic criteria. Br J Psychiatry. 2007;191(2):150–7.
75. British Psychological Society. Dementia and people with learning disabiliites. Guidance on the assessment, diagnosis, treatment and support of people with learning disabilities who develop dementia. Cr 155; 2009
76. Sullivan WF, Berg JM, Bradley E, Cheetham T, Denton R, Heng J, Hennen B, Joyce D, et al. Primary care of adults with developmental disabilities; Canadian consensus guidelines. Can Fam Physician. 2011;2011(57):541–53.
77. Draheim CC, Williams DP, McCubbin JA. Physical activity, dietary intake, and the insulin resistance syndrome in nondiabetic adults with mental retardation. Am J Ment Retard. 2002;107:361–75.
78. McDermott S, Platt T, Krishnaswami S. Are individuals with mental retardation at high risk for chronic disease? Fam Med. 1997;29:429–34.
79. Cooper SA. Clinical study of the effects of age on the physical health of adults with mental retardation. Am J Ment Retard. 1998;102:582–9.
80. Henderson CM, Robinson LM, Davidson P, Haveman M, Janicki MP, Albertini G. Overweight status, obesity and risk factors for coronary heart disease in adults with intellectual disability. J Policy Pract Intellect Disabil. 2008;5:174–7.
81. Kapell D, Nightingale B, Rodriguez A, Lee J, Zigman W, Schupf N. Prevalence of chronic medical conditions in adults with mental retardation: comparison with the general population. Ment Retard. 1998;36:269–79.

82. Patja K, Molsa P, Iivanainen M. Cause-specific mortality of people with intellectual disability in a population-based, 35-year follow-up study. J Intellect Disabil Res. 2001;45:30–40.
83. Esbensen A, Seltzer M, Greenberg J. Factors predicting mortality in midlife adults with and without Down syndrome living with family. J Intellect Disabil Res. 2007;51:1039–50.
84. Janicki MP, Dalton AJ, Henderson C, Davidson P. Mortality and morbidity among older adults with intellectual disability: health services considerations. Disabil Rehabil. 1999;21:284–94.
85. Strauss D, Kastner T, Shavelle R. Mortality of adults with developmental disabilities living in California institutions and community care, 1985–1994. Ment Retard. 1998;36:360–71.
86. McGillycuddy NB. A review of substance use research among those with mental retardation. Men Retard Dev Disabil Res Rev. 2006;12:41–7.
87. Frey G. Comparison of physical activity levels between adults with and without mental retardation. J Phys Act Health. 2004;1:235–45.
88. de Winter CF, Bastiaanse LP, Hilgenkamp TI, Evenhuis HM, Echteld MA. Cardiovascular risk factors (diabetes, hypertension, hypercholesterolemia and metabolic syndrome) in older people with intellectual disability: results of the HA-ID study. Res Dev Disabil. 2012;33:1722–31.
89. Kennedy C. Screening for Helicobacter pylori in adults with developmental disabilities—prevalence of infection and testing considerations for urea breath test, serology and whole-blood methods. M.Sc. thesis. Department of CommunityHealth & Epidemiology, Queen's University, Kingston, Ontario; 2002.
90. Morad M, Merrick J, Nasri Y. Prevalence of Helicobacter pylori infection in people with intellectual disabilities in a residential care center in Israel. J Intellect Disabil Res. 2002;46:141–3.
91. Wallace R, Schluter P, Webb P. Environmental, medical behavioural and disability factors associated with Helicobacter pylori infection in adults with intellectual disability. J Intellect Disabil Res. 2002;46:51–60.
92. Böhmer CJ, Klinkenberg-Knol EC, Kuipers EJ, Niezen-De Boer MC, Schreuder H, Schuckink-Kool F, et al. The prevalence of Helicobacter pylori infection among inhabitants and healthy employees of institutes for the intellectually disabled. Am J Gastroenterol. 1997;92:1000–4.
93. Clarke D, Vermuri M, Gunatilake D, Tewari S. Brief report. Helicobacter pylori infection in five inpatient units for people with intellectual disability and psychiatric disorder. J f Appl Res Intellect Disabil. 2008;21:95–8.
94. Beange H, Lennox N. Physical aspects of health in the learning disabled. Curr Opin Psychiatry. 1998;11:531–4.
95. Duff M, Scheepers M, Cooper M, Hoghton M, Baddeley P. Helicobacter pylori: has the killer escaped from the institution? A possible cause of increased stomach cancer in a population with intellectual disability. J Intellect Disabil Res. 2001;45:219–25.
96. Wallace R, Schluter P, Webb P. Recurrence of Helicobacter pylori infection in adults with intellectual disability. Intern Med J. 2004;34:132–3.
97. International Foundation for Functional Gastrointestinal Disorders, Inc. (IFFGD). GI disorders in adults: gastroesophageal reflux disease; 2003. http://www.iffgd.org/GIDisorders/GIAdults.htm. Retrieved 27 Oct 2009
98. Böhmer C, Niezen-De Boer M, Klinkenberg-Knol E, Deville W, Nadorp J, Meuwissen S. The prevalence of gastrooesophageal reflux disease in institutionalised intellectually disabled individuals. Am J Gastroenterol. 1999;94:804–10.
99. Böhmer C, Niezen-De Boer M, Klinkenberg-Knol E, Meuwissen S. Review article. Gastroesophageal reflux disease in intellectually disabled individuals: how often, how serious, how manageable? Am J Gastroenterol. 2000;95:1868–72.
100. Evenhuis H, Henderson CM, Beange H, Lennox N, Chicoine B. Healthy ageing—adults with intellectual disabilities: physical health issues. Geneva, Switzedand: World Health Organization; 2000. Available at http://www.who.int/mental_health/media/en/21.pdf
101. Tracy JM, Wallace R. Presentations of physical illness in people with developmental disability: the example of gastrooesophageal reflux. Med J Aust. 2001;175:109–11.

102. Kronhead A, Moller M. Effects of physical exercise on bone mass, balance skill and aerobic capacity in women and men with low bone mineral density, after one year of training a prospective study. Scand J Med Sci Sports. 1998;8:290–8.
103. Heinonen A, Kannus P, Sievnan H, Pasanen M, Oja P, Vuori I. Good maintenance of high-impact activity-induced bone gain by voluntary, unsupervised exercises: an 8-month follow-up of a randomized controlled trial. J Bone Miner Res. 1999;14:25–8.
104. van Schrojenstein Lantman- de Valk H, Metsemakers J, Haveman M, Crebolder H. Health problems in people with intellectual disability in general practice: a comparative study. Fam Pract. 2000;17:405–7.
105. Angelopoulou N, Matziari C, Tsimaras V, Sakadamis A, Souftas V, Mandroukas K. Bone mineral density andmuscle strength in young men with mental retardation (with and without Down syndrome). Calcif Tissue Int. 2000;66:176–80.
106. Center J, Nguyen T, Pocock N, Eisman J. Volumetric bone density at the femoral neck as a common measure of hip fracture risk for men and women. J Clin Endocrinol Metab. 2004;89:2776–82.
107. Schrager S. Osteoporosis in women with disabilities. J Women's Health. 2004;13:431–7.
108. Tyler C, Snyder C, Zyzansky S. Screening for osteoporosis in community-dwelling adults with mental retardation. Ment Retard. 2000;38:316–21.
109. Lohiya GS, Crinella FM, Tan-Figueroa L, Caires S, Lohiya S. Fracture epidemiology and control in a developmental center. West J Med. 1999;170:203–9.
110. Glick NR, Fischer HM, Heisey MD, Leverson EG, Mann CD. Epidemiology of fractures in people with severe and profound developmental disabilities. Osteoporos Int. 2005;16:389–96.
111. Vonken MTH, Maaskant MA, van den Akker M. Aandoeningen van het bewegingsapparaat bij mensen met een verstandelijke handicap [Disorders of the movement system of people with intellectual disability]. Nederlands Tijdschrift voor de Zorg aan verstandelijk gehandicapten (Dutch Journal for Care to Persons with Intellectual Disabilities). 2006;32:98–111.
112. Burkle A, Caselli G, Franceschi C, Mariani E, Sansoni P, Santoni A, Witkowski W, Caruso I. Pathophysiology of ageing, longevity and age related diseases. Immun Ageing. 2007;4:4–11.
113. Effros R. Roy Walford and the immunologic theory of aging. Immun Ageing. 2005;2:7–10.
114. Cohen WI. Current dilemmas in Down syndrome clinical care: celiac disease, thyroid disorders and atlanto-axial instability. Am J Med Genet. 2006;142(3):141–8.
115. Hansson T, Dahlbom I, Rogberg S, Nyberg B, Dahlstrom J, Anneren G, Klareskog L, Dannaeus A. Antitissue transglutaminase and antithyroid autoantibodies in children with Down syndrome and celiac disease. J Pediatr Gastroenterol Nutr. 2005;40:170–4.
116. Kinik ST, Ozcay F, Varan B. Type 1 diabetes mellitus, Hashimotos' thyroiditis and celiac disease in an adolescent with Down syndrome. Pediatr Int. 2006;48:433–5.
117. Prada N, Nasi M, Troiani L, Roat E, Pinti M, Nemes E, et al. Direct analysis of thymic function in children with Down's syndrome. Immun Ageing. 2005;2:4–10.
118. Ugazio AG, Maccario R, Notarangelo LD, Burgio GR. Immunology of Down syndrome: a review. Am J Med Genet. 1990;7:204–12.
119. Boker LK, Merrick J. Cancer incidence in persons with Down syndrome in Israel. Downs Syndr Res Pract. 2002;8(1):31–6.
120. Sullivan SG, Hussain R, Threlfall T, Bittles AH. The incidence of cancer in people with intellectual disabilities. Cancer Causes Control. 2004;15:1021–5.
121. Hollins S, Attard MT, von Fraunhofer N, McGuigan S, Sedgwick P. Mortality in people with learning disability: risks, causes and death certificate findings in London. Dev Med Child Neurol. 1998;40:50–6.
122. Hogg J, Tuffrey-Wijne I. Cancer and intellectual disability: a review of some key contextual issues. J Appl Res Intellect Disabil. 2008;21(6):509–18.
123. Maaskant M, Gevers J, Wierda H. Mortality and life expectancy in Dutch residential centres for individuals with intellectual disability, 1991–1995. J Appl Res Intellect Disabil. 2002;15:200–12.

124. Satgé D, Vekemans M. Down syndrome patients are less likely to develop some (but not all) malignant solid tumours. Clin Genet. 2011;79(3):289–90.
125. European Association for Palliative Care. EAPC Definition of palliative care; 2014. http://www.eapcnet.eu/Corporate/AbouttheEAPC/Definitionandaims.aspx. Accessed 04 Dec 2017.
126. McCallion P, Hogan M, Santos FH, McCarron M, Service K, Stemp S, Keller S, Fortea J, Watchman K, Janicki MP, The Working Group of the International Summit on Intellectual Disability and Dementia. Consensus statement of the international summit on intellectual disability and dementia related to advanced dementia and end-of-life care. J Appl Res Intellect Disabil. 2017;30(6):977–1164. https://doi.org/10.1111/jar.12349.
127. Kadam UT, Croft PR; North Staffordshire GP Consortium Group. Clinical multimorbidity and physical function in older adults: a record and health status linkage study in general practice, Family Practice; 2007.
128. Fortin M, Bravo G, Hudon C, Vanasse A, Lapointe L. Prevalence of multimorbidity among adults seen in family practice. Ann Fam Med. 2005;3:223–8.
129. Kirchberger I, Meisinger C, Heier M, Zimmermann AK, Thorand B, Autenrieth CS, et al. Patterns of multimorbidity in the aged population. Results from the KORA-age study. PLoS One. 2012;7:e30556.
130. van den Akker M, Buntinx F, Metsemakers JF, Roos S, Knottnerus JA. Multimorbidity in general practice: prevalence, incidence, and determinants of co-occurring chronic and recurrent diseases. J Clin Epidemiol. 1998;51:367–75.
131. Britt HC, Harrison CM, Miller GC, Knox SA. Prevalence and pattern of multimorbidity in Australia. Med J Aust. 2008;189(2):72–7.
132. Marengoni A, Winblad B, Karp A, Fratiglioni L. Prevalence of chronic diseases and multimorbidity among the elderly population in Sweden. Am J Public Health. 2008;98:1198–200.
133. Hermans H, Evenhuis HM. multimorbidity in older adults with intellectual disabilities. Res Dev Disabil. 2014;35(4):776–83.
134. Axmon A, Björne P, Nylander L, Ahlström G. Psychiatric diagnoses in older people with intellectual disability in comparison with the general population: a register study. Epidemiol Psychiatr Sci. 2017:1–13. https://doi.org/10.1017/S2045796017000051.
135. Janicki MP, Henderson CM, Rubin L. Neurodevelopmental conditions and aging: report on the Atlanta study group charrette on neurodevelopmental conditions and aging. Disabil Health J. 2008;1:116–24.
136. Trinity College Dublin. IDS TILDA. The intellectual disability supplement to the Irish longitudinal study on ageing; 2016. Available at: http://www.idstilda.tcd.ie/. Accessed 05 Dec 5 2017.
137. McCarron M, Swinburne J, Burke E, McGlinchey E, Carroll R, McCallion P. Patterns of multimorbidity in an older population of persons with an intellectual disability: results from the intellectual disability supplement to the Irish longitudinal study on aging (IDS-TILDA). Res Dev Disabil. 2013;34(1):521–7.
138. van Timmerena EA, Waningea A, van Schrojenstein Lantman-De Valk HMJA, van der Putten AJ, van der Schansade CP. Patterns of multimorbidity in people with severe or profound intellectual and motor disabilities. Res Dev Disabil. 2017;67:28–33.
139. Doos L, Roberts EO, Corp N, Kadam UT. Multi-drug therapy in chronic condition multimorbidity: a systematic review. Fam Pract. 2014;31:654–63.
140. Robertson J, Emerson E, Gregory N, et al. Receipt of psychotropic medication by people with intellectual disability in residential settings. J Intellect Disabil Res. 2000;44:666–76.
141. Stortz JN, Lake JK, Cobigo V, et al. Lessons learned from our elders: how to study polypharmacy in populations with intellectual and developmental disabilities. Intellect Dev Disabil. 2014;52:60–77.
142. O'Dwyer M, Peklar J, McCallion P, McCarron M, Henman MC. Factors associated with polypharmacy and excessive polypharmacy in older people with intellectual disability differ from the general population: a cross-sectional observational nationwide study. BMJ Open. 2016;6:e010505. https://doi.org/10.1136/bmjopen-2015-010505.

143. Doan TN, Lennox NG, Taylor-Gomez M, et al. Medication use among Australian adults with intellectual disability in primary healthcare settings: a cross-sectional study. J Intellect Dev Disabil. 2013;38:177–81.
144. Lunsky Y, Klein-Geltink JE, Yates EA, Cobigo V, Ouellette-Kuntz H, Lake JK, et al. Medication use. In: Lunsky Y, Klein-Geltink JE, Yates EA, editors. Atlas on the primary care of adults with developmental disabilities in Ontario. Toronto, Canada: Institute for Clinical Evaluative Sciences and Centre for Addiction and Mental Health; 2013. http://www.ices.on.ca/~/media/Files/Atlases-Reports/2013/Atlas-on-developmental-disabilities/Full-Report.ashx.
145. Haveman M, Stöppler R. Gesundheit und Krankheit bei Menschen mit geistiger Behinderung. Stuttgart: Verlag W. Kohlhammer; 2014.
146. Lennox N, Bain C, Rey-Conde T, Purdie D, Bush R, Pandeya N. Effects of a comprehensive health assessment programme for Australian adults with intellectual disability: a cluster randomized trial. Int J Epidemiol. 2007;36:139–46.
147. Felce D, Baxter H, Lowe K, Dunstan F, Houston H, Jones G, et al. The impact of repeated health checks for adults with intellectual disabilities. J Appl Res Intellect Disabil. 2008;21:585–96.
148. Strydom A, Lee LA, Jokinen N, Shooshtari S, Raykar V, Torr J, Tsiouris JA, Courtenay K, Bass N, Sinnema M, Maaskant MA. Report on the state of science on dementia in people with intellectual disabilities. IASSID special interest research group on ageing and intellectual disabilities; 2009.

Psychotropic Polypharmacy

16

Michelle Cornacchia and Priya Chandan

16.1 Introduction

Polypharmacy is a major issue for individuals with intellectual disability. However, given the lack of consensus regarding the definition of polypharmacy, it has been challenging to characterize and study this phenomenon in order to improve health care for this population. Polypharmacy has been described in the literature utilizing a variety of definitions, including the use of five or more medications, using more medications than is medically necessary, and the use of more than one medication for the same indication [1, 2]. In this chapter, we have adopted the definition of using five or more medications.

16.2 Significance

Though a variety of definitions of polypharmacy are used in the literature, it is clear that individuals with intellectual disability are at high risk for polypharmacy. Previous studies have shown the prevalence of polypharmacy in individuals with intellectual disability ranges between 11% to 60% [2, 3]. There are multiple reasons for this, including the fact that individuals with intellectual disability often have multiple co-morbidities that may require pharmacotherapy, such as, neurologic, endocrine, cardiovascular, gastrointestinal conditions and mental health/behavioral issues. Individuals with intellectual disability have 2.5 times the number of health problems reported compared to the general population [4].

M. Cornacchia (✉)
Department of Internal Medicine, Geisinger Medical Center, Danville, PA, USA

P. Chandan
Division of Physical Medicine and Rehabilitation, Department of Neurological Surgery, University of Louisville, Louisville, KY, USA

© Springer Nature Switzerland AG 2019
V. P. Prasher, M. P. Janicki (eds.), *Physical Health of Adults with Intellectual and Developmental Disabilities*, https://doi.org/10.1007/978-3-319-90083-4_16

In particular, pharmacotherapy for mental health, as well as for challenging behaviors, in persons with underlying drug treatment of physical disorders has been a major contributor to polypharmacy in this population. Tong and Einfeld [5] showed that 40% of children with intellectual disability had a psychiatric disorder, which is a three- to four-fold increase as compared to individuals without intellectual disability. In particular, there is a high prevalence of depression, anxiety, hyperactivity disorder, bipolar disorder, schizophrenia, and sleep disorders in this population [2]. Prevalence estimates of psychotropic drug use in people with intellectual disability range from 25% to 89% depending on the residential setting, with greater psychotropic drug use seen in individuals living in institutions or nursing homes as opposed to individuals living in a community setting [6, 7]. Deb et al. [6] documented that 89% of individuals with intellectual disability were on psychotropic medications, and of these individuals, 45% had polypharmacy. This study also showed that the most common prescribed medication was antipsychotics for behavioral issues [6], which is not surprising given the high prevalence of challenging behaviors within this population. Behaviors such as aggression, over activity, and self-injurious acts were reported up to 62% in individuals with intellectual disability [4].

Another study tracking the prescribing patterns for individuals with intellectual disability showed that the majority of medications prescribed (52%) were psychoactive drugs including anticonvulsants, antipsychotics, and antidepressants [8]. The study also supported the presence of polypharmacy: 62% of participants were given more than one psychoactive medication and 36% received three or more psychoactive medications [8]. The majority of indications given for prescribing antipsychotics included psychotic illness, anxiety, and aggressive behaviors [9]. Another study showed that 31.5% of participants were prescribed five to nine medications and 20.1% were prescribed ten or more medications [4]. The large amount of medications taken increases the risk for adverse drug reactions.

Other factors that have impacted polypharmacy within this population include severity of intellectual disability, place of residence, and age. Individuals with severe/profound intellectual disability were more likely to be exposed to polypharmacy [4]. In one study, individuals with mild intellectual disability had a polypharmacy prevalence of 16.2% versus 39.2% for individuals with profound intellectual disability [2]. This may be explained by the increased diagnosis of neurologic and psychiatric conditions in over 90% of individuals with severe intellectual disability [10]. Other studies showed that institutionalized (residential facility or nursing home) individuals have higher rates of psychotropic medication use than community dwelling counterparts [11]. Lastly, age is an important risk factor for polypharmacy for adults with intellectual disability. Given medical advances, life expectancy has improved for individuals with intellectual disability. As a result, there is a growing population of older adults with intellectual disability which increases the risk for multiple co-morbidities such as dementia, cataracts, hearing disorders, diabetes, hypertension, osteoarthritis, and osteoporosis that increase use of drugs and/or sensitivity to drugs. Some of these co-morbidities may be due to the sedentary lifestyle that is seen in more than 60% of older adults with intellectual disability [9]. Also, use of psychotropic drugs within this group is controversial, given the lack of evidence to support its benefits, along with significant evidence of harm. Therefore, it is important to take into account the severity of intellectual disability, residence of the individual with intellectual disability, and the age of the patient when evaluating them in the office.

16.3 Prescribing Patterns in Patients with Intellectual/Developmental Disabilities

Prescribed medication lists of people with intellectual disability may reflect several trends. First, people with intellectual disability may be on a large number of medications. For example, a study by Schieffer et al. (2016) noted that the average number of prescription drugs per patient in their sample was 5.2 drugs, with a range from 1 drug to 15 drugs [7]. Second, people with intellectual disability may be on combinations of drugs. In a study by Deb et al. [6], the most common combination for polypharmacy was an atypical antipsychotic (usually risperidone) and an SSRI antidepressant (usually fluoxetine, paroxetine, citalopram, or sertraline) [6]. The second most common combination was an antipsychotic and a mood stabilizer (usually carbamazepine or sodium valproate). Other combinations included antipsychotics and psychostimulants (primarily methylphenidate and atomoxetine in one case) and beta-blockers (such as propranolol) [6]. Third, indications for prescribed medications are often absent or unclear [7, 12]. Finally, studies have shown that psychotropic medications tend to be prescribed at high doses and for longer time periods in people with intellectual disability as compared to the general population [13].

Of note, as expressed by Deb et al. [6], there is public concern regarding the use of psychotropic medications in people with intellectual disability for the management of problem behavior in the absence of a diagnosed psychiatric disorder [6]. Reasons for this concern include an overall lack of evidence to support the effectiveness of psychotropic medications to manage problem behaviors, especially aggressive behavior; adverse events such as somnolence, weight gain, and other metabolic syndromes caused by new generation antipsychotics; use of medication without explicit patient consent; and difficulty in obtaining necessary blood work such as serum levels or blood tests for other adverse effects [6].

Common medication classes prescribed for people with intellectual disability include antiepileptics, antipsychotics, antidepressants, medications for gastroesophageal reflux disease (GERD) and/or peptic ulcer disease (PUD), and laxatives. In the Deb et al. [6] study, atypical antipsychotics were the most frequently prescribed psychotropic medication, followed by antiepileptics/mood stabilizers, followed by new generation antidepressants, and lastly by typical antipsychotics [6]. Below, we discuss the literature base around a few of these commonly used medication classes in greater detail.

16.4 Antiepileptics

Antiepileptics may be used in people with intellectual disability for the management of seizures. While approximately 3% of the general population is diagnosed with epilepsy at some point in their life, estimates in people with intellectual disability range from 14% to 44% [14]. While a systematic review supported the use of antiepileptics in people with intellectual disability and epilepsy, it also called for further research, as higher quality studies are needed to better understand the effects of pharmacological interventions for people with intellectual disability and epilepsy [14]. Current evidence does not allow for comment on the relative efficacy of medications, which is problematic for clinical decision-making [14]. As a result, providers often rely on side effect profiles when deciding which antiepileptic to use in this population.

In addition to epilepsy as an indication for antiepileptics, people with intellectual disability may be prescribed antiepileptics for aggressive behavior and/or mood stabilization [6]. Evidence regarding efficacy of antiepileptics for this indication is limited.

16.5 Antipsychotics

Antipsychotics are the most frequently prescribed class of psychotropic drugs in the population of people with intellectual disability [6, 15]. This class of medications is used for a variety of indications, including psychotic symptoms, aggressive behavior disorders, self-injurious behavior, vocal and motor tics, and stereotyped behaviors [16]. In general, atypical antipsychotics (risperidone, olanzapine, clozapine, quetiapine, and aripiprazole) are preferred to classic antipsychotics due to less side effects and better tolerance [16].

Within this class of medications, risperidone is the most studied and appears to be effective in reducing problem behaviors in children with intellectual disability in the short term [16, 17], although evidence in adults is inconclusive [18]. In general, the literature regarding the use of antipsychotics in people with intellectual disability is limited. A systematic review conducted in 2015 highlighted the fact that although clozapine is recommended for treatment-resistant psychosis, there are no randomized control trials that assess the efficacy and side effects of clozapine in people with a dual diagnosis of intellectual disability and psychosis [19]. Similarly, another review examining the use of aripiprazole for problem behaviors noted that the overall quality of studies was poor, as there were only two randomized control trials, both of which were performed by the pharmaceutical company that produces aripiprazole [1].

Thus, although antipsychotics are commonly used in people with intellectual disability for a variety of indications, further studies, particularly randomized control trials, are needed to truly understand the efficacy and safety of these medications in this population.

16.6   Antidepressants

Antidepressants are used for a variety of indications, including depression, anxiety, obsessive-compulsive spectrum disorders, and behavioral disorders (stereotypies, aggression, self-injurious behavior) [16]. However, the literature base for these medications remains limited. Another systematic review noted that the existing literature regarding pharmacotherapy for self-injurious behavior in adults with intellectual disability is sparse, lacks power, and has a high risk of bias, resulting in an inability to draw conclusions about the benefits or safety of any antidepressant, antipsychotic, or mood stabilizing medications for self-injurious behavior in adults with intellectual disability [20].

Thus, although antidepressants are commonly used in people with intellectual disability for a variety of indications, further studies, particularly employing randomized control trials, are needed to truly understand the efficacy and safety of these medications in this population.

16.7   Side Effects of Common Medications Prescribed to People with Intellectual Disability

It is important to note that some people with intellectual disability may respond to drugs at lower doses as compared to the general population [16] and that the occurrence of side effects tends to be more frequent as compared to the general population [16, 18]. A recent Cochrane systematic review of the use antiepileptics in people with intellectual disability and epilepsy found that reported adverse effects were similar to those seen in people without intellectual disability [14]. Given this fact and the lack of evidence regarding relative efficacy of antiepileptics in people with intellectual disability, clinical decision making is often guided by adverse event profiles [14].

Several resources exist regarding assessing side effects commonly seen in people with intellectual disability. Here, we highlight three resources for clinicians. First, Selph and Cosca [21] created a helpful table regarding commonly used medications (antidepressants, antipsychotics, anticonvulsants, benzodiazepines, Alzheimer's/dementia medications, mood stabilizers) and their corresponding side effects, which include sedation, insomnia, nausea, constipation, diarrhea, and weight gain [21]. Similarly, Special Olympics International has developed a Medication Watch List, which highlights long QT syndrome (a disorder of the heart's electrical system), obesity, constipation, sun sensitivity, and osteoporosis as potential side effects of medications commonly used in people with intellectual disability [22].

While these resources focus on clinical decision-making, resources are also needed to systematically characterize side effects over time. The Matson Evaluation of Side Effects (MEDS) is a psychotropic drug side effect scale that was specifically developed to assess side effects in people with intellectual disability [23]. This 90-item instrument assess nine categories of side effects: cardiovascular/hematologic, gastrointestinal, endocrine/genitourinary, eye/ear/nasal/throat, skin/allergies/

temperature, central nervous system (CNS)-general, CNS-dystonia, CNS-parkinsonism/dyskinesia, and CNS-akathisia [23].

16.8   Polypharmacy as a Risk Factor for Negative Outcomes

Polypharmacy is an important topic for clinicians to be aware of because it can lead to increased risk for negative outcomes, such as adverse drug reactions, drug–drug interactions, noncompliance/nonadherence, and inappropriate use of medications [2]. For example, Zaal et al. [24] identified polypharmacy as a risk factor for drug-related problems, including use of potentially unnecessary or inappropriate drugs [24]. Modi et al. [25] found that psychotropic polypharmacy significantly predicted specialized inpatient admissions for individuals with intellectual disability who received outpatient services as a psychiatric hospital [25].

16.9   Solutions and Strategies

Given the significant risks of polypharmacy, it is important for providers to identify and apply strategies/solutions to reduce polypharmacy and its negative impact on individuals with intellectual disability. Zaal et al. [24] created the Systematic Tool to Reduce Inappropriate Prescribing (STRIP) [24]. The method includes obtaining pharmacotherapeutic history (which includes experiences and expectations of the patient), analysis of potential drug-related problems using START and STOPP methods, proposing a pharmaceutical care plan by the physician and the pharmacist, concordance between physician and patient on the care plan, and follow up [24]. Another study from Scheifes et al. [7] looked at a structured medication review, which includes structured review of current medications, preparation of a pharmaceutical care plan based on drug related problems that were detected and actions planned, and follow up and monitoring [7]. Both methods involve the physician, pharmacist, and patient. Therefore, providers would benefit from adopting a multidisciplinary approach to reducing polypharmacy and its risks for the intellectual disabled population.

Another important method includes empowering individuals with intellectual disability and/or their caregiver. Recommendations include encouraging individuals to know their medications and why they are taking them; bringing their medication list, medication passport, and/or pill bottles to office visits; using organizers (such as blister packs, dosette boxes, and/or alarm systems) to help with taking the correct medications at the right time; planning when to take the medications to prevent or lessen side effects; keeping medications where they will be remembered to be taken; and tracing the effect of the medication. For individuals that do not have decision-making capacity, decisions need to be made using the most appropriate legal and ethical framework. A person will need to be designated for medication management and given the complex care network of individuals with, intellectual disability all members within that individual's care network need to be made aware of any pharmacologic changes.

For the providers, some general principles warrant consideration, especially for medications involving behaviors. Providers should first trial behavioral modification before starting pharmacotherapy and exhaust monotherapy options before combination therapy is applied. A general rule of thumb is to "start low and go slow". Individuals with intellectual disability may be sensitive to the medications and could benefit from low initial doses, which can also reduce the possibility of side effects. It is recommended to trial a short course of medication and arrange appropriate follow up. At each follow up visit, the medication list needs to be evaluated to determine if there has been any response to the medication, or any side effects. Providers should also document the length of therapy, consider the epileptogenic potential of the medication, and obtain appropriate instrumental (i.e., EKG) or laboratory examinations to monitor side effects or drug levels in order to evaluate the need to adjust or discontinue medications. Tools that can be used to monitor side effects for antipsychotics include the "Dyskinesia Identification System Condensed User Scale" (DISCUS) [26] or the "Matson Evaluation of Drug Side Effects Scale" (MEDS) [23]. Other strategies to consider include additional provider training in pharmacotherapy for adults with intellectual disability, creation of developmental medicine as a specialty, and implementation of electronic medical records that can help with identifying drug–drug interactions.

Next, it is important to discuss care for specific groups of individuals with intellectual disability (syndromes and etiologies) based on age and comorbidities. Consideration for caring for older individuals with intellectual disability is important. Newer antipsychotics are relatively contraindicated in individuals with dementia or history of cerebro-vascular disease given increased risk of stroke. Another important point is that olanzapine and quetiapine have potential anti-muscarinic activity, which can cause alteration in mental status, changes in gastrointestinal motility, urinary retention, and narrow-angle glaucoma in older individuals, especially if combined with other medications with anti-muscarinic activity. In an individual is already on anti-hypertensive medications or has a history of hypotension, one should be cautious when also prescribing clozapine, quetiapine, olanzapine, or risperidone since they can cause hypotension. Also, because atypical antipsychotics have been known to cause metabolic syndrome, one needs to monitor blood sugar, weight, body mass index, HbA1c, electrolytes, and liver function tests before starting and during medication use. This monitoring is also important if individuals are already obese and/or have diabetes mellitus. For individuals with epilepsy, providers need to be cautious in prescribing other medications that lower the seizure threshold such as clozapine, tricyclic antidepressants, and venlafaxine [27]. In individuals with hypertension, providers should avoid medications that are known to further elevate blood pressure, such as venlafaxine, desvenlafaxine, duloxetine, and various central nervous stimulants, such as methylphenidates. Respiratory difficulties and dysphagia are also commonly seen in some patients with intellectual disability, such as those with co-existing cerebral palsy. In these individuals, medications should be avoided that are sedating and can exacerbate respiratory failure or increase swallowing difficulties such as clozapine, olanzapine, risperidone, and quetiapine [27].

Though there few studies discussing first line therapy for individuals with concomitant diagnoses of intellectual disability and psychiatric disorder. Trollor et al. [27] discuss some guidelines for this population. For treating anxiety and depression in adults with intellectual disability, SSRIs are recommended as first line medications. Benzodiazepines for anxiety should only be used for the short term because they can cause agitation and impulsivity. When prescribing mood stabilizers or antipsychotics for bipolar disorder or schizophrenia, it is important to limit the use of medications that require multiple blood draws if the person will not tolerate this necessary safety monitoring. As noted, it is important to "start low and go slow" in titrating up these medications.

Lastly, it's important to recognize that individuals with intellectual disability may not present with the same clinical manifestations as the general population. Guidelines to help diagnosis these disorders are available, such as the "Practice Guidelines for the Assessment and Diagnosis of Mental Health Problems in Adults with Intellectual Disability" [28]. Though psychotropic medications are commonly prescribed for individuals with intellectual disability, many individuals do not have specific diagnosis; in such cases, these medications are used to treat a certain symptom such as aggression, hyperactivity, or social withdrawal. Therefore, it is important to understand why medications are prescribed, and when possible, apply the appropriate diagnostic framework to make sure the individual is being treated appropriately.

16.10 Conclusion

Polypharmacy is a major issue for the intellectual disabled population. As we have discussed, there are several definitions of polypharmacy in the literature. In this chapter, we adopted the definition of using five or more medications, which people with intellectual disability are at increased risk for, given the presence of multiple co-morbidities. Commonly prescribed medications for persons with intellectual disability include antipsychotics, anti-epileptics, and antidepressants, all of which have common adverse effects including sedation, insomnia, nausea, constipation, and weight gain. Tools such as the Matson Evaluation of Side Effects (MEDS), a psychotropic drug side effect scale, can be used to assess side effects in people with intellectual disability [23].

Overall, it is important to (1) "start low and go slow" when adding a new medication to a patient's regimen and to (2) determine the indication for each medication on a patient's medication list, as indications for medications prescribed for individuals with intellectual disability are often absent or unclear. Importantly, there are strategies that can help reduce polypharmacy and its negative effects, including medication reconciliation tools and processes such as the Systematic Tool to Reduce Inappropriate Prescribing (STRIP). To improve the quality of medical care for adults with intellectual disability, more research is needed to further define and understand the phenomenon of polypharmacy and to reduce polypharmacy's role in negative outcomes for this population.

References

1. Deb S, Farmah BK, Arshad E, Deb T, Roy M, Unwin GL. The effectiveness of aripiprazole in the management of problem behaviour in people with intellectual disabilities, developmental disabilities and/or autistic spectrum disorder – a systematic review. Res Dev Disabil. 2014;35:711–25.
2. Haider SI, Ansari Z, Vaughan L, Matters H, Emerson E. Prevalence and factors associated with polypharmacy in Victorian adults with intellectual disability. Res Dev Disabil. 2014;35:3071–80.
3. Stortz JN, Johanna KL, Cobigo V, Ouellette-Kuntz HMJ, Lunsky Y. Lessons learned from our elders: How to study polypharmacy in populations with intellectual and developmental disabilities. Intellect Dev Disabil. 2014;52:60–77.
4. O'Dwyer M, Peklar J, McCallion P, McCarron M, Henman MC. Factors associated with polypharmacy and excessive polypharmacy in older people with intellectual disability differ from the general population: a cross-sectional observational nationwide study. BMJ Open. 2016;6:e010505.
5. Tonge B, Einfeld S. The trajectory of psychiatric disorders in young people with intellectual disabilities. Aust N Z J Psychiatry. 2000;34:80–4.
6. Deb S, Unwin G, Deb T. Characteristics and the trajectory of psychotropic medication use in general and antipsychotics in particular among adults with an intellectual disability who exhibit aggressive behaviour. J Intellect Disabil Res. 2015;59:11–25.
7. Scheifes A, Egberts TCG, Stolker JJ, Nijman HLI, Heerdink ER. Structured medication review to improve pharmacotherapy in people with intellectual disability and behavioural problems. J Appl Res Intellect Disabil. 2016;29:346–55.
8. Lott IT, McGregor M, Engelman L, Touchette P, Tournay A, Sandman C, Walsh D. Longitudinal prescribing patterns for psychoactive medications in community-based individuals with developmental disabilities: Utilization of pharmacy records. J Intellect Disabil Res. 2004;48:563–71.
9. Eady N, Courtenay K, Strydom A. Pharmacological management of behavioral and psychiatric symptoms in older adults with intellectual disability. Drugs Aging. 2015;32:95–102.
10. Arvio M, Sillanpaa M. Prevalence, aetiology, and comorbidity of severe and profound intellectual disability (SPID) in Finland. J Intellect Disabil Res. 2004;48:429.
11. Häßler F, Thome J, Reis O. Polypharmacy in the treatment of subjects with intellectual disability. J Neural Transm (Vienna). 2015;122:S93–S100.
12. van der Heide DC, van der Putten AAJ, van den Berg PB, Taxis K, Vlaskamp C. The documentation of health problems in relation to prescribed medication in people with profound intellectual and multiple disabilities. J Intellect Disabil Res. 2009;53:161–8.
13. Mahan S, Holloway J, Bamburg JW, Hess JA, Fodstad JC, Matson JL. An examination of psychotropic medication side effects: Does taking a greater number of psychotropic medications from different classes affect presentation of side effects in adults with ID? Res Dev Disabil. 2010;31:1561–9.
14. Jackson C, Makin S, Marson A, Kerr M. Pharmacological interventions for epilepsy in people with intellectual disabilities. Cochrane Database Syst Rev. 2015;3(9):CD005399.
15. Matson JL, Mahan S. Antipsychotic drug side effects for persons with intellectual disability. Res Dev Disabil. 2010;31:1570–6.
16. Molina-Ruiz RM, Martín-Carballeda J, Asensio-Moreno I, Montañés-Rada F. A guide to psychopharmacological treatment of patients with intellectual disability in psychiatry. Int J Psychiatry Med. 2017;52:176–89.

17. McQuire C, Hassiotis A, Harrison B, Pilling S. Pharmacological interventions for challenging behaviour in children with intellectual disabilities: a systematic review and meta-analysis. BMC Psychiatry. 2015;15:303. https://doi.org/10.1186/s12888-015-0688-2.
18. Ji NY, Findling RL. Pharmacotherapy for mental health problems in people with intellectual disability. Curr Opin Psychiatry. 2016;29:103–25.
19. Ayub M, Saeed K, Munshi TA, Naeem F. Clozapine for psychotic disorders in adults with intellectual disabilities. Cochrane Database Syst Rev. 2015;23(9):Cd010625.
20. Rana F, Gormez A, Varghese S. Pharmacological interventions for self-injurious behaviour in adults with intellectual disabilities: abridged republication of a Cochrane systematic review. J Psychopharmacol. 2014;28:624–32.
21. Selph C, Cosca B. Less is more: preventing polypharmacy in individuals with intellectual disabilities. Impact. 2016;29:28–9. Retrieved from https://ici.umn.edu/products/impact/291/291.pdf.
22. Special Olympics International. MedFest medication watch list. Retrieved from http://resources.specialolympics.org/Taxonomy/Health/_Catalog_of_MedFest.aspx.
23. Matson JL, Cervantes PE. Current status of the matson evaluation of drug side effects (MEDS). Res Dev Disabil. 2013;34:1849–53.
24. Zaal RJ, Ebbers S, Borms M, de Koning B, Mombarg E, Ooms PE, M H. Medication review using a systematic tool to reduce inappropriate prescribing (STRIP) in adults with an intellectual disability: A pilot study. Res Dev Disabil. 2016;55:132–42.
25. Modi M, McMorris C, Palucka A, Raina P, Lunsky Y. Predictors of specialized inpatient admissions for adults with intellectual disability. Am J Intellect Dev Disabil. 2015;120:46–57.
26. Kalachnik JE, Sprague RL. The dyskinesia identification system condensed user scale (DISCUS): relability, validity, and a total score cut-off for mentally ill and mentally retarded populations. J Clin Psychiatry. 1993;49:177–89.
27. Trollor JN, Salomon C, Franklin C. Prescribing psychotropic drugs to adults with an intellectual disability. Aust Prescr. 2016;39:126–30.
28. Deb S, Matthews T, Holt G, Bouras N. Practice guidelines for the assessment and diagnosis of mental health problems in adults with intellectual disability. Res Dev Disabil. 2002;23:234–5.

Health Self-Management

17

Jaclyn K. Schwartz, Carmen E. Capó-Lugo,
and Patricia C. Heyn

17.1 Introduction

While intellectual disability is at times included under health conditions, persons with these disabilities are not "sick." In theory, these adults should have health outcomes comparable to adults in the general population. Unfortunately, persons with intellectual disability experience disparities across all categories of health [1]. Consequently, such adults and their older adult parents and other family members must simultaneously manage their disabilities and a multiplicity of secondary and comorbid health conditions [2]. In this chapter we describe health conditions commonly experienced by adults with intellectual disability, suggest tools to evaluate health-related self-management, and describe different intervention activities to promote health and wellbeing.

17.2 What Is Health-Related Self-Management?

Self-management is the "active management by individuals of their treatment, symptoms, lifestyle, physical and psychological consequences inherent with living with a chronic condition" [3]. Health care providers can play a valuable role

J. K. Schwartz (✉)
Occupational Therapy Department, Nicole Wertheim College of Nursing and Health Sciences, Florida International University, Miami, FL, USA
e-mail: jschwart@fiu.edu

C. E. Capó-Lugo
Department of Physical Therapy, School of Health Professions, University of Alabama at Birmingham, Birmingham, AL, USA

P. C. Heyn
Department of Physical Medicine and Rehabilitation, School of Medicine, University of Colorado Denver Anschutz Medical Campus, Aurora, CO, USA

© Springer Nature Switzerland AG 2019
V. P. Prasher, M. P. Janicki (eds.), *Physical Health of Adults with Intellectual and Developmental Disabilities*, https://doi.org/10.1007/978-3-319-90083-4_17

in supporting self-management in adults with intellectual disability, aimed at empowering individuals which can enhance their health and improve outcomes.

Health empowerment is a social process of recognizing, promoting, and enhancing the client's patient's' abilities to meet their own needs, solve their own problems, and mobilize necessary resources to take control of their own lives. In other words, patient empowerment is a process of helping people to assert control over factors that affect their health. Increasing empowerment enhances their potential for their participation, in concert along with their clinicians to, in the prevention and treatment of diseases that are dependent on a change in personal behavior. It is a critical aspect of the continuum of care and the goal to achieve a higher state of wellness that begins in the clinical setting, followed by transition to the community, and ultimately to the person's lifestyle. Knowledge is power, therefore communication and education is the central key factor in the process of self-health management and empowerment. Empowerment requires an individual to take care of one's self and be well-informed to make choices about care from the among the all available options identified in concert with the healthcare team. To successfully empower adults with intellectual disability, providers must work with them to develop an interdisciplinary comprehensive plan and then work collaboratively towards a seamless transition.

17.3   Health Outcomes in Adults with Intellectual Disability

Reichard et al. [1] found that persons with intellectual disability demonstrate higher rates of multiple chronic health conditions and reported worse health status than age peers in the general population. Further, research has found that adults with ID are less likely to receive needed health care services [1]. These disparities persist across domains of health (i.e., physical, sensory, mental, and oral).

17.3.1 Physical Health Conditions

Adults with intellectual disability are more likely to have both chronic health conditions and susceptibility to episodic illnesses [4]. They are more likely to experience conditions such as fractures, skin conditions, respiratory disorders, intestinal obstruction, pneumonia, and trauma [5] and they s are significantly more likely to be at abnormal body weight [6]. A review of studies related to the weight found that approximately half of study subjects were overweight or obese [4]. Additionally, such adults have higher rates of chronic health conditions, including cardiac disease, high blood pressure, high cholesterol, diabetes, stroke, arthritis, and asthma [1]. One feature is that even as adults are more likely a chronic health condition, they are also more likely to have multiple chronic conditions at once [1].

Persons aging with intellectual disability are also at increased risk for secondary health conditions. For example, older adults with Down syndrome experience accelerated aging associated with increased rates of cataracts, hearing loss, hypothyroidism, osteoporosis, epilepsy, sleep apnea, and Alzheimer's disease [7]. Persons with intellectual disability who also have cerebral palsy have a greater risk of accelerated musculoskeletal system aging, which can result in a loss of mobility, osteoporosis, chronic fatigue, and chronic pain [7]. While these health conditions are common in older adults, when added to the conceptual, social, and practical impairments of intellectual disability, common age-related conditions can become more disabling.

17.3.2 Sensory Conditions

Persons with intellectual disability are also at higher risk to have vision and hearing impairments [5]. When researchers screened Special Olympic athletes, they found 40% of athletes had ocular abnormalities [8]. Visual impairments were so intense; researchers estimated 14% of athletes would meet the diagnostic criteria for a visual impairment even after correction. Similarly for hearing impairments, Evenhuis et al. [9] found that 21% of persons with intellectual disability under the age of 50 had a hearing impairment and 6% required hearing aids. In persons over 50, approximately 80% of older adults had a hearing impairment. Vision and hearing impairments were also found to be co-occurring' approximately 20% of the sample had both vision and hearing impairment.

17.3.3 Mental Health Conditions

Adults with intellectual disability are also more likely to have a mental health condition compared to persons in the general population [5]. Cooper et al. [10] found that 40% of people with intellectual disability had a diagnosable mental illness or psychiatric condition, including psychosis, and anxiety, affective, obsessive compulsive and personality disorders, alcohol and substance abuse, or attention deficit hyperactivity. In older adulthood, mental illness prevalence rates can reach 70% when dementia is included [11].

Because of the high rates of mental illness, adults with intellectual disability are also more likely to be on psychiatric medications such as antidepressants, antipsychotics, and antiepileptic medications [12]. Lewis et al. [13] found that approximately one third of their sample of adults with intellectual disability was prescribed psychotropic medications. Unfortunately, psychiatric medications can lead to weight gain and poor oral health, thereby also affecting other health outcomes.

17.3.4 Oral Health Conditions

Persons with intellectual disability are at risk to have poorer oral health than the general population [5]. Krahn et al. [5] found that persons with intellectual disability were more likely to have missing or decayed teeth, and fillings. Anders and Davis [14] found individuals in this population were more likely to have periodontal disease and untreated cavities.

17.3.5 Mortality

Given the high rates of physical, sensory, mental, and oral health conditions, it's not surprising the standardized mortality rates for persons with intellectual disability are also higher than the general population [4]. Tyrer et al. [15] found that the mortality rate for persons with intellectual disability was three times higher than the rate of age peers in the general population. The results were more pronounced when they looked at adults in their twenties. Tyrer and colleagues found that the mortality rate was nine times higher for men and seventeen times higher for women with intellectual disability between age 20 and 29.

17.4 Factors Affecting Health Outcomes

As evidenced by the Person-Environment-Occupation model, one's ability to engage in regular health management and maintenance activities is shaped by the dynamic interaction among the person, environment, and occupation (i.e. activity) [16]. Unfortunately, persons with intellectual disability experience barriers across domains, and subsequently have difficulty managing their health. Figure 17.1 demonstrates the factors affecting health in each domain.

17.4.1 Personal Factors Affecting Health Outcomes

Impairments associated with intellectual disability can impact a person's ability to receive needed health care. According to the Diagnostic and Statistical Manual of Mental Disorders (DSM-5), intellectual disorders impair general mental abilities [17]. Specifically, impairments are noted in three domain areas:

1. Conceptual: Skills in language, reading, writing, math, reasoning, knowledge, and memory.
2. Social: Skills in empathy, social judgement, interpersonal communications skills, the ability to make and maintain friendships, and similar capacities.
3. Practical: Skills in personal care, job responsibilities, money management, recreation, and organizing school and work tasks.

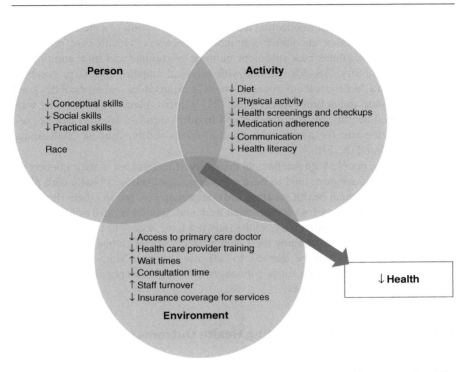

Fig. 17.1 Person-, environment-, and activity-based factors affecting health outcomes in adults with intellectual disability

Impairments associated with a diagnosis of intellectual disability can limit an adult's ability to request and thus receive needed health care. For example, an adult with intellectual disability may be unable to effectively communicate with caregivers and health care professionals to describe constipation, leading to small bowel obstruction. At times, a person's level of conceptual, social, and practical skills may inhibit him or her from full participation in health self-advocacy and health-related management.

17.4.2 Environmental Factors Affecting Health Outcomes

Environmental factors may also affect health disparities related to adults with intellectual disability. Many individuals have difficulty identifying a primary care or specialty physician who is able to meet their needs as they age [4, 18]. Research reveals that persons with intellectual disability may continue to receive care by a pediatrician or services through a children's hospital well into their 40s or later [18]. While pediatric health care providers may have good rapport with the client, they may miss the diagnosis and treatment for adult-specific conditions, an area which may not always be within their area of expertise.

When individuals with intellectual disability do go to adult oriented health care practitioners, they often encounter a number of barriers. Health care providers across various disciplines lack sufficient training to evaluate and treat adults with intellectual disability [18–20]. Adults with physical impairments (e.g. cerebral palsy) often find the physical environment (such as exam tables and medical devices) to be problematic and at times inaccessible [21]. Further, barriers such as long wait times, a rushed health care atmosphere, and frequent turnover by staff can be particularly problematic for adults with intellectual disability, causing challenging behaviors to flare [18, 20].

Additionally, people with intellectual disability, if recognized in their country as eligible for public support, tend to have a government-sponsored health care plan. In some countries, such health schemes are comprehensive, but in others they may lack components that pay for services such as dental, mental health, or habilitation therapy [4, 19]. In such situations, adults may not have access to the services they need to be successful in managing their own health. Even when health schemes are comprehensive, there may be barriers to self-management. Many aspects of the health care schemes may present self-management barriers to people with intellectual disability and their families.

17.4.3 Activity Factors Affecting Health Outcomes

Occupations and activities, or the execution of tasks by an individual, can also affect health outcomes [22]. Failure to correctly complete an important health function, like brushing teeth, can lead to poor health due to dental cavities and gum disease. Unfortunately, as many as 90% of adults with ha intellectual disability have health behaviors that fail to meet provider recommended standards [23].

1. **Diet.** An unhealthy diet can lead to obesity and other adverse health conditions. The research literature demonstrates a significant portion of community-dwelling adults with intellectual disability have "nutritionally poor" diets that are inadequate in some essential nutrients, not drawn from recommended food groups (e.g. fruits, vegetables, and dairy), and are excessive in other foods (e.g. fats, sweets, and junk food) [24]. Robertson et al. [23] found that only 8% of adults with intellectual disability in their study had a balanced diet. Poor diet not only results in obesity and metabolic disease, but it can also lead to other health conditions, such as constipation/bowel obstruction and pressure sores. Experts suggest that a lack of involvement in selecting meals, poor cooking skills, and gaps in dietary knowledge may lead to nutritional impairment [25]. Interventions are needed to help adults with intellectual disability better understand making sound decisions about food, increasing cooking skills, and in making healthy nutritional choices.

2. **Physical Activity.** A lack of physical activity and conditioning can affect the health of adults with intellectual disability. Robertson et al. [23] found that in their study sample, 84% of men and 88% of women with intellectual disability

were classified as physically inactive. Melville et al. [12] found that adults with ID were not only inactive, but significantly less active than age-peers in the general population. Interventions are needed to help adults with intellectual disability engage in more physically active lives and improve conditioning.

3. **Health Screenings and Preventative Care.** Persons with intellectual disability are significantly less likely to receive important screenings and preventative care than persons in the general population [1]. Further, the observed screening rates for adults with intellectual disability are below the standards of care suggested by the U.S. Preventative Task Force [1]. For example, when compared to the general population persons with intellectual disability are less likely to have:

- An optometric or eye examination [8, 26]
- A hearing exam [9, 26]
- A teeth cleaning [27]
- Receive a flu shot [13]
- Visit a gynecologist [27]
- Received cervical screening or mammograms [27]
- Subsequently, when researchers investigate health conditions in this population, they find many persons with intellectual disability have undiagnosed or underdiagnosed health conditions [9]. Advocacy and intervention are needed to help adults with intellectual disability receive health screenings and preventative services at the recommended rates.

4. **Medication Adherence.** Because of the number of secondary and comorbid health conditions, many adults with intellectual disability require regular medication to manage their health condition(s). In a study of 598 individuals with intellectual disability, Kerr et al. [26] found that 96% of participants were prescribed two or more medications and 22% were prescribed seven or more. Unfortunately, only half of people with intellectual disability take their medications as prescribed [28]. Education and interventions are needed to help people with intellectual disability better adhere to schedules for taking their prescribed medications.

5. **Communication.** When persons with intellectual disability receive health services, the person (and/or family member) are required to communicate with the medical staff and advocate for their needs. Unfortunately, many adults may be limited in their ability to describe their needs and to understand complex health information [29]. When people with intellectual disability are unable to communicate with their care teams, this often results in poor quality of care [18, 20]. Education and interventions are needed to help people with ID better communicate with health care providers to improve their quality of care (see [30]).

6. **Oral Hygiene.** Adults with intellectual disability have worse oral hygiene than age peers in the regular population. A study of the oral health of persons with intellectual disability demonstrated poor oral hygiene evidenced by heavy plaque

accumulation on 1 in 3 subjects [31]. Such adults are also less likely to receive oral health services. Only 36.5% adults with severe disabilities reported a dental visit compared to 53.4% of adults without disabilities [32].

17.5   Impact of Diversity on Health Outcomes

Lewis et al. [13] found that adults with intellectual disability are a diverse population and that the demographics of adults with intellectual disability mirrored the demographics of their state (California). Specifically, Californians with intellectual disability identified as African American (10%), Hispanic (20%), other (11%), white non-Hispanic (59%). Unfortunately, in addition to disparities due to their disability, preliminary data suggests that in the United States racial disparities also persist in adults with intellectual disability for health behaviors and health outcomes. Yang et al. [33] found that in the United States persons with Down syndrome from non-European ethnic communities have higher mortality rates compared to persons with Down syndrome of traditional European heritage. In terms of health behaviors, Pruchno and McMullen [34] found individuals with intellectual disability of African heritage were more likely to have unmet health needs for dental services, occupational therapy, psychological services, and social work. Similarly, Patel et al. [35] found that racially diverse individuals with intellectual disability had worse medication adherence than homogenous European-heritage persons with. intellectual disability. While many individuals with intellectual disability have difficulty communicating with health professionals, Ward et al. [18] found communications was even more difficult for non-English speaking families when the families resided in predominantly English-speaking communities. In some countries, racial and language barriers can negatively affect the health care experiences of adults with intellectual disability.

17.6   Importance of Self-Management

Adults with intellectual disability generally demonstrate worse self-management abilities and have more health conditions. Therefore, health care professionals should evaluate and treat for discordance between the nature of health conditions and health-care self-management.

17.7   Evaluating Health and Self-Management Skills

Assessment of health behaviors should be a standard part of practice across the continuum of care. Assessments can inform the care team about the client's strengths and need for client- and family-centered intervention. Health assessment should include a holistic approach that promotes self-empowerment by educating the adult with intellectual disability about his or her illness and treatment options. Evaluation and treatment should emphasize the importance of adult's active participation in

Table 17.1 Assessments for health conditions and health self-management

Assessment Name	Reference	Type of Assessment	What does it measure?
Health Self-Management			
Chronic Disease Self-Management Program Questionnaire	[36]	Survey	Chronic health conditions, insurance, general health, health impact on daily activities, physical activity, symptoms of chronic disease, recent health, medication adherence, mental health, communicating with medical staff, health care utilization
Dietary Screener	[37]	Survey	Foods one had ate or drank in the past month including meals and snacks
Oral Health Questionnaire	[38]	Survey	Frequency of brushing, frequency of flossing, use of toothpaste, duration of brushing, knowledge of the risks and benefits of oral hygiene, knowledge of impact of food on oral health
Self-efficacy	[39]	Survey	Confidence in exercising, communicating, obtaining help, talking with a doctor, managing disease, doing chores, engaging in recreational activity, managing symptoms, managing shortness of breath, managing depression
Health			
Body Mass Index	[40]	Observed	Height and weight
Pure-Tone Testing	[41]	Performance-based	The faintest tones a person can hear at select pitches (frequencies)
Sloan Letter Near Vision Card	[42]	Performance-based	Visual acuity
Oral Health Assessment Tool	[43]	Observed	Health of the lips, tongue, gums and tissues, saliva, natural teeth/dentures, oral cleanliness, and dental pain

treatment decisions as well as to empower confidence in them to take control over his or her health. Table 17.1 illustrates assessments for health and health self-management.

17.8   Interventions to Improve Self-Management in Adults with Intellectual Disability

Once health and self-management skills are quantified, health care providers can work to improve the health and or self-management abilities of adults with intellectual disability and their families. A person-focused approach for health and wellness can has the goal of enhancing patients, physicians, caregivers, and the community by delivering health information and resources tailored to support individualized health care needs, while promoting adherence to a healthy lifestyle. Successful person-focused programs are collaborative, multi-disciplinary, and attentive to the individual needs of the client. While these concepts may already exist occur in a traditional health care setting, opportunities exist to include this approach in non-traditional situations such as incorporating a "personal deliverable" or "health passport" for participants in clinical research protocols, or providing "personal coaching" in community outreach program.

17.8.1 Diet and Exercise

The majority of research has focused on diet and exercise [44, 45]. The research demonstrates that physical activity and exercise interventions can improve fitness, reduce weight, reduce maladaptive behaviors, improve adaptive behaviors, and improve life satisfaction [44, 45]. Some nutrition interventions were able to decrease participants' body mass index [45]. The most effective interventions were complex comprehensive interventions, meaning that they targeted a variety of approaches such as increasing physical activity and addressing diet.

17.8.2 Physical Activity

These goals can be addressed by (1) preventing prolonged inactivity and (2) increasing cardiovascular fitness. For example, prolonged physical inactivity behavior in a person with mild stroke can be avoided by increasing his or her long-term participation in any type of leisure-time physical activity. However, for the person to increase their cardiovascular and aerobic fitness the physical activity prescription needs to include prolonged, structured, repetitive, and somewhat effortful exercises. Rehabilitation professionals have a critical role in the promotion, adherence, maintenance, and success of active lifestyles for persons with mild stroke that start during acute care and expands throughout the continuum of care.

17.8.3 Healthy Lifestyle Change Program (HLCP)

The HLCP is a "twice-weekly education and exercise program to increase knowledge, skills, and self-efficacy regarding health, nutrition, and fitness among adults with intellectual disability" ([46], p. S201). The HLCP dedicates significant focus on increasing exercise time, improving nutritional habits, and reducing weight. Bazzano et al. [46] reported that adults with intellectual disability who participated in this program felt better prepared to manage their own health.

17.8.4 Comprehensive Self-Assessment Programme (CHAP)

CHAP is an intervention designed to enhance interactions between adults with intellectual disability, their caregiver, and their doctor via a systematic health history, guided health review, and development of a health action plan ([47], p. 139). Outcomes for the CHAP program include increased incidence of screening and preventative examinations and immunization rates.

17.8.5 The Advocacy Skills Kit (ASK)

ASK is an education intervention designed to improve communication between patients, general practitioners, and advocates for adults with intellectual disability. ASK was developed through a research-driven participatory action process, but lacks final outcomes testing. The ASK has four components:

(a) A diary of personal details about the patient.
(b) Health advocacy tips describing how to prepare for the doctor's visit.
(c) Tips for doctors on working with persons with intellectual disability, including a checklist of health problems associated with different intellectual syndromes.
(d) A medical records section describing diagnoses, medication, immunizations, allergies, family history of disease, and medical consultations.

17.9 Conclusion

Health-related self-management has the potential to increase participation in health surveillance and adherence to healthy life practices. Its applications will entail a lifespan commitment to health education and the integration of provider advice, assessment, and interventions with the native and instilled ability of adults with intellectual disability about concerns about personal health status and involvement in health treatment and advocacy.

References

1. Reichard A, Stolzle H, Fox MH. Health disparities among adults with physical disabilities or cognitive limitations compared to individuals with no disabilities in the United States. Disabil Health J. 2011;4:59–67.
2. Greenberg JS, Seltzer MM, Greenley JR. Aging parents of adults with disabilities: the gratifications and frustrations of later-life caregiving. Gerontologist. 1993;33:542–50. https://doi.org/10.1093/geront/33.4.542.
3. Boger EJ, Demain S, Latter S. Self-management: a systematic review of outcome measures adopted in self-management interventions for stroke. Disabil Rehabil. 2013;35:1415–28.
4. Scheepers M, Kerr M, O'Hara D, Bainbridge D, Cooper S-A, Davis R, Wehmeyer M. Reducing health disparity in people with intellectual disabilities: a report from health issues special interest research group of the international association for the scientific study of intellectual disabilities 1. J Policy Pract Intellect Disabil. 2005;2:249–55.
5. Krahn GL, Hammond L, Turner A. A cascade of disparities: health and health care access for people with intellectual disabilities. Ment Retard Dev Disabil Res Rev. 2006;12:70–82.
6. Yamaki K. Body weight status among adults with intellectual disability in the community. Ment Retard. 2005;43:1–10.

7. Perkins EA, Moran JA. Aging adults with intellectual disabilities. JAMA. 2010;304:91–2. Retrieved from http://jama.jamanetwork.com/article.aspx?articleid=186147

8. Woodhouse JM, Adler P, Duignan A. Vision in athletes with intellectual disabilities: the need for improved eyecare. J Intellect Disabil Res. 2004;48:736–45.

9. Evenhuis HM, Theunissen M, Denkers I, Verschuure H, Kemme H. Prevalence of visual and hearing impairment in a Dutch institutionalized population with intellectual disability. J Intellect Disabil Res. 2001;45:457–64.

10. Cooper S-A, Smiley E, Morrison J, Williamson A, Allan L. Mental ill-health in adults with intellectual disabilities: prevalence and associated factors. Br J Psychiatry. 2007;190:27–35.

11. Torr J, Chiu E. The elderly with intellectual disability and mental disorder: a challenge for old age psychiatry. Curr Opin Psychiatry. 2002;15:383–6.

12. Melville CA, Hamilton S, Hankey CR, Miller S, Boyle S. The prevalence and determinants of obesity in adults with intellectual disabilities. Obes Rev. 2007;8:223–30. https://doi.org/10.1111/j.1467-789X.2006.00296.x.

13. Lewis MA, Lewis CE, Leake B, King BH, Lindemann R. The quality of health care for adults with developmental disabilities. Public Health Rep. 2002;117:174–84. https://doi.org/10.1016/S0033-3549(04)50124-3.

14. Anders PL, Davis EL. Oral health of patients with intellectual disabilities: a systematic review. Spec Care Dentist. 2010;30:110–7. Retrieved from http://www.ncbi.nlm.nih.gov/pubmed/20500706

15. Tyrer F, Smith LK, McGrother CW. Mortality in adults with moderate to profound intellectual disability: a population-based study. J Intellect Disabil Res. 2007;51:520–7. Retrieved from http://www.ncbi.nlm.nih.gov/pubmed/17537165

16. Law M, Cooper BA, Strong S, Stewart D, Rigby P, Letts L. The person-environment-occupation model: a transactive approach to occupational perfomance. Can J Occup Ther. 1996;63:9–23.

17. American Psychiatric Association. Diagnostic and Statistical Manual of Mental Disorders. Arlington: American Psychiatric Association; 2013. https://doi.org/10.1176/appi.books.9780890425596.744053.

18. Ward RL, Nichols AD, Freedman RI. Uncovering health care inequalities among adults with intellectual and developmental disabilities. Health Soc Work. 2010;35:280–90.

19. Fenton SJ, Hood H, Holder M, May PB Jr, Mouradian W. The American Academy of Developmental Medicine and Dentistry: eliminating health disparities for individuals with mental retardation and other developmental disabilities. J Dent Educ. 2003;67:1337–44.

20. Iacono T, Davis R. The experiences of people with developmental disability in Emergency Departments and hospital wards. Res Dev Disabil. 2003;24:247–64.

21. Mudrick NR, Breslin ML, Liang M, Yee S. Physical accessibility in primary health care settings: results from California on-site reviews. Disabil Health J. 2012;5:159–67. https://doi.org/10.1016/j.dhjo.2012.02.002.

22. World Health Organization. International classification of functioning, disability and health. Geneva: World Health Organization; 2001. Retrieved from http://www.who.int/classifications/icf/en/

23. Robertson J, Emerson E, Gregory N, Hatton C, Turner S, Kessissoglou S, Hallam A. Lifestyle related risk factors for poor health in residential settings for people with intellectual disabilities. Res Dev Disabil. 2000;21:469–86. https://doi.org/10.1016/S0891-4222(00)00053-6.

24. Humphries K, Traci MA, Seekins T. Nutrition and adults with intellectual or developmental disabilities: systematic literature review results. Intellect Dev Disabil. 2009;47:163–85. https://doi.org/10.1352/1934-9556-47.3.163.

25. Melville CA, Boyle S, Miller S, Macmillan S, Penpraze V, Pert C, Hankey CR. An open study of the effectiveness of a multi-component weight-loss intervention for adults with intellectual disabilities and obesity. Br J Nutr. 2011;105:1553–62.

26. Kerr AM, McCulloch D, Oliver K, McLean B, Coleman E, Law T, Prescott RJ. Medical needs for people with intellectual disability require regular reassessment, and the provision of client- and carer-held reports. J Intellect Disabil Res. 2003;47:134–45. https://doi.org/10.1046/j.1365-2788.2003.00453.x.

27. Havercamp SM, Scandlin D, Roth M. Health disparities among adults with developmental disabilities, adults with other disabilities, and adults not reporting disability in North Carolina. Public Health Rep. 2004;119:418–26.
28. Vacek JL, Hunt SL, Shireman T. Hypertension medication use and adherence among adults with developmental disability. Disabil Health J. 2013;6:297–302.
29. Lennox N, Taylor M, Rey-Conde T, Bain C, Boyle FM, Purdie DM. ASK For it: development of a health advocacy intervention for adults with intellectual disability and their general practitioners. Health Promot Int. 2004;19:167–75.
30. Bishop KM, Hogan M, Janicki MP, Keller SM, Lucchino R, Mughal DT, Perkins EA, Singh BK, Service K, Wolfson S, Health Planning Work Group of National Task Group on Intellectual Disabilities and Dementia Practices. Guidelines for dementia-related health advocacy for adults with intellectual disability and dementia: National Task Group on Intellectual Disabilities and Dementia Practices. Intellect Dev Disabil. 2015;53:2–29. https://doi.org/10.1352/1934-9556-53.1.2.
31. Altun C, Guven G, Akgun OM, Akkurt MD, Basak F, Akbulut E. Oral health status of disabled individuals attending special schools. Eur J Dent. 2010;4:361–6.
32. Glassman P, Miller CE. Preventing dental disease for people with special needs: the need for practical preventive protocols for use in community settings. Spec Care Dentist. 2003;23:165–7. https://doi.org/10.1111/j.1754-4505.2003.tb00305.x.
33. Yang Q, Rasmussen SA, Friedman JM. Mortality associated with Down's syndrome in the USA from 1983 to 1997: a population-based study. Lancet. 2002;359(9311):1019–25.
34. Pruchno RA, McMullen WF. Patterns of service utilization by adults with a developmental disability: type of service makes a difference. Am J Ment Retard. 2004;109:362–78. https://doi.org/10.1352/08958017(2004)109<362:POSUBA>2.0.CO;2.
35. Patel I, Erickson SR, Caldwell CH, Woolford SJ, Bagozzi RP, Chang J, Balkrishnan R. Predictors of medication adherence and persistence in Medicaid enrollees with developmental disabilities and type 2 diabetes. Res Social Adm Pharm. 2015;12:592–603. https://doi.org/10.1016/j.sapharm.2015.09.008.
36. Stanford Patient Education Research Center. Chronic Disease Self-management Questionnaire. Palo Alto, CA: Stanford University; 2007. Retrieved from http://patienteducation.stanford.edu/research/
37. National Cancer Institute. Dietary Screener Questionnaire (DSQ). Bethesda, MD: National Institutes of Health; 2016. Retrieved from http://epi.grants.cancer.gov/nhanes/dietscreen/questionnaires.html#inter
38. Crest, Oral-B, Ambulatory Healthcare Services, Abu Dhabi Health Services Co.. Oral health questionnaire. Retrieved from http://schoolsforhealth.haad.ae/media/28695/questionnaire.pdf.
39. Lorig K, Stewart A, Ritter P, González V, Laurent D, Lynch J. Outcome measures for health education and other health care interventions. Thousand Oaks, CA: Sage Publications; 1996.
40. National Institutes of Health. Calculate your body mass index. Retrieved from http://www.nhlbi.nih.gov/health/educational/lose_wt/BMI/bmicalc.htm.
41. American Speech-Language-Hearing Association. Pure-tone testing. Retrieved from http://www.asha.org/public/hearing/Pure-Tone-Testing/.
42. Sloan LL. New test charts for the measurement of visual acuity at far and near distances. Am J Ophthalmol. 1959;48(6):807–13.
43. Chalmers J, King P, Spencer A, Wright F, Carter K. The Oral Health Assessment Tool – Validity and reliability. Aust Dent J. 2005;50:191–9. https://doi.org/10.1111/j.1834-7819.2005.tb00360.x.
44. Hamilton S, Hankey CR, Miller S, Boyle S, Melville CA. A review of weight loss interventions for adults with intellectual disabilities. Obes Rev. 2007;8:339–45. Retrieved from http://www.ncbi.nlm.nih.gov/pubmed/17578383
45. Heller T, McCubbin JA, Drum C, Peterson J. Physical activity and nutrition health promotion interventions: what is working for people with intellectual disabilities? Intellect Dev Disabil. 2011;49:26–36.

46. Bazzano AT, Zeldin AS, Diab IRS, Garro NM, Allevato NA, Lehrer D. The Healthy Lifestyle Change Program: a pilot of a community-based health promotion intervention for adults with developmental disabilities. Am J Prev Med. 2009;37:S201–8.
47. Lennox N, Bain C, Rey-Conde T, Purdie D, Bush R, Pandeya N. Effects of a comprehensive health assessment programme for Australian adults with intellectual disability: A cluster randomized trial. Int J Epidemiol. 2007;36:139–46. https://doi.org/10.1093/ije/dyl254.

Health Promotion and People with Intellectual Disability

18

Beth Marks, Jasmina Sisirak, and Tamar Heller

18.1 Introduction-Expectations for Health Promotion

More than 30 years have passed since the World Health Organization (WHO) adopted the Ottawa Charter of 1986 [1, 2], often seen as "health promotion's founding document" [3]. Health promotion is a fundamental function of public health and contributes to the work of addressing communicable and non-communicable diseases and other threats to health [4]. Operationalizing the Ottawa Charter's core pre-requisites to improve health, "Advocate–Enable–Mediate" [1], has a more recent history among researchers, practitioners, and policy makers working with people with intellectual disability. In 2001, the Aging Special Interest Research Group of the International Association for the Scientific Study of Intellectual and Developmental Disabilities (IASSIDD) in collaboration with the WHO developed formal international guidelines, which created a significant impetus for increased awareness regarding the value of health promotion [5]. The IASSIDD-WHO joint report resulted in a call-to-action to develop health promotion initiatives inclusive of active participation of people with intellectual disability [6]. Following the IASSIDD/WHO 2001 report, two significant reports published in the United States (U.S.) highlighted the critical need for research, education, and practice to improve culturally relevant care, reduce barriers to health and health promotion services, and facilitate access to decrease health disparities.

B. Marks (✉) · J. Sisirak · T. Heller
Department of Disability and Human Development, University of Illinois at Chicago, Chicago, IL, USA

© Springer Nature Switzerland AG 2019
V. P. Prasher, M. P. Janicki (eds.), *Physical Health of Adults with Intellectual and Developmental Disabilities*, https://doi.org/10.1007/978-3-319-90083-4_18

In 2002, the *2002 Closing the Gap: A National Blueprint to Improve the Health of People with Mental Retardation* [7] was published following input from a US Surgeon General's Listening Session on Health Disparities and Mental Retardation held on October 10, 2001 [8]. In 2005, the *Surgeon General's Call to Action to Improve the Health and Wellness of Persons with Disabilities* [9] was published based on a need to promote accessible, available, and appropriate health care and health promotion services for people with disabilities.

Today, targeted health promotion programming is even more relevant and urgently needed for adults with intellectual disability to be able to live, work, learn, and recreate in communities and settings of their choice. With an increased availability of diagnostic technology, medication therapies, surgical interventions, and improved access to health care, adults with intellectual disability (ID) are experiencing improved health outcomes and decreased mortality rates [10]. Over the next two to three decades, more adults with intellectual disability (ID) are expected to live into their 70s and 80s and beyond. Unfortunately, with advanced age, they also are experiencing more complex health conditions, earlier onset of age-related conditions, and premature age-related changes in their health compared to their age peers without a disability [11–14]. In comparison to people without a long-term disability, people with intellectual disability (ID) in most countries, are often the most underserved with regard to health care services [15]. Additionally, because people with intellectual disability (ID) frequently live in settings devoid of inclusive and accessible health promoting environments and communities, they experience a number of issues related to negative determinants of health (e.g., genetics, environmental exposures, social circumstances, poor healthcare access, poor health behaviors) [16, 17]. With respect to risk factors, for people with intellectual disability, the prevalence of being overweight and obese is documented as equal or higher compared to the general population [18, 19]. Conditions, such as high cholesterol, hypertension, cardiovascular disease, and multiple chronic conditions are also more common among people with intellectual disability (ID) [20]. Given select societal factors, such as the increased burden of non-communicable diseases, aging populations, and obstacles related to determinants of health, a need exists for more epidemiological data, along with more proactivity in addressing political challenges and changing in health policy [21].

Article 25 and the other articles within the 2007 UN Convention on the Rights of Persons with Disabilities ([CRPD]; [22]) provide a global impetus to secure community-integrated, sustainable health promotion initiatives so people with intellectual disability can enjoy optimal health without discrimination. This chapter provides an overview of the determinants of health and health promotion for people with intellectual disability. Additionally, it will introduce and discuss an ecological framework that can engage people with intellectual disability and their supporters in various health promotion activities. Lastly, examples of successful health promotion initiatives are presented, along with exploration of future directions for promoting health among people with intellectual disability and their supports.

18.2   People with Intellectual Disability Living Long, Healthy Lives

Today's global health concerns reflect a 'triple burden of diseases' perspective related to an ongoing agenda of communicable diseases, newly emerging and re-emerging diseases, as well as the unprecedented rise of non-communicable chronic conditions [23]. Challenges to public health initiatives include global climate change, sedentary lifestyles, and frequency and severity of natural disasters, financial crises, and security risks. Because health is heavily influenced by factors, such as social, economic and political forces, outside the domain of the health sector, policy makers, practitioners, and researchers increasingly recognize the limitations of biomedical interventions which might result in better health [23]. For people with intellectual disability, health promotion is *even more* imperative today given global public health issues, as they are a traditionally underserved group and becoming more vulnerable while living in turbulent communities.

The implementation of health promotion for people with intellectual disability requires an examination of the determinants of health and a review of evidence as to what works in health promotion [24]. Organizations including IASSIDD, in its official role with the World Health Organization (WHO), and Special Olympics International, the largest global sports organization for people with intellectual disability, have stimulated international political action to nurture health promotion for people with intellectual disability. The Ottawa Charter 1986 [2] clearly positions political action for redressing health inequities and the need for increasing power to access necessary resources to control health determinants [24]. Distinguishing between primary health care (PHC) and primary care (see Table 18.1 for Glossary of Terms) is important in being able to develop and implement health promotion and disease prevention activities for people with intellectual disability. PHC is basic health care that is universally accessible and acceptable to people with intellectual disability and their families located within their communities at an affordable cost [27]. PHC is an approach to health policy and service provision that includes services, such as, individual care from a primary care provider (primary care services) and population-level "public health-type" functions [28, 29]. Primary care is person-focused with a sustained partnership with adults over time [28, 30, 31]. PHC includes core components of universal access to care and coverage based on need; commitment to health equity oriented to social justice; community participation in developing and implementing health goals; and intersectoral approaches to health [28, 32]. The goal of PHC is "health care for all."

Because health outcomes for people with intellectual disability vary based on age, socioeconomic status, access to care, as well as, disability and health status, PHC addresses health policy and services that are delivered to both individuals and populations. Incorporating both PHC and PC can ensure that health promotion is a multisectoral action rather than located within the sole domain of the medical sector. Additionally, it can ensure that PHC's commitment to health equity is of equal importance to primary medical care.

Table 18.1 Glossary of terms

Health	The World Health Organization (WHO) defined human health in its broader sense in its 1948 constitution as "a state of complete physical, mental, and social well-being and not merely the absence of disease or infirmity".
Health Promotion	Health promotion "is the process of is the process of enabling people to increase control over their health and its determinants, and thereby improve their health" ... [4]. Health promotion is based on this critical human right and offers a positive and inclusive concept of health as a determinant of the quality of life and encompassing mental and spiritual well-being.
Disease Prevention	"Disease prevention covers measures not only to prevent the occurrence of disease, such as risk factor reduction, but also to arrest its progress and reduce its consequences once established" [25]. Disease prevention focuses on prevention strategies to reduce the risk of developing chronic conditions and other morbidities.
Ecological Public Health	Ecological public health emphasizes commonalities between achieving health and sustainable development [25]. The increased importance of ecological public health is due to the changing nature of health issues and their interface with emerging global environmental problems (e.g., destruction of the ozone layer, uncontrolled and unmanageable air and water pollution, and global warming). Global environmental problems impacts health as models of causality and intervention are not always known. The focus is on economic and environmental determinants of health and strategies to guide economic investments towards producing positive population health outcomes, greater health equity, and sustainable use of resources.
Health Communication	Health communication is used to inform the public about health concerns and to keep key health issues on the public agenda. Mass media and multimedia, along with technological innovations are used to disseminate health information to the public and to increases awareness of specific issues related to individual and collective health concerns.
Health Education	Health education provides health information and knowledge to people and communities along with skills to support the adoption of healthy behaviors voluntarily [23]. Health education consists of opportunities for learning through some modality of communication to improve health literacy, including improving knowledge and developing life skills, which promote individual and community health [25]. Previously, the term health education included a wider range of actions including social mobilization and advocacy. These methods are now encompassed in the term health promotion.
Health Literacy	"Health literacy is a shared function of social and individual factors. Individuals' health literacy skills and capacities are mediated by their education, culture, and language. Equally important are the communication and assessment skills of the people with whom individuals interact regarding health, as well as the ability of the media, the marketplace, and government agencies to provide health information in a manner appropriate to the audience" [26].
Primary care	The provision of primary care is often conducted on an individual level and includes services, such as, health promotion, disease prevention, health maintenance, counselling, patient education, diagnosis and treatment of acute and chronic illnesses in a variety of health care settings (e.g., office, inpatient, critical care, long-term care, school, worksites, home care, day care) (AAFP, retrieved from www.aafp.org/about/policies/all/primary-care.html).
Primary health care	Primary health care (PHC) is essential health care made accessible at a cost a country and community can afford, with methods that are practical, scientifically sound and socially acceptable [27]. PHC is a broader term derived from core principles articulated by the World Health Organization and an approach to health policy and service provision that includes the following types of services: (1) individuals (primary care services) and (2) population-level "public health-type" functions [28].
Wellness	Wellness is defined as the state of being in good health, especially as an actively pursued goal. Six multidimensional domains, including social, occupational, spiritual, physical, intellectual, emotional, often are used to encompass wellness.

Like people without disabilities, optimal health among people with intellectual disability, requires access to food, housing, education, income, sustainable resources, social justice, equity, and safety [33]. Major determinants of preventable illness and premature death are not limited to physiological and physiological factors, but are often the result of inadequate access to care and health literacy skills, lack of disability knowledge among health professionals, limited social support, poverty, and unemployment. People with disabilities may age differently based on their health behaviors across their lifetime, the nature and severity of their disability, co-existing health conditions, and chronic health conditions. Many age-related problems across the lifespan are attributed to a "high-risk lifestyle." Hence, health promotion activities are a way to age well by lowering the risk for disease and illness later in life by having control over determinants of health. WHO states "health promotion usually addresses behavioral risk factors such as tobacco use, obesity, diet and physical inactivity, as well as the areas of mental health, injury prevention, drug abuse control, alcohol control, health behavior related to HIV, and sexual health" [34].

Broadly, health determinants are categorized into four areas: (1) biological factors (e.g., syndrome and sex-related conditions, the only immutable factors); (2) socioeconomic and environmental factors; (3) factors related to health care (e.g., physical, communication, programmatic aspects); and, (4) behavioral factors (e.g., lifestyle choices health promotion, disease prevention practices).

18.3   Social Economics and Environments

As health begins in our homes, schools, workplaces, neighborhoods, and communities, creating social and physical environments that promote good health for all is critical for people with intellectual disability [35]. Socioeconomic and environmental factors which affect health status, include "rapid and often adverse social, economic and demographic changes that affect working conditions, learning environments, family patterns, and the culture and social fabric of communities" [4]. However, the vulnerability and exclusion of people with intellectual disability across the lifespan who are isolated and marginalized in many communities remains a challenge [36, 37]. Where people with intellectual disability live, work, and recreate matters. Financial stability and money also matters, as poverty (economic deprivation) is one of the most prevalent risk factors of poor health [38]. For example, in a study with a nationally representative cross-sectional sample of 7070 British families supporting children aged 0–16 years in 2002, families supporting a child with intellectual disability were 42% more likely to be living in poverty, 70% more likely to have no savings and to worry about money "all the time," and over twice as likely to be in debt and experience material hardship [38].

For people with intellectual disability, living in specific residential settings and participating in day programs, such as those in schools, worksites, group activity programs can affect their health status. As an example, in the U.S. adults living in the least restrictive community settings have the highest rates of obesity and often a low intake of fruits and vegetables [39, 40].

Limited social support, disruption of personal ties, loneliness, violence against people with intellectual disability, and conflicted interactions with peers and caregivers can be major sources of stress for people with intellectual disability [41, 42]. The quantity and quality of social relationships affect mental health and physical health, as well as, health behaviors, physical health, and mortality risk [43, 44]. Supportive social connections and intimate relations are vital sources of emotional strength and can have a positive effect on health status [43].

18.4   Access to Health Care

According to the United Nations, being able to enjoy the "highest attainable standard of health" without discrimination is one of the "fundamental rights of every human being." Access to health care, health promotion, and disease prevention is vital in being able to achieve and sustain community engagement to improve their health [45]. For a variety of reasons, including complex developmental trajectories and unique communication and cognitive skills, people with intellectual disability are often challenged in obtaining services that are accessible (i.e., affordable, available) and acceptable (i.e., culturally relevant, appropriate, satisfactory) health services.

With few professional health care training programs addressing disability issues in their curricula [46–48], people with intellectual disability do not have adequate access to health services which are culturally sensitive and developmentally appropriate. Researchers suggest that people with intellectual disability struggle with access to culturally and linguistically relevant health services [49, 50]. Nurses report knowledge gaps regarding the health needs of people with intellectual disability and limited training in communicating with people with intellectual disability [51]. Studies with health professionals also document reports of stress, lack of confidence, fear and anxiety, and different treatment with a lack of support for autonomy in caring for people with intellectual disability [52]. Across a range of professional groups, training needs have been categorized into areas of (1) general communication, (2) knowledge/information, and (3) profession-specific needs to reduce the high prevalence of poor physical and mental health among people with intellectual disability [53]. Training programs should focus on increasing confidence in specific skills, such as, managing associated challenging behaviors [54].

People with intellectual disability experience a "cascade of disparities" including a higher prevalence of adverse conditions, inadequate attention to care needs, inadequate focus on health promotion, and poor access to quality health care services [55]. The following common problems have been reported across multiple levels within primary care: (1) communication issues impacting people with intellectual disability' understanding of treatment plans and risks; (2) inattention to patients' concerns about maintaining daily activities; and, (3) difficulties accommodating patients who require more time for office visits, including accessibility barriers that interfere with the timely and complete of physical examinations, diagnostic procedures, and screening and preventive care [49]. Attitudinal barriers may affect the quality of care [56]. Health systems may lack availability of personal assistants as well as accessible screening equipment, signage regarding, and washrooms [57].

Health educational materials are rarely presented in accessible formats or inclusive of people with a variety of learning styles necessitating alternative communication modalities. Alternate communication modalities include assistive technology; sign language interpreters for people who are deaf or hard of hearing; large print formats for people with low vision; readers for people who are blind or visually impaired; and, health literate materials written at an appropriate level of understanding [58].

Low health literacy impacts people with intellectual disability as they may be less able to manage their health, which can result high utilization of treatment services, increased hospitalization rates and use of emergency services, low utilization of preventive services, and high health care costs [59, 60]. In order to build capacity for people with intellectual disability to interact with health information, research is needed to identify what health literacy means, what it means to participate in health literacy practices, and the nature of health texts (that is, what they are and what they do for people with intellectual disability) [61]. Clear health communication using multimodal strategies to ensure access needs to be increased among people with intellectual disability, their supports, and health services providers [62]. Improving health literacy among people with intellectual disability has the potential to increase knowledge about one's body and the relationship between lifestyle factors (e.g., food choices, physical activity) and health outcomes, along with recognizing the need to seek care [57].

People with intellectual disability will likely experience improved health outcomes when the provision of health care becomes equitable and inclusive at the primary care level [63]. A need continues for rigorous mixed-methods descriptive quantitative and qualitative research, epidemiological studies, and multi-level intervention-based research. Moreover, to address issues related to ineffective or absent health care delivery for people with intellectual disability [64], the provision of evidence-based didactic and clinical preparation for health care professionals can increase their confidence in providing health care [47].

18.5   Behaviors

Key behavioral factors of health include physical activity, diet, hand washing, alcohol, tobacco, and other drug use [65]. Various studies continue to report low levels of physical activity, poor fitness, poor nutrition, and a higher risk of falls among people with intellectual disability. The prevalence of common health conditions, such as high cholesterol, hypertension, cardiovascular disease is reportedly higher among people with intellectual disability [66–69]. People with intellectual disability have a higher incidence of multiple chronic conditions [20, 55, 66, 70, 71]. People with intellectual disability experience either an equal or higher prevalence of being overweight and obese compared to the general population [69, 72]. For many adults with intellectual disability, the combination of sedentary lifestyles, high fat diets, and low fruit and vegetable diets is a major factor for the increased risk for acquiring chronic health conditions. Like for people without disabilities, health behaviors of people with intellectual disability can directly influence health status, along with environmental factors. Elimination or modification of behavioral risk factors associated with either the onset of a chronic conditions or the management of a chronic condition can mitigate more serious health issues related to multiple chronic conditions.

18.6   Biology

An identifiable etiological cause of disability may have associated medical conditions in an estimated 40–60% of adults with intellectual disability [73–75] and when intellectual disability is more significant, an identifiable etiology is more likely, as is the prevalence of physical co-morbidity [74, 76]. In addition, many people with intellectual disability who also have specific syndrome-related conditions (e.g., Down syndrome, Fragile X, Prader-Willi, Williams, Retts, Anglemans, tuberous sclerosis, cerebral palsy) may also be predisposed to a variety of health conditions based on their disability. Additionally, people with intellectual disability often have higher rates of epilepsy, psychiatric and gastrointestinal disorders, sensory impairment, and limited mobility compared to their non-disabled age peers [77].

Lennox [74] provides a limited list of syndrome-specific medical conditions in Tables 11.2a, b (see Chaps. 3 and 11). Additionally, Lennox [74] presents a list of unrecognized or poorly managed medical conditions of people with intellectual disability in Table 11.1. Understanding disability etiology, syndromes, and associated medical conditions may be crucial to the development of accessible health promotion interventions that are inclusive of people with intellectual disability and that can maximize the positive impact on a person's quality of life [74]. For example, syndrome-related conditions may result in health concerns, such as, difficulty eating or swallowing, dental problems, reduced mobility, bone demineralization, gastro-esophageal reflux, arthritis, decreased muscle tone, and progressive cervical spine degeneration [57, 78]. Many people with intellectual disability are frequently prescribed psychotropic and anti-seizure medications on a long-term basis for behavioral issues [79, 80]. Medications prescribed for people with intellectual disability can contribute to a higher risk of falling [81] and for osteoporosis (brittle bone disease), which may be compounded by lack of physical activity and a diet limited in calcium and vitamin D [82]. Initiating health promotion activities in infancy is even more imperative for people with intellectual disability who may have a higher risk of various health conditions across the lifespan.

18.7   Successful Health Promotion Initiatives

The *Ottawa Charter for Health Promotion* [2] continues to guide the global practice of health promotion and provides a strategy that incorporates the following five essential actions: (1) building healthy public policy; (2) creating supportive environments; (3) strengthening community action; (4) developing personal skills; and, (5) reorienting health services. Building on the Ottawa Charter statement that "health is created and lived by people within the settings of their everyday life; where they learn, work, play and love" [2], creating a foundation of supportive environments within settings can provide an infrastructure for comprehensive health promotion strategies [83]. Identification of health promotion strategies for people with intellectual disability to maintain optimal health across the lifespan, like for the general population, is a key element for bridging equity gaps and advocating for policies to achieve optimal health and wellness [45]. By enabling people to increase control over and to improve their health through health promotion activities, the focus moves beyond individual level behavioral change interventions. Because personal health practices are just one of the determinants of health, health promotion programs are increasingly addressing the socio-environmental, cultural, and access constraints that impact individuals with Pan American Health Organization [45] and their support persons.

18.8   Healthy Settings

A recent systematic review of health promotion programs for people with ID, which identified 13 studies evaluating ten different health promotion programs [84], documented that much of the intervention research has focused on individual level behavior change. The ten health promotion programs reviewed by Scott and Havercamp [84] focused primarily on behavioral change in the following areas: exercise, diet, nutrition, physical activity knowledge, skills and participation, and stress education. Health promotion programs need to move beyond an individual level approach and incorporate a range of social and environmental frameworks using a settings-based approach, so as to improve health status and to mitigate the early onset of age-related chronic conditions. Achieving the fundamental aim of health promotion involves enabling people to increase control over and improve their health through action that is facilitated in community settings such as schools, homes, and work places [85].

The settings approach to health promotion is emerging and is being implemented by health promotion researchers and practitioners to reach people with intellectual disability and their supports in a variety of places. A settings approach also engages stakeholders to promote sustainable health activities and decrease inequities. Healthy settings involve a holistic and multi-disciplinary method, which integrates action across risk factors. The goal is to maximize disease prevention via a "whole system" approach. Principles include community participation, partnership, empowerment and equity [33]. Unfortunately, despite the extensively documented benefits of health promotion and education to maintain health and control risk factors, people with intellectual disability face continued exclusion within community-based programs. Initiation of health promotion over a 'whole system' for people with intellectual disability must include the following: (1) establishment of state-wide community practices for health; (2) development of multisectoral community collaboratives; (3) documentation of participation and outcomes in health-related initiatives (primary care, health promotion, disease prevention); and, (4) creation of "cultures of health" within communities and organizations providing services for people with intellectual disability [86].

18.9   Research-to-Practice Networks

Parallel to health promotion efforts in the general population, progress has been made in the areas of science and research [21] within the population of people with intellectual disability. Health promotion and disability is now an academic subject with publication of numerous articles, scoping reviews, textbooks, and chapters as well as the emergence of new journals. Additionally, many scientific conferences, symposiums, and discussion groups have convened. Using Google Scholar to search the terms "intellectual disability" and "health promotion," 423 articles were retrieved for the years between the Ottawa Charter [1] and the IASSIDD WHO report (2000). For the period 2001 to 2018, the number of articles increased to 9700. Future work should address strategies for achieving sustainable practices and the integration of health policy beyond the health sector to include all sectors and a multi-level approach ranging from local, state, national, and international arenas.

With the development of evidence-based health promotion programs for people with intellectual disability, implementation and sustainability on a large-scale remains challenging as providers and practitioners must sustain these programs and the needs are tremendous. Due to the demand for these programs in multiple community settings, such as schools, day programs, work, and residential settings, meeting the need for this demand presents unique opportunities. Providers and practitioners also struggle to maintain fidelity and program success of a evidence-based programs (EBPs), as many programs are developed without input from people who will ultimately implement and use a particular program [87]. The process of *collaborative design* can foster a collaborative partnership between researchers and practitioners to ensure that an EBP is adapted to the "real-world." Collaborative design has practitioner feedback and adaptation built in to the design-time development, which in turn enhances practitioner adaptation of an EBP [87].

Another methodology that aims to address the research to practice gaps that hinder the implementation of an EBP is *implementation science* [87, 88]. With implementation science, researchers are encouraged to adopt a "make it happen" approach versus the typical "let it happen" dissemination approach. The "make it happen" approach involves several strategies: (1) collaborating with community organizations capable of empowering practitioners to implement an EBP; (2) defining EBP components clearly; (3) using training methods that effectively teach practitioners to implement the EBP with fidelity; (4) providing organizational support for implementation; and, (5) fostering leadership throughout the organization, from adaptive leadership that champions the change to technical leadership that ensures long-term sustainability.

One example is the Autism Model of Implementation (AMI) for community-based organizations, which provided treatment for children diagnosed with autism spectrum disorder (ASD). It was designed and tested through a community-academic collaboration [88]. With an aim to assist the ASD community based organizations to assess and find EBPs to their meet service needs, the AMI facilitated the identification, adoption, and use of EBPs.

By researchers engaging community stakeholders as partners, community-academic partnerships (CAPs) can improve the research process, outcomes, and yield benefits for the community and researchers [89]. CAP engage community stakeholders as partners in research to shift research from being unidirectional, which is when researchers conceptualize research projects with minimal (or no) community stakeholder input, to a bidirectional approach which involves collaboration between community stakeholders and academic researchers [90, 91]. With CAPs, research questions, design, methods, sustainability plans, and dissemination modalities are developed collaboratively with the community organizations providing services to people with intellectual disability. CAPs can increase the speed and success of translation of research findings and practices from university based to "real world" settings [90]. Community-academic research-to-practice networks for health promotion hold potential to enhance bidirectional investment among community stakeholders and researchers to provide EBP or evidence-informed health promotion programs and activities to improve health participation and health outcomes among people with intellectual disability.

18.10   Future Directions for Promoting Health

The action areas outlined by the Ottawa Charter [1] continue to provide a structure for implementing health promotion initiatives through actions that build healthy public policy, create supportive environments, strengthen community actions, develop personal skills, and reorient health services. As health promotion for people with intellectual disability moves beyond the health sector, globally key stakeholders and policy makers across many sectors and system levels will become more aware of how their decisions impact health outcomes. With more direct involvement of key stakeholders, they may be more likely to assume greater responsibility for the health of all populations, including those people with intellectual disability.

18.11   Health Promotion Beyond the Health Sector

Building a healthy public policy for people with intellectual disability combines a variety of complementary approaches including legislative approaches, fiscal measures, tax policy, organizational change, and community support. The overall aim is to *make the healthier choices for people with ID and their supports the easiest choice*. The *HealthMatters Scale-Up Initiative* aims to support community organizations to build policies that support *health-friendly services and environments* across community sectors and local and state municipalities [86]. The *HealthMatters Initiative* is a multi-state research project in the U.S. that is identifying the facilitating "drivers" and processes to scale-up health promotion programming in each state, building health promotion capacity within participating community-based organizations (CBOs), and training CBO staff to implement the evidence-based 12-week *HealthMatters Program* for people with intellectual disability [92]. The *HealthMatters Initiative* leverages two national networks including the network of University Centers for Excellence in Developmental Disabilities (UCEDDs) and the Centers for Disease Control and Prevention (CDC) *State Disability and Health Programs*. Each U.S. state and territory has at least one UCEDD in every US state and territory that has a unique position to work with state and local government agencies, community providers, and people with intellectual disability in a variety of initiatives with a focus on building community capacity to serve people with disabilities [93]. Currently, the CDC funds 19 *State Disability and Health Programs* to improve health and quality of life among people with intellectual disability and other disabilities to adapt and implement evidence-based strategies in their communities [94].

Creating supportive environments requires an understanding that our communities are unique, complex, and interrelated. Health is interrelated with other goals. Hence, the links between people and their environments provide a foundation for including a socioecological approach to health. Similar to people without disabilities, work and leisure is a source of health for people with intellectual disability. Creating accessible environments that are inclusive of all people requires health promotion approaches to generate living and working conditions that are safe, stimulating, satisfying and enjoyable. Health promotion initiatives need to integrate systematic assessment of the health impact of an environment. Aspects of the environment impacted include those at work, home, recreation, and in business and commerce. For example, while the relationship between the built environment and physical activity has been documented for people in the general population, little is known about the impact of the built environment on physical activity for people with intellectual disability using valid and reliable measures inclusive of people with intellectual disability interacting within their environment [95]. The Community Health Inclusion Index (CHII) is the first instrument to operationalize community health inclusion using an assessment tool for public health professionals and community coalitions to assess needed supports to improve healthy, active living among people with disabilities [96].

Strengthening community actions to achieve better health outcomes occurs through ongoing priority setting, decision-making, strategic planning, and implementation. Empowerment of communities through ownership and control is central to this process. Community development utilizes existing human and material resources within the community to enhance self-care and social support through flexible systems that strengthen participation in and direction of health promotion. To achieve active involvement, all stakeholders need full, continuous, and equitable access to information, learning opportunities for health, and funding support. In the U.S., the *State Disability and Health Programs* are funded for either capacity building or core implementation programs. The "capacity building" states focus on developing an infrastructure to impact policy, systems, and environmental changes, while the states funded for "core implementation program" aim to strengthen the existing infrastructure to disseminate programmatic, policy, systems, and environmental changes [94].

Developing personal skills can occur through health promotion involving information, health literacy, education for health, and life skills. By developing personal and social skills, people with intellectual disability can have more options and control over their own health and their environments enabling them to make actual "choices" that are conducive to health. Because personal control and choice are often challenging for people with intellectual disability, developing advocacy skills is imperative for people with intellectual disability and their supports as it can be helpful to develop positive health behaviors in partnership. Lifelong learning can support people with intellectual disability to make plans and decisions throughout all stages across the life course and to manage their disability, chronic conditions, illnesses, and injuries as they age. Facilitating lifelong learning must incorporate a settings approach in school, home, work, and community settings. Health promotion strategies require action through educational, professional, and commercial and voluntary bodies. Programs with strong study designs that focus on health education and behavior change [84] include *Steps to Your Health* [97, 98], *HealthMatters Program* [92, 99, 100], *Bergstrom Diet and Physical Activity Program* [101], *Women Be Healthy* [102, 103], and the ASK Health Diary [104].

Reorienting health services is essential to shared responsibility for health promotion and the pursuit of health among individuals, community groups, health professionals, health service institutions and governments. The health sector must push for more health promotion activities and move beyond its responsibility for providing clinical and curative services. To reorient health services and provide holistic care for people with intellectual disability, changes are required in health research and professional education and training to shift attitudes and organization of health services. One example of a new training program is the New Hampshire Disability and Public Health Project's online, on-demand, free training for mammography Radiologic Technologists [105]. Another example is the "Health Care for Adults with Intellectual and Developmental Disabilities: Toolkit for Primary Care Providers," which is an excellent tool for providers and caregivers to address the cascade of health disparities among people with intellectual disability [106]. This toolkit provides guidelines for people with intellectual disability who may be experiencing one or more of the following: (1) a range of complex or difficult-to-treat medical conditions; (2) difficulty accessing health care; (3) inadequate health care; (4) difficulties expressing their symptoms and pain; and, (5) little attention given to wellness, preventive care, and health promotion.

18.12 Multilevel, Multisectoral Stakeholders

In moving forward, stakeholders across all sectors need to incorporate a guiding principle that, in each phase of planning, implementation and evaluation of health promotion activities, people with intellectual disability should become equal partners. Health is not created within a medical model approach based on illness care. Rather health is fulfilled and lived by people within their everyday life, such as where they live, learn, work, play and love. Contemporary health promotion initiatives must continue to expand beyond exercise and diets through systematic studies examining technology such as internet, social media, and cell telephone usage patterns among children and adults with intellectual disability [107]. Opportunities and risks associated with technology have implications for community engagement through education, employment, recreation, health behaviors, and health outcomes. As people with intellectual disability are living longer, future efforts need to address men and women's reproductive health, sexuality, relationships, abuse issues, and violence [108, 109].

18.13 Health as an Everyday Resource

Health promotion incorporating the key messages and approaches of the Ottawa Charter has yet to be implemented on a large scale for the general population [3]. For people with intellectual disability, health promotion leaders are in the early stages of rethinking health as a positive concept emphasizing social and personal resources and situating health as a resource for everyday life. As noted by Pettersson [21], what remains to be achieved is the process of making research findings more accessible to readers outside the academic community. For example, using the five action areas beyond the health care sector for health promotion, researchers and practitioners need to develop, test, and implement programs that operationalize the three core strategies of the Ottawa Charter, "advocate, enable, and mediate," for people with intellectual disability.

The prerequisites and prospects for health cannot be ensured by the health sector alone. People with intellectual disability can only achieve their optimal health potential when they are able to do the following: (1) advocate for political, economic, social, cultural, environmental, behavioral and biological factors that promote health; (2) control matters that determine their health (supportive environment, access to information, life skills and opportunities for making healthy choices); and (3) mediate between differing interests in society for the pursuit of health. Health promotion strategies and programs should be adapted to the local needs and possibilities of individual countries and regions accounting for unique social, cultural and economic systems. Professional groups, social networks, and health providers have a responsibility to mediate the practice of health promotion between differing interests and to involve people across all levels as individuals, families and communities. Pettersson [21] notes the disparity in the proportion of intervention and implementation research in public health research in that only 5% is spent on "how to actually do it." Research agendas must invest in developing strategies that document success in "scaling up" evidence-based health promotion interventions rather than merely documenting successes with small samples.

Within the context of changing health agendas, media, and globalization for practice, the three core strategies of the Ottawa Charter, "advocate, enable, and mediate," are even more relevant today [110]. While a major challenge for the general population is the engagement of community advocates, this is critical for people with intellectual disability and their supports across all settings. Moreover, "enabling" requires greater sensitivity to power relations and the role of health literacy; and, "mediating" has a central role in bridging the interests of stakeholder [110].

Acknowledgement   The chapter authors would like to thank the following for their contribution and support in the preparation of this chapter:

Judith Stych, DNP, RN, CDDN
Nurse Consultant
Wisconsin Department of Health Services
Bureau of Adult Long Term Care Services
1 West Wilson St. Room 518, Madison, Wisconsin 53707 USA

Michele A. (Micki) Hill, RN BSN CPN
Helen Denne Schulte Nursing Scholar and Adjunct Faculty
University of Wisconsin-Madison
School of Nursing
Nurse Consultant
Wisconsin Department of Health Services
Madison, Wisconsin 53707 USA

References

1. World Health Organization [WHO]. The Ottawa charter for health promotion; 2018. Retrieved from http://www.who.int/healthpromotion/conferences/previous/ottawa/en/
2. World Health Organization. The Ottawa Charter for Health Promotion. Geneva, Switzerland: WHO; 1986. Available from: http://www.who.int/healthpromotion/conferences/previous/ottawa/en/index.html
3. Potvin L, Jones C. Twenty-five years after the Ottawa charter: the critical role of health promotion for public health. Can J Public Health. 2011;102:244–8.
4. World Health Organization. The Bangkok Charter for Health Promotion in a Globalized World. 6th global conference on health promotion. Paper presented at the WHO, Bangkok, Thailand; 2005.
5. Evenhuis H, Henderson C, Beange H, Lennox N, Chicoine B. Healthy ageing – adults with intellectual disabilities: physical health issues. J Appl Res Intellect Disabil. 2001;14:175–94.

6. World Health Organization. Ageing and intellectual disabilities - improving longevity and promoting healthy ageing: summative report. Geneva, Switzerland: World Health Organization; 2000. Accessed from: http://www.who.int/mental_health/media/en/20.pdf
7. US Department of Health and Human Services. Closing the gap: a national blueprint to improve the health of persons with mental retardation; 2002. Retrieved from Rockville.
8. US Department of Health and Human Services. The surgeon General's call to action to prevent and decrease overweight and obesity; 2001. Retrieved from Rockville: http://www.surgeongeneral.gov/sgoffice.htm.
9. US Department of Health and Human Services. The surgeon General's call to action to improve the health and wellness of persons with disabilities; 2005. Retrieved from Rockville.
10. Bittles A, Glasson E. Clinical, social, and ethical implications of changing life expectancy in Down syndrome. Dev Med Child Neurol. 2004;46:282–6.
11. Bowers B, Webber R, Bigby C. Health issues of older people with intellectual disability in group homes. J Intellect Develop Disabil. 2014;39:261–9. https://doi.org/10.3109/13668250.2014.936083.
12. Carmeli E, Imam B. Health promotion and disease prevention strategies in older adults with intellectual and developmental disabilities. Front Public Health. 2014;2:31. https://doi.org/10.3389/fpubh.2014.00031.
13. Esbensen A. Health conditions associated with aging and end of life of adults with Down syndrome. Int Rev Res Ment Retard. 2010;39:107–26. https://doi.org/10.1016/S0074-7750(10)39004-5.
14. Krahn GL, Fox MH. Health disparities of adults with intellectual disabilities: what do we know? What do we do. J Appl Res Intellect Disabil. 2014;27:431–46. https://doi.org/10.1111/jar.12067.
15. Scott HM, Havercamp SM. Race and health disparities in adults with intellectual and developmental disabilities living in the United States. Intellect Dev Disabil. 2014;52:409–18. https://doi.org/10.1352/1934-9556-52.6.409.
16. Scheepers M, Kerr M, O'Hara D, Bainbridge D, Cooper SA, Davis R, et al. Reducing health disparity in people with intellectual disabilities: a report from Health Issues Special Interest Research group of the International Association for the Scientific Study of Intellectual Disabilities. J Policy Pract Intellect Disabil. 2005;2:249–55. https://doi.org/10.1111/j.1741-1130.2005.00037.x.
17. Sisirak J, Marks B, Heller T, Ronneberg C, McDonald K, Ailey S. People with IDD: health and wellness for all critical issues in intellectual and developmental disabilities: contemporary research, practice, and policy. Washington, DC: AAIDD; 2016.
18. Marks B, Sisirak J. Nurse practitioners promoting physical activity: people with intellectual and developmental disabilities. J Nurse Pract. 2017;13:e1–5. https://doi.org/10.1016/j.nurpra.2016.10.023.
19. Rimmer JH, Yamaki K, Davis BM, Wang E, Vogel LC. Obesity and overweight prevalence among adolescents with disabilities. Prev Chronic Dis. 2011;8:A41.
20. Reichard A, Stolzle H, Fox MH. Health disparities among adults with physical disabilities or cognitive limitations compared to individuals with no disabilities in the United States. Disabil Health J. 2011;4:59–67. https://doi.org/10.1016/j.dhjo.2010.05.003.
21. Pettersson B. Some bitter-sweet reflections on the Ottawa Charter commemoration cake: a personal discourse from an Ottawa rocker. Health Promot Int. 2011;26(Suppl 2):ii173–9. https://doi.org/10.1093/heapro/dar080.
22. United Nations. Convention on the rights of persons with disabilities; 2018. Accessed from: https://www.un.org/development/desa/disabilities/convention-on-the-rights-of-persons-with-disabilities.html
23. Kumar S, Preetha G. Health promotion: an effective tool for global health. Indian J Community Med. 2012;37:5–12.
24. Sparks M. Acting on the social determinants of health: health promotion needs to get more political. Health Promot Int. 2009;24:199–202. https://doi.org/10.1093/heapro/dap027.

25. World Health Organization (WHO). Health promotion glossary. Geneva: World Health Organization; 1998.
26. Institute of Medicine. Health literacy: a prescription to end confusion. Washington, DC: The National Academies Press; 2004.
27. World Health Organization [WHO]. Declaration of Alma-Ata international conference on primary health care, Alma-Ata, USSR; 1978.
28. Muldoon L, Hogg W, Levitt M. Primary care (PC) and primary health care (PHC). What is the difference? Can J Public Health. 2006;97:409–11.
29. Awofeso N. What is the difference between "primary care" and "primary healthcare"? Qual Prim Care. 2004;12:93–4.
30. Institute of Medicine (IOM). Primary care: America's health in a new era. In: Molla S, Donaldson K, Yordy D, Lohr K, Vanselow N, editors. Report of a study by a Committee of the Institute of Medicine. Washington, DC: Division of Health Care Services, National Academy Press; 1996.
31. Starfield BNYOOUP. Primary care: balancing health needs, services and technology. 2nd ed.. New York and Oxford: Oxford University Press; 1998;8–9.
32. World Health Organization (WHO). Health systems: principled integrated care world health report 2003, Geneva, Switzerland; 2003.
33. World Health Organization [WHO]. Healthy settings; 2018. Retreived from: http://www.who.int/healthy_settings/en
34. World Health Organization [WHO]. Health promotion and disease prevention through population-based interventions, including action to address social determinants and health inequity; 2018. Accessed from: www.emro.who.int/about-who/public-health-functions/health-promotion-disease-prevention.html.
35. Office of Disease Prevention and Health Promotion [ODPHP]. Determinants of health. In Healthy people 2020; 2016. Retrieved from: www.healthypeople.gov/2020/about/foundation-health-measures/Determinants-of-Health and https://www.healthypeople.gov/2020/topics-objectives/topic/heart-disease-and-stroke.
36. Cummins R, Lau A. Community integration or community exposure? A review and discussion in relation to people with an intellectual disability. J Appl Res Intellect Disabil. 2003;16:145–57. https://doi.org/10.1046/j.1468-3148.2003.00157.x.
37. Wilson N, Jaques H, Johnson A, Brotherton M. From social exclusion to supported inclusion: adults with intellectual disability discuss their lived experiences of a structured social group. J Appl Res Intellect Disabil. 2017;30:847–58. https://doi.org/10.1111/jar.12275.
38. Emerson E, Hatton C. Poverty, socio-economic position, social capital and the health of children and adolescents with intellectual disabilities in Britain: a replication. J Intellect Disabil Res. 2007;51:866–74. https://doi.org/10.1111/j.1365-2788.2007.00951.x.
39. Hsieh K, Rimmer J, Heller T. Obesity and associated factors in adults with intellectual disability. J Intellect Disabil Res. 2014;58:851–63. https://doi.org/10.1111/jir.12100.
40. Sisirak J, Marks B, Heller T, Riley B. Dietary habits of adults with intellectual and developmental disabilities residing in community-based settings. Paper presented at the American Public Health Association, 135rd annual meeting & exposition, Washington, DC; 2007, Nov 6.
41. Hartley S, MacLean W. Stressful social interactions experienced by adults with mild intellectual disability. Am J Intellect Dev Disabil. 2009;114:71–84. https://doi.org/10.1352/2009.114.71-84.
42. Petroutsou A, Hassiotis A, Afia A. Loneliness in people with intellectual and developmental disorders across the lifespan: a systematic review of prevalence and interventions. J Appl Res Intellect Disabil. 2018; https://doi.org/10.1111/jar.12432.
43. Umberson D, Crosnoe R, Reczek C. Social relationships and health behavior across life course. Annu Rev Sociol. 2010;36:139–57. https://doi.org/10.1146/annurev-soc-070308-120011.
44. Umberson D, Montez J. Social relationships and health: a flashpoint for health policy. J Health Soc Behav. 2010;51(Suppl):S54–66. https://doi.org/10.1177/0022146510383501.

45. Pan American Health Organization (PAHO). Promoting health in the Americas. Annual report of the Director 2001; 2001.
46. Havercamp SM, Scott HM. National health surveillance of adults with disabilities, adults with intellectual and developmental disabilities, and adults with no disabilities. Disabil Health J. 2015;8:165–72. https://doi.org/10.1016/j.dhjo.2014.11.002.
47. Holder M, Waldman H, Hood H. Preparing health professionals to provide care to individuals with disabilities. Int J Oral Sci. 2009;1:66–71. https://doi.org/10.4248/ijos.09022.
48. Thierer T, Meyerowitz C. Education of dentists in the treatment of patients with special needs. J Calif Dent Assoc. 2005;33:723–9.
49. Minihan PM, Robey KL, Long-Bellil LM, Graham CL, Hahn JE, Woodard L, Eddey GE. Desired educational outcomes of disability-related training for the generalist physician: knowledge, attitudes, and skills. Acad Med. 2011;86(9):1171–8. https://doi.org/10.1097/ACM.0b013e3182264a25.
50. Phillips A, Morrison J, Davis RW. General practitioners' educational needs in intellectual disability health. J Intellect Disabil Res. 2004;48:142–9.
51. Melville C, Finlayson J, Cooper SA, Allan L, Robinson N, Burns E, Morrison J. Enhancing primary health care services for adults with intellectual disabilities. J Intellect Disabil Res. 2005;49:190–8.
52. Pelleboer-Gunnink H, Van Oorsouw WJ, Van Weeghel J, Embregts P. Mainstream health professionals' stigmatising attitudes towards people with intellectual disabilities: a systematic review. J Intellect Disabil Res. 2017;61:411–34. https://doi.org/10.1111/jir.12353.
53. Hemm C, Dagnan D, Meyer T. Identifying training needs for mainstream healthcare professionals, to prepare them for working with individuals with intellectual disabilities: a systematic review. J Appl Res Intellect Disabil. 2015;28:98–110. https://doi.org/10.1111/jar.12117.
54. Ong N, McCleod E, Nicholls L, Fairbairn N, Tomsic G, Lord B, Eapen V. Attitudes of healthcare staff in the treatment of children and adolescents with intellectual disability: a brief report. J Intellect Develop Disabil. 2017;42:295–300. https://doi.org/10.3109/13668250.2016.1236368.
55. Krahn GL, Hammond L, Turner A. A cascade of disparities: health and health care access for people with intellectual disabilities. Ment Retard Dev Disabil Res Rev. 2006;12:70–82. https://doi.org/10.1002/mrdd.20098.
56. Lewis S, Stenfert-Kroese B. An investigation of nursing staff attitudes and emotional reactions towards patients with intellectual disability in a general hospital setting. J Appl Res Intellect Disabil. 2010;23(4):355–65. https://doi.org/10.1111/j.1468-3148.2009.00542.x.
57. Marks B, Sisirak J. Community health promotion programmes. In: Taggart L, Cousins W, editors. Health promotion for people with intellectual and developmental disabilities. Maidenhead, Berkshire, UK: Open University Press: McGraw Hill Education; 2013. p. 138–48.
58. Marks B. Cultural competence revisited: nursing students with disabilities. J Nurs Educ. 2007;46(2):70–4.
59. Baur C. Health literacy and adults with I/DD: achieving accessible health information and services. Paper presented at the state of science in aging with developmental disabilities, Atlanta, GA; 2007.
60. National Center for Education Statistics. National assessment of adult literacy; 2003. Retrieved from https://nces.ed.gov/naal/health_results.asp.
61. Chinn D. Critical health literacy health promotion and people with intellectual disabilities. Asia-Pacific J Health Sport Phys Educ. 2014;5(3):249–65. https://doi.org/10.1080/18377122.2014.940811.
62. Selden CR, Zorn M, Ratzan S, Parker RM. Health literacy, January 1990 through October 1999. Bethesda, MD: National Library of Medicine; 2000.
63. Lennox N, Van Driel M, van Dooren K. Supporting primary healthcare professionals to care for people with intellectual disability: a research agenda. J Appl Res Intellect Disabil. 2015;28:33–42. https://doi.org/10.1111/jar.12132.

64. Ali A, Scior K, Ratti V, Strydom A, King M, Hassiotis A. Discrimination and other barriers to accessing health care: perspectives of patients with mild and moderate intellectual disability and their carers. PLoS One. 2013;8:e70855. https://doi.org/10.1371/journal.pone.0070855.
65. Healthy People 2020 [Internet]. Washington, DC: U.S. Department of Health and Human Services, Office of Disease Prevention and HealthPromotion. Accessed 13 Feb 2018. Available from: https://www.healthypeople.gov/2020/about/foundation-health-measures/Determinants-of-Health.
66. Draheim CC. Cardiovascular disease prevalence and risk factors of persons with mental retardation. Ment Retard Dev Disabil Res Rev. 2006;12:3–12.
67. Hilgenkamp T, Reis D, van Wijck R, Evenhuis H. Physical activity levels in older adults with intellectual disabilities are extremely low. Res Dev Disabil. 2012;33:477–83. https://doi.org/10.1016/j.ridd.2011.10.011.
68. Sundahl L, Zetterberg M, Wester A, Rehn B, Blomqvist S. Physical activity levels among adolescent and young adult women and men with and without intellectual disability. J Appl Res Intellect Disabil. 2016;29:93–8. https://doi.org/10.1111/jar.12170.
69. Yamaki K. Body weight status among adults with intellectual disability in the community. Ment Retard. 2005;43:1–10.
70. Bodde AE, Seo DC. A review of social and environmental barriers to physical activity for adults with intellectual disabilities. Disabil Health J. 2009;2:57–66. https://doi.org/10.1016/j.dhjo.2008.11.004.
71. Tyler CV, Schramm SC, Karafa M, Tang AS, Jain AK. Chronic disease risks in young adults with autism spectrum disorder: forewarned is forearmed. Am J Intellect Dev Disabil. 2011;116:371–80. https://doi.org/10.1352/1944-7558-116.5.371.
72. Melville CA, Hamilton S, Hankey CR, Miller S, Boyle S. The prevalence and determinants of obesity in adults with intellectual disabilities. Obes Rev. 2007;8(3):223–30.
73. Battaglia A, Bianchini E, Carey J. Diagnostic yield of the comprehensive assessment of developmental delay/mental retardation in an insitute of child neuropsychiatry. Am J Med Genet. 1991;82:60–6.
74. Lennox N. Health promotion and disease prevention. In: Prasher V, Janicki M, editors. Physical health of adults with intellectual disabilities. New York: John Wiley & Sons, Inc.; 2002. p. 230–51.
75. Majnemer A, Shevell M. Diagnostic yield of the neurologic assessment of the developmentally delayed child. J Pediatr. 1995;127:193–9.
76. Gustavson K-H, Hagberg G, Sars K. Severe mental retardation in a Swedish county. I. Epidemiology, gestational age, birth weight and associated CNS handicaps in children born 1959–1970. Acta Paediatr Scand. 1977;66:373–9.
77. Traci MA, Seekins T, Szalda-Petree A, Ravesloot C. Assessing secondary conditions among adults with developmental disabilities: a preliminary study. Ment Retard. 2002;40:119–31. https://doi.org/10.1352/0047-6765(2002)040<0119:ascaaw>2.0.co;2.
78. White-Scott S. Health care and health promotion for aging individuals with intellectual diabilities. Paper presented at the state of science in aging with developmental disabilities, Atlanta, GA; 2007.
79. Bowring DL, Totsika V, Hastings RP, Toogood S, McMahon M. Prevalence of psychotropic medication use and association with challenging behaviour in adults with an intellectual disability. A total population study. J Intellect Disabil Res. 2017;61:604–17. https://doi.org/10.1111/jir.12359.
80. Perry BI, Cooray SE, Mendis J, Purandare K, Wijeratne A, Manjubhashini S, Kwok HF. Problem behaviours and psychotropic medication use in intellectual disability: a multinational cross-sectional survey. J Intellect Disabil Res. 2018;62:140–9. https://doi.org/10.1111/jir.12471.
81. Hsieh K, Rimmer J, Heller T. Prevalence of falls and risk factors in adults with intellectual disability. Am J Intellect Dev Disabil. 2012;117:442–54.

82. Bolton JM, Morin SN, Majumdar SR, et al. Association of mental disorders and related medication use with risk for major osteoporotic fractures. JAMA Psychiat. 2017;74:641–8. https://doi.org/10.1001/jamapsychiatry.2017.0449.
83. Dooris M. Healthy settings: challenges to generating evidence of effectiveness. Health Promot Int. 2006;21:55–65. https://doi.org/10.1093/heapro/dai030.
84. Scott HM, Havercamp SM. Systematic review of health promotion programs focused on behavioral changes for people with intellectual disability. Intellect Dev Disabil. 2016;54:63–76.
85. Bloch P, Toft U, Reinbach H, Clausen L, Mikkelsen B, Poulsen K, Jensen B. Revitalizing the setting approach – supersettings for sustainable impact in community health promotion. Int J Behav Nutr Phys Act. 2014;11:118. https://doi.org/10.1186/s12966-014-0118-8.
86. Sisirak J, Marks B, Mullis L, Sheppard-Jones K, Tew L, Krok K, Grosso C HealthMatters for people with intellectual and developmental disabilities: building communities of practice for health; 2016. Retrieved from Washington, DC.
87. Lucyshyn J. Bridging the research to practice gap; 2016. Retrieved from https://www.psychologytoday.com/blog/psyched/201608/bridging-the-research-practice-gap.
88. Drahota A, Aarons GA, Stahmer AC. Developing the autism model of implementation for autism spectrum disorder community providers: study protocol. Implement Sci. 2012;7:1–10.
89. Meza R, Drahota A, Spurgeon E. Community-academic partnership participation. Community Ment Health J. 2016;52:793–8. https://doi.org/10.1007/s10597-015-9890-4.
90. Drahota A, Meza RD, Brikho B, Naaf M, Estabillo JA, Gomez ED, Aarons GA. Community-academic partnerships: a systematic review of the state of the literature and recommendations for future research. Milbank Q. 2016;94:163–214. https://doi.org/10.1111/1468-0009.12184.
91. Stahmer AC, Aranbarri A, Drahota A, Rieth S. Toward a more collaborative research culture: extending translational science from research to community and back again. Autism. 2017;21:259–61. https://doi.org/10.1177/1362361317692950.
92. Marks B, Sisirak J, Heller T. Health matters: the exercise, nutrition, and health educational curriculum for people with developmental disabilities. Baltimore: Paul H. Brookes Publishing Co.; 2009.
93. Association of University Centers on Disability. UCEDD Directory – display all; 2011. Accessed from: https://www.aucd.org//directory/directory.cfm.
94. Center for Disease Control and Prevention (CDC). State disability and health programs; 2017. Accessed from: https://www.cdc.gov/ncbddd/disabilityandhealth/programs.html.
95. Eisenberg Y, Vanderbom KA, Vasudevan V. Does the built environment moderate the relationship between having a disability and lower levels of physical activity? A systematic review. Prev Med. 2017;95s:S75–s84. https://doi.org/10.1016/j.ypmed.2016.07.019.
96. Eisenberg Y, Rimmer JH, Mehta T, Fox MH. Development of a community health inclusion index: an evaluation tool for improving inclusion of people with disabilities in community health initiatives. BMC Public Health. 2015;15:1050. https://doi.org/10.1186/s12889-015-2381-2.
97. Mann J, Zhou H, McDermott S, Poston MB. Healthy behavior change of adults with mental retardation: attendance in a health promotion program. Am J Ment Retard. 2006;111:62–73.
98. McDermott S, Whitner W, Thomas-Koger M, Mann J, Clarkson J, Barnes T, Meriwether R. An efficacy trial of 'Steps to Your Health', a health promotion programme for adults with intellectual disability. Health Educ J. 2012;71:278–90. https://doi.org/10.1177/0017896912441240.
99. Heller T, Hsieh K, Rimmer JH. Attitudinal and psychological outcomes of a fitness and health education program on adults with Down syndrome. Am J Ment Retard. 2004;109:175–85.
100. Marks B, Sisirak J, Chang Y. Efficacy of the HealthMatters program train-the-trainer model. J Appl Res Intellect Disabil. 2013;26:319–34. https://doi.org/10.1111/jar.12045.
101. Bergstrom H, Hagstromer M, Hagberg J, Elinder LS. A multi-component universal intervention to improve diet and physical activity among adults with intellectual disabilities in community residences: a cluster randomised controlled trial. Res Dev Disabil. 2013;34:3847–57. https://doi.org/10.1016/j.ridd.2013.07.019.

102. Lunsky Y, Straiko A, Armstrong S. Women be healthy: evaluation of a women's health curriculum for women with intellectual disabilities. J Appl Res Intellect Disabil. 2003;16:247–53. https://doi.org/10.1046/j.1468-3148.2003.00160.x.
103. Parish SL, Rose RA, Luken K, Swaine JG, O'Hare L. Cancer screening knowledge changes: results from a randomized control trial of women with developmental disabilities. Res Soc Work Pract. 2012;22:43–53.
104. Lennox N, Bain C, Rey-Conde T, Taylor M, Boyle F, Purdie D, Ware R. Cluster randomized-controlled trial of interventions to improve health for adults with intellectual disability who live in private dwellings. J Appl Res Intellect Disabil. 2010;23:303–11. https://doi.org/10.1111/j.1468-3148.2009.00533.x.
105. Institute of Disability/UCED. Responsive practice; 2018. Accessed from: http://responsive-practice.org/.
106. Vanderbilt University. Health care for adults with intellectual and developmental disabilities; 2018. Accessed from: https://vkc.mc.vanderbilt.edu/etoolkit/
107. Jenaro C, Flores N, Cruz M, Pérez M, Vega V, Torres V. Internet and cell phone usage patterns among young adults with intellectual disabilities. J Appl Res Intellect Disabil. 2018;31:259–72. https://doi.org/10.1111/jar.12388.
108. Addlakha R, Price J, Heidari S. Disability and sexuality: claiming sexual and reproductive rights. Reprod Health Matters. 2017;25:4–9. https://doi.org/10.1080/09688080.2017.1336375.
109. Merrick J, Morad M, Carmeli E. Intellectual and developmental disabilities: male health. Front Public Health. 2014;2:208.
110. Saan H, Wise M. Enable, mediate, advocate. Health Promot Int. 2011;26(Suppl 2):ii187–93. https://doi.org/10.1093/heapro/dar069.

Barriers to Health Care Services and the Role of the Physician

19

Harriet Slater, Helen Baxter, and Mike Kerr

19.1 Introduction

People with intellectual disability experience poorer physical and mental health compared with the general population [1]. This is partly because people with intellectual disability are more likely to have additional health problems [2–5], however significant differences in health status are also directly attributable to deficits in their quality of health care received. These differences represent health inequalities which are primarily caused by barriers to accessing timely, appropriate, and effective medical care [1, 6–8].

There is growing worldwide evidence about the health inequalities that people with intellectual disability face. Numerous thought-provoking reports, such as the United Kingdom's charity Mencap's [9] report: 'Death by Indifference,' have also raised awareness of this issue to a wider audience. A 2013 confidential inquiry into premature deaths of people with intellectual disability (CIPOLD) in the United Kingdom, revealed not only a significantly decreased life expectancy for people with intellectual disability compared with the general population (some 20 years earlier for women and 13 years for men), but also a significantly higher proportion of deaths due to avoidable causes (38% vs 9%; [10]). In other words, people with intellectual disability were over four times more likely to die of causes related to

H. Slater
Mental Health and Learning Disabilities Delivery Unit, Abertawe Bro Morgannwg University Health Board, Cardiff, UK

H. Baxter
Centre for Academic Primary Care, Population Health Sciences, Bristol Medical School, University of Bristol, Bristol, UK

M. Kerr (✉)
Psychiatry at Cardiff University, Wales and an Honorary Professor at the School of Medicine, Swansea University, Swansea, Wales, UK
e-mail: KerrMP@cardiff.ac.uk

© Springer Nature Switzerland AG 2019
V. P. Prasher, M. P. Janicki (eds.), *Physical Health of Adults with Intellectual and Developmental Disabilities*, https://doi.org/10.1007/978-3-319-90083-4_19

poor quality healthcare. Furthermore, studies have found, when compared to the general population, (1) a high number of untreated common conditions amongst patients with intellectual disability [11–15] and (2) a low level of health promotion and preventative care [16–19]. The gap between need and outcome is further widened by the special conditions and additional health care needs that individuals with ID often have as a result of etiology.

A number of barriers have been identified that may be preventing people with intellectual disability from accessing health services appropriate to their needs. Patient-based issues include physical difficulties, behavior problems, and communication difficulties. Physician-based issues include a lack of specialist knowledge about health issues and the need for additional service time and resources to see patients with intellectual disability. People with intellectual disability should be able to expect that reasonable adjustments be made by their health providers to facilitate their access to care [20, 21].

Physicians have a pivotal role in overcoming these barriers and maintaining patient access to health care, through their knowledge of the patient's health, and their understanding of their country's health care system. This chapter addresses the barriers to the delivery of health care to individuals with intellectual disability through an analysis of five issues.

19.2   Accessibility, Mobility and Sensory Impairment

19.2.1 Accessibility

Globally, people with intellectual disability are usually poorer and more often dependent on social systems for underwriting their care [22, 23]. They are more unlikely to have a personal means of transport and will often need to be taken to health care visits. Lack of transport can present an impediment to physically accessing health services, particularly in areas where a high proportion of people with intellectual disability live in rural areas, where services are scarce [24, 25]. Thus, accessibility may encompass not only awkwardly sited health care resources, but difficulties encountered in attempts to get to them.

In certain developing countries, the urban drift of people into the towns and cities may reduce the ability of the extended family to care for an individual, thus removing a valuable source of support. This may not always be the case, as Piachaud [24] notes, there also is the phenomenon of extended families, resulting in a network of relations across the country. This may in turn have other advantages for individuals living in rural areas, who by utilizing this family network may be able to access services by staying with relations in towns with services. A family discussion with the physician on options and opportunities for obtaining services can ensure continuous access to care and a reduction in anxiety for family members.

In developed countries individuals may be able to use social systems of care for transport and assistance to attend appointments or treatment. This may require an increase in organizational support and redeployment of personnel. Chambers et al. [26], in a study on the care of adults with intellectual disability moving into the community, found that doctors believed that additional home visits for these patients were due to the unavailability of staff to assist individuals in attending the practitioner's office or surgery. Awareness that patients and their caregivers may need more planning time to arrange consultations and the option of different appointment times could make the process easier to manage. It may also be beneficial for staff teams and family members to have a discussion with the physician regarding possible arrangements when the individual is unable to attend alone.

19.2.2 Mobility

Maintenance of acquired skills through the use of assistive devices, such as sensory aids and wheelchairs, can enable adults to be more independent. However, for these devices to help an adult, health service buildings and accommodation also need to be physically accessible and barrier free. A study conducted in Boston in the USA found that 614 physicians reported that 12% of their offices were inaccessible to their patients with mobility problems [27]. Whilst improvements have been made in the physical accessibility of health services, due in part to increased awareness of disability and equality legislation, progress has not been universal and physical access to many services still falls short [28]. Early intervention or treatment of mobility impairment can reduce the risk of secondary illness and mortality for individuals with chronic constipation, incontinence, gastro-esophageal reflux, deterioration of pulmonary function, and coronary heart disease [29]. Evenhuis [29] has included physical activity, control of dietary calcium, adequate treatment and control of childhood mobility impairment, surgical treatment of hip fractures and active mobilization, as well as appropriate design and adequate walking devices in her recommendations for prevention of mobility impairment.

19.2.3 Sensory Impairment

People with intellectual disability are more likely to have sensory impairment, with prevalence rates of visual and hearing deficits increasing with increased age and severity of the disability [1]. Sensory impairment is also associated with specific syndromes. In addition, people with autism and more severe intellectual disability are more likely to have distorted sensory profiles, meaning that they could be overly sensitive in one sensory modality (e.g. to noise), but under-stimulated by another modality (e.g. touch). Sensory impairment may reduce the ability of the patient to attend appointments alone and increase patient distress during consultations and physical examinations, as communication and comprehension are reduced. Assistive devices, such as glasses and hearing aids, can help to reduce impairment and have been used successfully by people with intellectual disability once they are diagnosed [30, 31]. Early detection and treatment for sensory impairment has also been advocated to reduce further handicap and increase an individual's acceptance and use of sensory aids [30]. Consideration may also need to be made regarding the health care setting in which the person is seen as; for example, it may be preferable to book medical appointments for quieter times in order to minimize the effects of sensory overstimulation.

19.3   Behavioral Problems

The prevalence of behavioral problems that obstruct physicians in examining or treating a patient is difficult to judge. Behaviors are classified as problematic if they are of a sufficient intensity, frequency or duration so as to cause harm to the individual, others, or property, or if they significantly restrict an individual's ability to access community facilities (e.g., stereotypic behavior, sexually inappropriate behavior) [32]. Behaviors may be classed as 'challenging' if they impinge on the individual's activities (e.g., severe stereotypic behavior); however, these may not prove an obstacle for physical examination. Likewise, an usually compliant individual may be extremely distressed by a visit to a physician and express this inappropriately, thus, making an examination virtually impossible. Minihan and Dean [33] found 20% of adults with intellectual disability could only be examined or treated after supportive measures, such as pre-medication or pre-visits for desensitization.

Rates of challenging behavior in people with intellectual disability have been found to be around 22% in the United Kingdom [2]. Prevalence rates can be much higher however in certain syndromes which may have a specific behavioral phenotype. Whilst the etiology for the behavior may be multifactorial and include physical, psychiatric and environmental factors, particular risk factors for challenging behaviors include sensory impairment, sleep problems and mental health problems. Rates of psychiatric disorder have been found at 40.9% [2] in a population of adults with intellectual disability. Additionally, Moss et al. [34] discovered a particular association between patients exhibiting challenging behavior and the prevalence of depression, compared with the other mental health disorders. Although levels of challenging behavior in general have been found to reduce with increasing age [35], other studies have shown aggressive behavior, to be persistent throughout the lifespan [36, 37]. With the life expectancy of patients with intellectual disability increasing and the improved longevity for individuals with Down syndrome, dementia prevalence is likely to increase in this population, which may impact upon the future prevalence of challenging behaviors. Thus, challenging behavior could still prove to be a barrier to care as individuals age into their later years.

Behavioral problems may hinder diagnosis of conditions. This is emphasized by Aylward et al. [38] who discussed the problems of diagnosing dementia in individuals with a history of abnormal behaviors. The authors noted that such behaviors could mask the symptoms of dementia and for this reason recommended an evaluation of adults before the age of 25 years to obtain a baseline for behavior and functioning from which to measure change. Also, when in diagnosing epilepsy, challenging behavior may mimic some forms of seizures and hamper the process

[39]. Problems in interpreting a person's behavior, due to unusual response patterns [40], and distinguishing fear of a medical procedure and a patient's legal right to refuse treatment [27], have also been highlighted as causing difficulties for diagnosis and treatment. Only one in five primary care physicians reported that they felt well prepared to handle a patient refusing to cooperate with an examination or treatment [27]. The potential benefits of early evaluation in measuring some of the difficulties in diagnosis are highlighted by the findings of Lennox et al. [40] who found three quarters of physicians were unsure of their patient's baseline health and behavior.

Studies examining the views of physicians [27, 38, 40] indicate that barriers due to behavior arise from concerns with giving accurate diagnosis and issues around consent. The studies note that only 19% of physicians rated the maladaptive behaviors of patients in the office setting as a major obstacle to health care [27] and in the study by Lennox et al. [40] maladaptive behavior in the surgery was not mentioned at all. Kerr [41] suggested that an individual's difficult behavior may be more of a problem for parents or staff that may be embarrassed and therefore reduce visits to the doctor. Physicians can do much to alleviate the worries of the family or caregivers by reassurance, arranging visits at quiet times so that others are not disturbed, and also through treatment. Diagnosis of an underlying psychiatric illness that can be treated medically will obviously be of benefit; however, involving psychologists and specialists in behavioral problems may also help in reducing the incidence of difficult behavior.

19.4   Communication

Numerous studies have found high levels of unmet health needs across all health settings [16, 42], which is testament to the fact that identification of a health need is more difficult in the intellectual disability population. Communication is a major factor, both in terms of the individual's ability to communicate his or her symptoms to caregivers and clinicians and in the health providers role to communicate effectively with people regarding health promotion and appropriate health-seeking behaviors.

Research has shown that some people with intellectual disability may not always be able to recognize when they are unwell as they may have poor body awareness [43] and some may even have depressed pain responses [44]. Adults with a mild intellectual disability, are more apt to be able to indicate pain when using a body map and locate pain [45]. Whilst some adults may be able to inform the physician of their symptoms directly, others may need some basic aids and additional time to express themselves. Others with more severe intellectual disability may be unable to communicate verbally and thus be entirely reliant on caregivers to notice changes in their behavior. Evenhuis [29] found that people with intellectual disability tended to tolerate symptoms or express them atypically via irritability, inactivity, loss of appetite, and problems with sleep, particularly for conditions such as visual impairment, hearing loss, chest pain, dyspnea, dyspepsia, and micturition. Kinnell [46] has suggested that adults who cannot communicate well due to limited vocabulary and speech may have learned to suppress mention of bodily functions, or may not be given the opportunity to express themselves, especially if the family is under stress. It is difficult in this situation for the physician to obtain the relevant information, as the adult may well have not expressed his or her discomfort to others. It is therefore advisable for physicians to ensure that checks are done for medical conditions that have a high prevalence in adults with intellectual disability, even in the absence of obvious symptoms. It is also imperative that healthcare systems have a mechanism for identifying and flagging individuals who have intellectual disability so that targeted interventions can be undertaken.

People with intellectual disability are often reliant on their family or caregivers to communicate their health needs on their behalf. Even when a caregiver knows the person very well, it still may be difficult to detect a health problem when the individual's communication skills are limited. This is especially evident in cases where a change in the health need is gradual (e.g., sensory loss). The reliance on caregivers to communicate health needs has been cited as a major barrier to care. Beange et al. [16] studied a group of adults with intellectual disability and found that despite a mean of 5.4 medical problems per patient, 65% of patients and 24% of the caregivers reported no symptoms. In their study of adults with intellectual disability attending a day center, Wilson and Haire [15] noted that health problems had been overlooked in instances when caregivers believed the person to be in good health. In the same study, the authors found that caregivers failed to predict sensory impairment in 50% of patients who had difficulties in hearing or vision. This was happening even in adults who had been given hearing aids and who did not receive check-ups for any further problems. An additional problem with being reliant on a caregiver to advocate for a patient's health needs is the caregiver's individual views, beliefs, and culture regarding health and health-seeking behaviors. Studies have shown that caregivers can inadvertently become barriers to care because they may not perceive that a person with intellectual disability' health needs warrant an assessment. This could be due to a false assumption that the complaint is 'trivial' or that the patient would not benefit (e.g., recommending glasses for a someone who doesn't read) [15].

Time constraints can also impact on the quality of the history taking as there is an increased risk that, if adults with intellectual disability cannot speak for themselves or are slow at getting information across, physicians may be forced to ignore the patient in order to elicit information quickly from the caregiver [41, 47]. This is often a source of frustration to patients [21, 48]. With this method, there is an additional risk that the caregiver's reporting of the patient's symptoms can be biased towards the caregiver's own interpretation and views about diagnosis and treatment [49]. Research suggests that caregivers can be valuable advocates for the people they support and that they should be included more often in consultations; however, the research also notes that their views are often disregarded by clinicians [48]. Lennox et al. [40] found that perceived difficulties with history taking and communication were most prominent in primary care physicians' responses to an open-ended question on barriers to care. However, an Australian qualitative study of general practitioner's (GPs) views regarding the piloting of a health screening tool found that anticipated concerns about communication and cooperation with patients directly were not borne out, whereas matters concerning support worker engagement were an area of concern [50]. The problem with poor quality history taking can also be exacerbated for adults in residential services, if due to staff turnover, there is no one with adequate knowledge of the adult with whom to communicate [40, 51]. Numerous authors have highlighted the need for the patient to be accompanied by someone who knows them well. This may be difficult for the physician to influence unless there is an existing relationship with the staff group. Strategies in primary care, such as keeping accurate medical records [51], using validated objective screening tools, and seeking an alternative collaborative history if required, can reduce many of the difficulties for the physician in having to base a diagnosis on information that may be unreliable. Liaison with community intellectual disability services may also be helpful in cases where diagnosis is unclear.

In contrast to primary care, people with intellectual disability are more likely to access secondary health care compared to the general population [52]. Admission to hospital can be a hazardous time for patients where the transition of important health information can easily get lost without effective communication. Health passports or Hospital Traffic Light systems are strategies that are becoming more widely utilized in the UK to improve communication among adults with intellectual disability, their caregivers, and health professionals. These are written documents containing an overview of the person's important medical information, alongside information about their baseline functioning, communication, and support needs, and their likes and dislikes. They are designed to be a concise snapshot of individuals so that they can be better supported in unfamiliar, acute healthcare settings [52]. NHS Wales' [52] '1000 Lives' campaign resulted in specific care bundles for people with intellectual disability in secondary care; these can be a useful resource.

Healthcare providers also have a responsibility to ensure that they communicate effectively with people with intellectual disability in order to ensure that their service is inclusive and is promoting and supporting the person to make autonomous decisions about the care that they receive, as much as it is feasible. Allerton and Emerson [53] analyzed large scale data from the UK and found that 40% of people with intellectual disability report difficulties with using health services, compared with 18% of people without a chronic health condition or impairment. Organizational barriers which impair access could include rigid appointment systems and non-attendance policies, reliance on written forms of communication, a lack of awareness of the patient's needs regarding interpreter services, and poor signage, which people with low literacy and visual problems may find difficult to follow. Strategies to promote equity could include addressing the above points. A simplified example would be use of easy-read materials in order to improve access to health information.

People with intellectual disability receive fewer health promotion measures than their non-disabled counterparts. These include relatively simple procedures such as weight and blood pressure measurement and more complex processes such as mammography and cervical smears. In a large survey of half of the primary care practices in England, cervical screening in women with intellectual disability is approximately half that of the general population (30.2% vs 73.5%). Breast cancer screening uptake was marginally better with 50% of women with intellectual disability undergoing screening vs >66% of the general population [18]. Studies have suggested that uptake rates could be lower among adults with intellectual disability as not all of the eligible women were invited to attend; this could possibly be due to assumptions made by general practitioners and caregivers about the appropriateness of performing the tests. Additionally, the use of inappropriate communication methods to invite eligible women to attend has been observed as a cause for non-attendance [54, 55]. The introduction of annual health checks in general practice across the UK has been a major strategy in order to facilitate health promotion and has been found to be an effective way of identifying unmet health needs [11].

19.5   Knowledge, Attitudes and Accessing Specialist Services

The physician's role in caring for people with intellectual disability can vary according to the health care system of the country, and the specialism adopted. In many countries de-institutionalization has increased the primary care physician's role as the first contact with health services for people with intellectual disability. In the literature, GPs agree that the routine healthcare of people with intellectual disability is now primarily their responsibility [56–58]. This has raised some concern as to whether the providers of services in the community have the concentration of specialist knowledge previously found in institutions.

Aulagnier et al. [59] found that 21% of general practitioners reported discomfort in treating patients with intellectual disability. Negative attitudes were positively correlated with GPs who reported less experience managing people with disabilities, no medical training about disabilities, a lack of assistance during consultations, and inadequate consultation time. Both the lack of knowledge and confidence about treating people with intellectual disability have been identified in earlier studies [40, 60]. However, in one study, confidence in treating people with intellectual disability improved to 95% in GPs who had some previous specialist training [60]. People with intellectual disability can have specific health needs and so without the appropriate knowledge there is a risk of inadequate care and even diagnostic overshadowing, where an individual's symptoms are attributed to being entirely behavioral or inherent to their intellectual disability rather than due to a co-existing physical or mental health problem. Dissemination of knowledge, particularly through practical resources such as handbooks, resource guides [40], lists of specialist physicians, referral guides, and policy documents regarding informed consent [27] have all been highlighted as useful by primary care physicians. Innovations such as online educational resources and toolkits for GPs have been made widely available in the UK [61]. Specialist education on managing people with intellectual disability should not be restricted to primary care physicians. There is also a need for research and knowledge to broaden into other areas of medicine and allied health care professions [62].

Research has demonstrated that some healthcare providers exhibit negative attitudes and discriminatory behaviors towards people with intellectual disability. This can be an intentional or inadvertent cause of sub-optimal care or even care denial. Cases of clinicians' questioning a person with intellectual disability' suitability to receive surgery, based on discriminatory beliefs about the person's quality of life, has been reported in more than one study [63, 64]. This demonstrates the importance of education about the lives of people with intellectual disability so as to increase understanding and effect attitudinal change. It is vital that people with intellectual disability are encouraged and supported to make treatment decisions for themselves, as long as they have been provided with understandable information and have the mental capacity to make this decision. In cases where mental capacity is lacking, decisions made in the patient's best interests should require consultation with the multidisciplinary team, caregivers, family members, and even advocacy services. A lack of knowledge about informed consent procedures for people with intellectual disability has previously been an area of concern [27, 65], and is of particular importance for health professionals in areas such as dentistry and gynecology. In the United Kingdom, legislation such as the Mental Capacity Act [66] has sought to provide clarity regarding how to assess a person's mental capacity to make decisions for themselves and how to proceed if a person is unable to make such decisions.

In order for health care providers to feel supported to treat people with intellectual disability, there needs to be effective liaison and inter-agency working arrangements between primary and secondary care services, a clear demarcation of clinician's roles and responsibilities, and clear referral pathways. Beange et al. [16] found that 74% of 202 individuals with intellectual disability had conditions for which specialist care was needed. This specialist care had not always been received, and half of the identified conditions were found to be inadequately managed. The same Australian study identified that GPs felt that they lacked backup resources to work with patients with disabilities and felt restricted by a secondary health service that is not designed to meet the needs of this group [67]. In the intervening 20 years, service reform has been slow with many studies concluding that secondary care services are still failing to make reasonable adjustments in order to serve the needs of the intellectual disability population [20, 48, 62]. This is particularly evident regarding access to secondary mental health care [68, 69]. Qualitative studies provide insight into the struggles that patients and caregivers have faced regarding access to healthcare services, which include difficulties with finding out which services are available locally and how these services are structured, confusion about referral pathways and a lack of clarity regarding service eligibility and clinicians' responsibilities [48]. Organizational barriers to inter-professional working, such as data protection laws, ineffective liaison between healthcare professionals and the absence of clear lines of responsibility and accountability, have also been found to be a barrier to adults with intellectual disability receiving adequate healthcare within the inpatient care system [62]. Specialty intellectual disability liaison nurses have been introduced into some acute hospitals in the UK in order to bridge some of these barriers to care, however their effectiveness is reliant, in part, on the backing of hospital managers in order to give them sufficient powers to change the hospital's culture and practice.

19.6   Time and Resources

It has long been recognized that financial considerations can be a significant barrier to accessing health care for adults with intellectual disability [33, 70]. In insurance based healthcare systems, such as the United States, people with intellectual disability have often expressed experiences of being discriminated against and refused care due to their health insurance status, which in many cases is funded via the state. Minihan et al. [27] suggested that accessibility to services seemed, in part, to be a function of the willingness of some physicians to provide uncompensated or under compensated care. Lennox et al. [40] noted that Australian GPs stated that they would be willing to see more patients with intellectual disability if this brought greater remuneration. As patients with intellectual disability are often dependent on the social system of care for their finances [22] or, in less developed countries, reliant on other family members [24], this is likely to continue to be a significant barrier to care unless governments intervene.

Whilst it is recognized that people with intellectual disability underutilize primary care services, studies have shown a greater level of unmet needs and significantly higher outpatient attendances and contact with specialist services than age and sex matched controls [17]. Chambers et al. [26] investigated consultation rates for 136 adults with intellectual disability being discharged from a long stay hospital and found that the workload involved exceeded by 3.9 times that for age and non-disabled controls matched by age and sex. Walsh et al. [71] demonstrated that people with intellectual disability had a higher number of hospital admissions and a greater average length of stay than the general population. However, the mean length of hospital stays reduced to levels comparable with that for the general population when care was coordinated [72]. This study found that care coordination (e.g., organizing referrals, maintaining and communicating medical record information, and assisting and supporting patients to access health care services appropriately) was associated not just with reductions in length of hospital stay, but also with readmission rates and hospital charges.

Adults with intellectual disability, due to mobility, and sensory and communication difficulties, may well need longer or even additional consultations to address certain medical problems. Although this may increase workload initially, early diagnosis and treatment of conditions could reduce the need for more complicated medical procedures later on, as well as giving obvious benefits for the adult. The benefits of early detection and treatment in a population that has been shown to have a high rate of unmet health needs has been one of the strong arguments for the use of health checks with adults with intellectual disability [14, 41, 73, 74]. Evenhuis [29] noted that, although adults with disabilities may fail to report symptoms, conditions can be diagnosed as accurately as for adults in the general population as long as health professionals use routine diagnostic screenings employing their knowledge of risk factors and atypical presentations, and take account of caregiver observations. Studies of GP attitudes regarding the use of annual health checks has been met with mixed reviews, with most recognizing their value in reducing health inequalities; however, there were concerns about the financial implications, both in terms of the additional time and staffing that these additional checks would incur [56, 75, 76]. In 2008, the UK introduced primary care led annual health checks for people with intellectual disability with the government providing financial remuneration. Despite this financial incentive, GP compliance with this initiative is not universal and many patients do not receive the annual health check due to a multitude of organizational and patient factors [77].

19.7 Conclusion

The barriers to accessing health care services facing people with intellectual disability can be reduced through support and awareness from health professionals and through changes to address health inequalities at a national governmental level. Where there are problems with mobility, assistive devices can be used to foster and maintain independence and both buildings housing health care services and providing residential accommodations can be made more accessible. Developing flexible approaches to provide health care to patients with additional sensory needs should become standard practice. With a high prevalence of psychiatric disorders among adults with intellectual disability there may be additional behavioral issues that need to be addressed due to underlying mental illness. As problem behaviours can mask some morbidities (e.g., dementia and epilepsy) and hinder diagnosis, this could be of particular concern for physicians. Early behaviour evaluation at a younger age may benefit health professionals by providing a historical baseline level of behaviour from which to judge any future changes. Although physicians have expressed concerns that behaviour can be difficult to interpret, especially in considering the adult's right to refuse to consent to treatment, disruptive or embarrassing behaviors in medical offices seems to be of more concern to caregivers than to physicians.

Research has highlighted the reliance of many people with intellectual disability on caregivers to communicate their health needs. This can both facilitate and hinder a patient's access to and assessment in the health setting and so clinicians should have a low threshold for taking concerns seriously. Patients with mild intellectual disability who have some communication assets can tolerate rather that report symptoms [29]. For individuals living in staffed homes this could be of particular concern as residents are often accompanied by different members of staff who may or may not be familiar with the medical history or complaints of the person brought for examination or service. There may be an increased need therefore, for particular attention to be paid in obtaining the past medical notes for individuals with intellectual disability and for ensuring access to these notes for any specialists involved with their care. Clinicians should also aim to promote inclusive practice by communicating with patients directly during consultations, as appropriate, and ensuring that information about health promotion and ongoing management is communicated in an equitable way.

Primary care physicians have expressed a concern over their lack of knowledge of the illnesses and conditions found to be more prevalent among adults with intellectual disability. This lack of confidence was reduced when physicians received some specialist training. In some countries GP curriculums are addressing gaps in specialist knowledge with additional online education and resources. In addition, physicians in the United Kingdom have requested that knowledge about intellectual disability become available to professionals in other health disciplines. In light of the lack of knowledge shown by physicians in many countries about specialist care available for adults with intellectual disability, broader dissemination of research about intellectual disability may be of benefit. Particularly, this would include information about the correct procedures for consent to treatment for patients with intellectual disability, which has clear importance for physicians across various medical disciplines. Over the coming years, physicians are likely to need adequate support from intellectual disability specialists until the modern-day healthcare workforce is sufficiently equipped to meet the needs of the intellectual disabled population within mainstream services.

Finally, the issues of finance and resources are obvious problems in treating people with intellectual disability. This group generally has a higher need for the use of medical resources than the general population due to additional health issues. Care coordination is one method, which has been found to make more efficient use of resources and therefore wherever possible should be maximised. In addition, successful diagnosis of conditions and early intervention could allow treatment at a younger age, which can be preventative to secondary illness and thus reduce use of resources. Similarly, the use of preventative medicine such as health checks and routine diagnostic screening is likely to benefit persons of all ages with intellectual disability.

The physician stands as the cornerstone of health care delivery, yet is dependent on others to ensure that individuals with intellectual disability can achieve health gain. The barriers will only be removed by individuals, caregivers, and professional's working together. In this context apparent "deficits" in care can be formulated as problems with health systems recognising need, rather that professional or other failure.

References

1. Emerson E, Baines S, Allerton L, Welch V. Health inequalities and people with learning disabilities in the UK: 2012. Durham: Improving Health & Lives: Learning Disabilities Observatory; 2012.
2. Cooper S-A, Smiley E, Morrison J, Williamson A, Allan L. Mental ill-health in adults with intellectual disabilities: prevalence and associated factors. Br J Psychiatry. 2007;190:27–35.
3. Haveman M, Heller T, Lee L, Maaskant M, Shooshtari S, Strydom A. Major health risks in aging persons with intellectual disabilities: an overview of recent studies. J Policy Pract Intellect Disabil. 2010;7:59–69.
4. McCarron M, Swinburne J, Burke E, McGlinchey E, Mulryan N, Andrews V, Foran S, McCallion P. Growing older with an intellectual disabilities in Ireland in 2011: first results

from the intellectual disability supplement of The Irish Longitudinal Study on Ageing. Dublin: School of Nursing and Midwifery, Trinity College Dublin; 2011.

5. Moseley D, Tonge B, Bereton A, Einfeld A. Psychiatric comorbidity in adolescents and young adults with autism. J Ment Health Res Intellect Disabil. 2011;4:229–43.

6. Emerson E, Baines S. Health inequalities and people with learning disabilities in the UK: 2010. Durham: Improving Health & Lives: Learning Disabilities Observatory; 2010.

7. Holly D, Sharp J. Addressing health inequities: coronary heart disease training within learning disabilities services. Br J Learn Disabil. 2014;42:110–6.

8. Townsend C. Developing a comprehensive research agenda for people with intellectual disabilities to inform policy development and reform. J Policy Pract Intellect Disabil. 2011;8:113–24.

9. MENCAP. Death by indifference. London: MENCAP; 2007.

10. Heslop P, Blair P, Fleming P, Hoghton M, Marriott A, Russ L. Confidential inquiry into premature deaths of people with learning disabilities (CIPOLD): final report. Bristol: Norah Fry Research Centre; 2013.

11. Baxter H, Lowe K, Houston H, Jones G, Felce D, Kerr M. Previously unidentified morbidity in patients with intellectual disability. Br J Gen Pract. 2006;56:93–8.

12. Beange H, Bauman A. Caring for the developmentally disabled in the community. Aust Fam Physician. 1990;19:1558–63.

13. Howells G. Are the medical needs of mentally handicapped adults being met. J R Coll Gen Pract. 1986;36:449–53.

14. Webb O, Rogers L. Health Screening for people with intellectual disability: The New Zealand experience. J Intellect Disabil Res. 1999;43:497–503.

15. Wilson DN, Haire A. Health care screening for people with mental handicap living in the community. Br Med J. 1990;301:1379–81.

16. Beange H, McElduff A, Baker W. Medical disorders of adults with mental retardation: a population study. Am J Ment Retard. 1995;99:595–604.

17. Kerr MP, Richards D, Glover G. Primary care for people with a learning disability – a Group Practice survey. J Appl Res Intellect Disabil. 1996;9:347–52.

18. NHS Digital. Health and care of people with learning disabilities: experimental statistics, 2014–15 report; 2016. Available at: www.digital.nhs.uk/pubs/LD1415. Accessed 26 Jan 2018.

19. Whitfield M, Langan J, Russell O. Assessing general practitioners' care of adult patients with learning disability: case-control study. Qual Health Care. 1996;5:31–5.

20. Michael J. Healthcare for all. Report of the independent inquiry into access to healthcare for people with learning disabilities. London: Department of Health; 2008.

21. Ward RL, Nichols AD, Freedman RI. Uncovering health care inequalities among adults with intellectual and developmental disabilities. Health Soc Work. 2010;35:280–90.

22. Beange H. Caring for a vulnerable population. Med J Aust. 1996;164:159–60.

23. Department for Work and Pensions. Fulfilling potential – outcomes and indicators framework: second annual progress report. London: Stationary Office; 2015.

24. Piachaud J. Strengths and difficulties in developing countries: the case of Zimbabwe. In: Bouras N, editor. Mental health in mental retardation: recent advances and practices. Cambridge: Cambridge University Press; 1994. p. 383–92.

25. Sonnander K, Claesson M. Classification, prevalence, prevention and rehabilitation of intellectual disabilities: an overview of research in the People's Republic of China. J Intellect Disabil Res. 1997;41:180–92.

26. Chambers R, Milsom G, Evans N, Lucking A, Campbell I. The primary care workload and prescribing costs associated with patients with learning disabilitiy discharged from long-stay care to the community. Br J Learn Disabil. 1998;26:9–12.

27. Minihan PM, Dean DH, Lyons CM. Managing the care of patients with mental retardation: a survey of physicians. Ment Retard. 1993;31:239–46.

28. Healthwatch England. Primary care: a review of local health watch reports; 2015. Available at: https://www.healthwatch.co.uk/resource/primary-care-review-local-healthwatch-reports. Accessed 26 Jan 2018.

29. Evenhuis H. Medical aspects of ageing in a population with intellectual disability: mobility, internal conditions and cancer. J Intellect Disabil Res. 1997;41:8–18.

30. Evenhuis H. Medical aspects of ageing in a population with intellectual disability: I. Visual impairment. J Intellect Disabil Res. 1995;39:19–25.
31. Evenhuis H. Medical aspects of ageing in a population with intellectual disability: II. Hearing impairment. J Intellect Disabil Res. 1995;39:27–33.
32. Emerson E. Challenging behaviour: analysis and intervention in people with severe intellectual disabilities. Cambridge: Cambridge University Press; 1995.
33. Minihan PM, Dean DH. Meeting the needs for health services of persons with mental retardation living in the community. Am J Public Health. 1990;80:1043–8.
34. Moss S, Emerson E, Kiernan C, Turner S, Hatton C, Alborz A. Psychiatric symptoms in adults with learning disability and challenging behaviour. Br J Psychiatry. 2000;177:452–6.
35. Moss SC. Age and functional abilities of people with a mental handicap: evidence for the Wessex Mental Handicap Register. J Ment Defic Res. 1991;35:430–45.
36. Davidson PW, Houser KD, Cain NN, Sloane-Reeves J, Quijano L, Matons L, Giesow V, Ladringan PM. Characteristics of older adults with intellectual disabilities referred for crisis intervention. J Intellect Disabil Res. 1999;43:38–46.
37. Day KA. The elderly mentally handicapped in hospital: a clinical study. J Ment Defic Res. 1987;31:131–46.
38. Aylward EH, Burt DB, Thorpe LU, Lai F, Dalton A. Diagnosis of dementia in individuals with intellectual disabilities. J Intellect Disabil Res. 1997;41:152–64.
39. Paul A. Epilepsy or stereotypy? Diagnostic issues in learning disabilities. Seizure. 1997;6:111–20.
40. Lennox NG, Diggens JN, Ugoni AM. The general practice care of people with intellectual disability: barriers and solutions. J Intellect Disabil Res. 1997;41:380–90.
41. Kerr MP. Primary health care and health gain for people with a learning disability. Tizard Learn Disabil Rev. 1998;3:6–14.
42. Kerr AM, McCulloch D, Oliver K, McLean B, Coleman E, Law T. Medical needs of people with intellectual disability require regular reassessment, and the provision of client- and carer-held reports. J Intellect Disabil Res. 2003;47:134–45.
43. March P. How do people with a mild/moderate mental handicap conceptualise physical illness and its cause? Brit J Ment Subnorm. 1991;37:80–91.
44. Gilbert-McLeod CA, Craig KD, Rocha EM, Mathias MD. Everyday pain responses in children with and without developmental delays. J Pediatr Psychol. 2000;25:301–8.
45. Bromley J, Emerson E, Caine A. The development of a self-report measure to assess the location and intensity of pain in people with intellectual disabilities. J Intellect Disabil Res. 1998;42:72–80.
46. Kinnell HG. Community medical care of people with mental handicaps: room for improvement. Ment Handicap Res. 1987;15:146–50.
47. Duckworth MS, Radhakrishnan G, Nolan ME, Fraser WI. Initial encounters between people with a mild handicap and psychiatrists: an investigation of a method of evaluating interview skills. J Intellect Disabil Res. 1993;37:263–76.
48. Ali A, Scior K, Ratti V, Strydom A, King M, Hassiotis A. Discrimination and other barriers to accessing health care: perspectives of patients with mild and moderate intellectual disability and their carers. PLoS One. 2013;8:e70855.
49. Alborz A, McNally R, Swallow A, Glendinning C. From the cradle to the grave: a literature review of access to health care for people with learning disabilities across the lifespan. London: National Co-ordinating Centre for NHS Service Delivery and Organisation; 2003.
50. Lennox NG, Brolan CE, Dean J, Ware RS, Boyle FM, Taylor Gomez M, van Dooren K, Bain C. General practitioners' views on perceived and actual gains, benefits and barriers associated with the implementation of an Australian health assessment for people with intellectual disability. J Intellect Disabil Res. 2013;57:913–22.
51. Crocker AC, Yankauer A. Basic issues. Ment Retard. 1987;25:227–32.
52. NHS Wales. How to guide 1000 Lives Plus. Improving general hospital care of patients who have a learning disabilities. Wales: NHS Wales; 2014.

53. Allerton L, Emerson E. British adults with chronic health conditions or impairments face significant barriers to accessing health services. Public Health. 2012;126:920–7.
54. Davies N, Duff M. Breast cancer screening for older women with intellectual disability living in community group homes. J Intellect Disabil Res. 2001;45:253–7.
55. Nightingale C. Barriers to health access: a study of cervical screening for women with learning disabilities. Clin Psychol Forum. 2000;137:26–30.
56. Bond L, Kerr M, Dunstan F, Thapar A. Attitudes of general practitioners towards health care for people with intellectual disability and the factors underlying these attitudes. J Intellect Disabil Res. 1997;41:391–400.
57. Dovey S, Webb OJ. General practitioners' perception of their role in care for people with intellectual disability. J Intellect Disabil Res. 2000;44:553–61.
58. Lennox NG, Diggens J, Ugoni A. Health care for people with an intellectual disability: general practitioners' attitudes, and provision of care. J Intellect Develop Disabil. 2000;25:127–33.
59. Aulagnier M, Verger P, Ravaud JF, Souville M, Lussault PY, Garnier JP, Paraponaris A. General practitioners' attitudes towards patients with disabilities: the need for training and support. Disabil Rehabil. 2005;27:1343–52.
60. Stanley R. Primary health care provision for people with learning disabilities: a survey of general practitioners. J Learn Disabil Nurs Soc Care. 1993;2:23–30.
61. Royal College of General Practitioners. Learning disabilities; 2018. http://www.rcgp.org.uk/learningdisabilities/. Viewed 26 Jan 2018.
62. Tuffrey-Wijne I, Giatras N, Goulding L, Abraham E, Fenwick L. Identifying the factors affecting the implementation of strategies to promote a safer environment for patients with learning disabilities in NHS hospitals: a mixed-methods study. Health Services and Delivery Research, No. 1.13. 2013.
63. Gibbs SM, Brown MJ, Muir WJ. The experiences of adults with intellectual disabilities and their carers in general hospitals: a focus group study. J Intellect Disabil Res. 2008;52:1061–77.
64. Webber R, Bowers B, Bigby C. Hospital experiences of older people with intellectual disability: responses of group home staff and family members. J Intellect Dev Disabil. 2010;35:155–64.
65. Turner NJ, Brown AR, Baxter KF. Consent to treatment and the mentally incapacitated adult. J R Soc Med. 1999;92:290–2.
66. Mental Capacity Act. London: The Stationery Office; 2005, c.9.
67. Alborz A, McNally R, Glendinning C. Access to healthcare for people with learning disabilities: mapping the issues and reviewing the evidence. J Health Serv Res Policy. 2005;10:173–82.
68. Moss S, Patel P. The prevalence of mental illness in people with intellectual disability over 50 years of age, and the diagnostic-importance of information from carers. Ir J Psychol. 1993;4:110–29.
69. Roy A, Martin DM, Wells MB. Health gain through screening – mental health: developing primary health care services for people with an intellectual disability. J Intellect Develop Disabil. 1997;22:227–39.
70. Flaskerud JH, Lesser J, Dixon E, Anderson N, Conde F, Kim S. Health disparities among vulnerable populations: evolution of knowledge over five decades in Nursing Research publications. Nurs Res. 2002;51:74–85.
71. Walsh KK, Kastner T, Criscione T. Characteristics of hospitalizations for people with developmental disabilities: utilization, costs and impact of care coordination. Am J Ment Retard. 1997;101:505–20.
72. Criscione T, Kastner TA, Walsh KK, Nathanson R. Managed health care services for people with mental retardation: impact on impatient utilization. Ment Retard. 1993;31:297–306.
73. Jones RG, Kerr MP. A randomised control trial of an opportunistic health screening tool in primary care for people with intellectual disability. J Intellect Disabil Res. 1997;41:409–15.
74. Martin DM, Roy A. A comparative review of primary health care models for people with learning disabilities: towards the provision of seamless health care. Br J Learn Disabil. 1999;27:58–63.

75. Bakker-van Gijssel EJ, Lucassen PLBJ, Olde Hartman TC, van Son L, Assendelft WJJ, van Schrojenstein Lantman-de Valk HMJ. Health assessment instruments for people with intellectual disabilities—a systematic review. Res Dev Disabil. 2017;64:12–24.
76. Stein K. Caring for people with learning disability: a survey of general practitioners' attitudes in Southampton and South-West Hampshire. Br J Learn Disabil. 2000;28:9–15.
77. Glover G, Niggebrugge A. The uptake of health checks for adults with learning disabilities 2008/9 to 2012/13. London: Public Health England; 2013.

Future Prospects: A Challenge to Promote Wellness

20

Vee P. Prasher, Matthew P. Janicki, and Seth M. Keller

20.1 Introduction

We began the overview of this text with a discussion of health disparities with the intent to use the expert knowledge of our authors to help build understanding and capacity to address the disparities. In our text, *Physical Health in Adults with Intellectual and Developmental Disabilities,* we have highlighted several clinical and practical areas of physical health affecting adults with intellectual disability, with a focus on their maturation, aging, and lifestyle practices associated with well-ness. The authors discussed a number of particular conditions which significantly affect many adults with intellectual disability; however, phenotypic physical problems (for example, septal heart defects in individuals with Down syndrome) were excluded and readers are referred to more specific books on such issues. Further, psychiatric and psychological concerns and extensive pondering of sex-based health issues were also excluded, as these have been discussed by other authors [1–6].

Much of our knowledge regarding physical health issues in adults with intellectual disability is based primarily on generalizations from clinical and research findings on the general population and secondarily from the limited research base on adults and children with intellectual and developmental disabilities. Some years ago, the then Surgeon General of the United States, spoke to the problem of accessibility at a major convening on health disparities and noted that "too many doctors and dentists either refuse to treat people with [intellectual and] developmental

V. P. Prasher (✉)
Neuro-Developmental Psychiatry, Birmingham, UK

M. P. Janicki
Department of Disability and Human Development, University of Illinois at Chicago, Chicago, IL, USA

S. M. Keller
Advocare Neurology of South Jersey, Lumberton, NJ, USA

© Springer Nature Switzerland AG 2019
V. P. Prasher, M. P. Janicki (eds.), *Physical Health of Adults with Intellectual and Developmental Disabilities*, https://doi.org/10.1007/978-3-319-90083-4_20

disabilities or they give them inferior care." He also noted that more studies were needed to document the extent and causes of the health problems that adults with intellectual disability face, as testimony from doctors, people with intellectual disability, and their families has shown that attending to such problems is a major weakness in many health systems. From his perspective, little had been done at the time to synthesize the extant literature on health and adults and even little more had been done to apply what is known to medical education.

It was noted that disparities in health knowledge and health care can stem from a number of sources, among them the vagaries of national health delivery systems, lack of sufficient research and information about the confluence of age, health and lifelong disability, the inadequate knowledge base of health practitioners, and the behavior of people with intellectual disability when in contact with the health system. Although the U.S. Surgeon General's remarks were prepared for an American audience, they apply to any place in the world. To what extend have remedies become universal is unknown, but given the expanded participation of people with intellectual disability within the fabric of local communities, it helps to better understand to what degree each of these factors contributes to the deficiencies that Dr. Satcher described and from this knowledge continue to develop strategies that will lead to a better understanding of the interaction of aging and health and to the mitigation of problems associated with access to and financing of health care.

20.2   A Framework for Understanding Research on Physical Health

With greater awareness and understanding of the variables that affect maturation and aging, we would expect that there would be a continued impetus to promote interest in the health of adults with intellectual disability, and there would be more specific and accurate information made available regarding the diagnosis, assessment, management and prevention of physical disease and secondary conditions in this population. While current clinical and research knowledge has improved since Dr. Satcher's pleading on health disparities, there remains a scarcity of in-depth information on implementation of social health policies, routine screening, health prevention and user involvement. It is our hope that behavioral and the non-medical management of health conditions may in the future prove to be of equal relevance to people with intellectual disability to that, of the general population. In many countries large-scale de-institutionalization programs have now been completed or are well under way and alternative care systems and programs have been put into place. Older generations have benefited from living in more freedom and with more choice, but at times may have lost access to routine and scrutinized medical care. Younger generations have now more freedom and choice and no experience with routinized care but may lack access to systematic health services and less health status surveillance. This can be a double-edged sword as one group lost routine access to health care and the other may never had developed an expectation for such care.

Research and clinical experience would suggest that the transfer of focus from institutional-based services to community-based services needs to be placed in context with regard to our understanding of the nature of the health of people with intellectual disability. This should be done for two reasons: the first being the response (and adherence) to published studies which examined and reported on the health status of persons who have been institutionalized and then deinstitutionalized, and the second, the shift of referent group from institutionalized adults to those who lives have always been spent in their community. Research has shown that proximity to systematic services, whether in congregate care or in-community and linked for formal services, increases the rate of physical visits and thus improves health status. Conversely, living distally in non-formalized settings (such as with family or on one own) tends to be associated with infrequent contact with health services and potentially lower health status (if select health conditions occur and are not caught early).

This first factor (reliance on institution-based research) has relevance to us as studies based on institutional populations have always been somewhat suspect as to their natural application to adults with intellectual disability who have never experienced institutionalization. One suspects that these institutional populations may have been subject to a cohort effect given that families and local authorities generally institutionalized those children or adults for whom they could not sufficiently care (and who were perceived as sufficiently deviant) either due to behavioral management issues, their physical condition, or simply a lack of alternative community supports extended to families in general. In the past, an extensive body of clinical knowledge was built on institutional populations, most likely since they were captive and easily served as a convenience sample. Thus, to what extent do these reports explain the optimal or true nature of health conditions among all persons with intellectual disability is questionable. Yet, not to minimize their import, since institutional cohorts historically represented a broad spectrum of functional abilities, these studies did have value and provided us with a great deal of information. However, the question is to what extent would have enriched and quality experiences in the community changed patterns of health problems and decline that were observed in these institutionalized adults and more truly been reflective of the optimal health status of adults with intellectual disability?

Thus, this brings us to the second factor. Clearly, in those nations with aggressive communitization policies coupled with well-thought out social care policies and well-financed community supports, there has been a sea change in the debate around health status and health services provision. One aspect of this is the debate regarding whether people with intellectual disability should access generic services for physical health issues, or whether a speciality service focussing on all health issues for people with intellectual disability should be developed. Another is to what extend can and do adults with intellectual disability access and receive needed health services as they become more like any other member of their community. Studies have shown that the more distance between formalized care and the adults, the less frequent are physician visits, routine medical care provision, and specialized surveillance for health conditions. Disability provider organizations generally do a very good job of looking after the health care needs of adults on their case rolls, particularly if the adults are residents of formal group living programs (such as group homes). When left on their own, as Edgerton [7] and others have reported, they tend not to see physicians or easily access formal health services. However, notwithstanding all of the difficulties reported regarding health care provision in community settings, it is now clear that community-dwelling adults with intellectual disability are the contemporary referent group of choice (with the exception of special subgroups, such as adults being treated for certain conditions, and so on). Certainly, it is our expectation that with appropriate planning and adequate financial support, adults with intellectual disability should be able to live comfortably in their communities and have the appropriate advocacy to allow them to live their lives to the best of their abilities. The expectation is also that health authorities will incorporate providing health services to persons with special needs within the generic health care system or recognize that specialist services may be needed to see select sub-populations. The work in some countries were specialty health practitioners (e.g., physicians and nurses) are brought in for specialty training and professional and licensing designation is an example of blending of these two. To what extent this approach has lessened disparities is left in question.

In the past when many adults with intellectual disability were living in public institutions where they were often receiving health services that were provided in-house by staff and clinicians who worked together and had experience with this population. In the United States, the American with Disabilities Act [8] and Olmstead decision [9], in association with changing cultural and social tenets, led to the closure and downsizing of most public institutions and led the way to having individuals live in the community. These monumental civil rights outcomes unfortunately did not equally prepare for providing similar and adequate access to healthcare in the community. Studies of the 'deinstitutionalization' process and its outcomes showed that while previous residents of these settings had more freedom and choice, they also experienced a lack of access to formal medical services [10]. This led to a further appreciation that there remained significant medical and oral health disparities in adults with intellectual disability.

The issue of health disparities which was highlighted by the Surgeon General's meeting did lead to a number of proactive efforts following the conference. There was the creation in the United States of the American Academy of Developmental Medicine and Dentistry (AADMD) as a direct response to the realization that there was not a specific professional healthcare organization that focussed on adult health needs. There was also the realization that healthcare professions students needed to be provided education and training in the areas relevant to the unique and pertinent needs seen in adults with intellectual disability; which would require the creation of curriculum, guidelines, and credentialing as well as a more focused transitioning of care model. The challenges of enabling healthcare practitioners to be able to care for this population is hampered by inadequate reimbursement policies. The presence of health disparities has been made clear and this has led to advocacy to have adults with intellectual disability formally designated as being a Medically Underserved Population (MUP) under the guidelines set forth by the US Health Resources Services Administration [11].

20.3   Medically Underserved Population

The US federal government defines "medically underserved populations" (MUP) according to a formula crafted in 1975 that weighs a population's lack of primary care providers, its experience with poverty and increased infant mortality, and its percentage of people age 65 and older. As a population, people with intellectual disability meet most of these criteria. Two Surgeons General reports [12, 13] and a report of the National Council on Disabilities [14] document that people with intellectual disability experience significant health disparities, poorer health, and lack access to care. To date there has been a number of federal, state and local efforts to get this designation applied, yet there has not been success at the federal level because of the narrow definition of what the MUP was intended to cover [15]. The original intent was to cover groups based on distance and geographical location from providers and not primarily based on direct assess to quality and knowledgeable providers of healthcare.

Another direction in tackling MUP is currently being undertaken at the state level. Working directly with a number of state governors and their associated state developmental disability authority leadership groups is being promoted. The MUP designation allows a variety of federal agencies and state health departments to qualify for J-1 visa waivers for physicians who are currently working outside of the USA. Under some programs, MUP designation provides for increased reimbursement for funding, and funding preference. Other federal agencies, including the National Institutes of Health (NIH) have concerned themselves with MUPs and have incorporated the designation into their work. NIH has also funded research and asked researchers to study and investigate medically under-served populations. NIH also provides a Health Disparities Research Loan Repayment Program (LRP) to "recruit and retain highly qualified health professionals to research careers that focus on minority health or other health disparity issues" [16]. These targeted grants and LRPs support and encourage grantees to develop professional careers in health disparities research with medically underserved populations. Individual states use the MUP designation in their own laws to provide additional benefits. For example, in the US state of Kansas, the Primary Care Safety Net Clinic Capital Loan Guarantee Act incorporates the MUP language directly from Section 330 of the PHSA as the criteria to qualify for loans for capital improvements to safety net clinics. States also use HRSA's MUP designation in RFAs as criteria to warrant preference for the state's own funding for those who will serve MUPs. Even private foundations and non-governmental organizations (NGOs) such as Susan G. Komen for the Cure [17] provide funding and preferences to fund "medically underserved populations".

National healthcare organizations which support their providers all have a vested interest and an appreciation of the current and long-standing health disparities which have existed within the population of adults with intellectual disability [18]. Direct attention and discussion with leaders of this group has led to a number of MUP designations and statements, for example, from the American Medical

Association [19] and the American Dental Association [20] to a range of other organizations [21].

20.4   Transitioning of Care

The healthcare of children with intellectual disability is often delivered by healthcare providers who have been trained and educated through well-established university and academic programs. These centers of training have based their programs on years of research and on well-established curricula, as well as expertise in the field. Pediatric care is often turned over to an adult oriented healthcare provider when an individual turns 18 to 21 years old [22]. There have been a number of well-established transition of care guidelines produced and disseminated to help with this process, including Got Transition [23], Transition of Care by the Child Neurology Foundation [24], and the Children's Hospital of Philadelphia Transitioning to Adult Care: Supporting Youth with Special Healthcare Needs [25]. It has been well established that transitioning of healthcare from pediatrics into adult care has been and remains a challenge in particular with those young adults with intellectual disability who have complex personal, social, and health needs [26, 27]. Transitioning into older adult age and geriatric care remains an area that has not yet received a lot of attention and focus [28]. The current transitioning efforts are pediatric centric and general and have not focused specifically on the intellectually disabled population as well as on the inadequacies in adult healthcare. Some of this focus is in areas of neurology and the transitioning from pediatric to adult neurology. Current work in this particular area is being done through the Child Neurology Foundation, the American Academy of Neurology, and the American Academy of Developmental Medicine and Dentistry [29].

20.5   A Framework for Health Promotion and Wellness

Given the above, we were pleased to see that contemporary studies are tackling diverse epidemiological issues and framing the status of epidemiological knowledge about the health status of adults with intellectual disability. To begin any effort at health promotion one must have a solid grounding in the epidemiology of conditions and knowledge of the factors that influence disease occurrence. When individuals have a lifelong condition and may be at significant risk of occurring secondary conditions, then epidemiological knowledge is even that more important for it lays the groundwork to our understanding the prevalence and nature of any condition. Among our contributors we have had many note the importance of this first step. Our contributors took the opportunity to synthesize what knowledge we have on how common are physical disorders in adults with intellectual disability. They pointed out that even with the number of studies investigating the prevalence of physical health that have now been reported, there remains a major absence of reported studies regarding the incidence, long term management and in the prognosis of the number of illnesses in adults with intellectual disability. This, in turn, raises the question of how best can the above-norm morbidity and mortality rates (compared to the general population) be reduced? Our contributors (as well as many others) have suggested several measures, including well-person checklists, improved screening, and better collaboration between heath and accommodation service providers, realizing that many of these issues are influenced by how well physical disorders can be reliably detected and to what extent the data are valid.

Following a solid grounding in epidemiological knowledge, we see the need for well-reasoned and tested approaches designed to provide accurate and prognostic assessment. With this in mind, our other contributors have given us a roadmap for something that we should all keep in mind: that although the assessment procedure is much the same irrespective of the underlying level of disability, there are important and highly significant differences when applied to people with lifelong disabilities. Many adults with intellectual disability are unable to communicate and as such rely considerably on surrogates to speak on their behalf. Means of improving health communication and health symptomatology need to be developed. Absent reliable self-informants, carers and advocates need better ways of being able to observe, detect and report problems in the people for whom they care. Cooperation and compliance among adults with intellectual disability when confronted by physical examinations and investigatory tests can be at times quite limited. We certainly agree with this position that alternative means need to be developed to improve health assessments. For example, pin-prick tests or saliva examinations may be ways of assessing bodily fluids for routine screening (e.g., for thyroid disease in individuals with Down syndrome, as well as for DNA studies).

Following assessment, we enter the specialized area of cataloguing syndromes, conditions, and diseases most prevalent among adults with intellectual disability. Historically, interest in this field has been focussed on the medical aspects of syndromes with articles and textbooks reporting on clinical features which now appear to have limited clinical significance (e.g., dermatoglyphs of Down syndrome, as noted by [30]). Over the last two decades, the social and human rights of people with lifelong disabilities have gained greater importance. However, with the completion of the Human Genome Project, medical issues affecting different syndromes will once again become the focus of future research interest. This also raises some obvious questions, such as: are there particular genes that predispose to, for example, premature cataracts or a form of epilepsy? In addition, considerable progress has been made in the management of conditions which affect adults with intellectual disability. These include hearing impairment, visual impairment, epilepsy, oral health, endocrine disorders, and nutritional-related problems. Also, contemporary work in biomarkers research may soon bear fruit as to being able to identify select individuals with a premorbid state condition – which may then be amenable to pharmacological treatment and potentially be ameliorative [31].

Adding to this is the work that has been developed in terms of international guidelines (e.g., [32–35]) as well as those with on-going support of the American Academy of Developmental Medicine and Dentistry (see [36]). However, implementation of widespread social surveillance and prevention policies requires continual research into the cost-analysis of such polices and their health status impact. Good health promotion and the difficulties people with intellectual disability face in assessing services are fundamental areas for future development. We also recognize outside contributions, like those of the series of reports emanating from the World Health Organization [37–41], the invitational research symposium on healthy aging and intellectual disability that was sponsored by the University of Illinois at Chicago [42], the charette conducted at the Centers for Disease Control and Prevention [43], and more recently the efforts undertaken at the International Summit on Intellectual Disabilities and Dementia [44]. Further, as advances in areas such as molecular genetics and drug therapy rapidly are leading to changes in the accepted management of disorders in individuals with intellectual disability, it is likely that 'biological markers' will soon be developed for particular disorders [45, 46]. It is important that such 'breakthroughs' are appropriately applied to people with intellectual disability; however, capacity and consent issues, and ethical considerations must be involved in all of these medical advances. We are convinced that both research and the efforts of such consensus meetings need to continue to play a major part in the development of good quality healthcare and the development of appropriate services for people with intellectual disability.

A few other thoughts warrant our consideration. As noted in the report of the Chicago Invitational Research Symposium on Healthy Aging and Intellectual Disabilities [42], physical health issues are significantly influenced by a number of factors. Three main life domains dominated this symposium and we see these as a good means of expanding our discussion of health and aging. First, is the consideration of the interaction of mental and physical health; second, is the consideration of nutrition and health; and third, is the consideration of physical conditioning and health. With regard to the first, clinical experience and the research literature support our belief that there is an interaction between mental and physical health and that it is important to identify key risk factors for disease that may bear on this interaction. With this in mind, a number of specific concerns should be raised, including considering the adverse effects of a number of exogenous factors affecting this interaction, such as the effects of physical and mental abuse on health both short and long term and predispositions for being affected by stress. While we recognize that there is an important link between the psyche and the body, we also recognize that there is a continuing need for more reliable, valid, and standardized screening tools for assessing health status and personal condition.

Given the above, a research agenda needs to include an examination of competence and consent aspects for participants in research, an assessment of the interaction of general life satisfaction and health status, and the impact of confident relationships and friends of substance, as well as a daily routine of meaningful activities, as a contributor to health and wellness. Other areas that warrant attention include the effects of staff knowledge and competence on identifying and maintaining health status, identifying effective means of promoting healthy lifestyles, the relationship of poverty and health status using cross-cultural studies to tease out culturally beneficial health practices, and identifying the key factors that make for "healthy agers" (as to who are the people who survive the longest and why do they survive in good health for as long as they do).

Regarding nutrition and wellness, we see a need to better understand some of the metabolic and dietary challenges facing older adults with intellectual disability as they age, including on the plus side the trend toward healthier nutrient intake and on the minus side the fact that many adults with intellectual disability may be over-weight and at-risk for significant health problems due to obesity. Interestingly, although one would imagine that nutrition and caloric intake would be a simple matter, even here, there are definitional difficulties beginning with a significant problem with data collection standardization on nutritional status and diet. In addi-tion, genetics play a role in metabolism and related factors, such that there are nota-ble differences in exercise and weight conditions among syndromes (for example, among adults with Down syndrome in contrast to most other etiologies of intellec-tual disability). In the area of nutrition and wellness, there are a number of research areas of importance, including examining nutritional issues through comparative studies of Down syndrome vs. other etiologies of intellectual disability, identifying factors that significantly contribute to obesity and weight difficulties, examining the meaning of food and it implications on mental health, and the effects of staff and carer role models on eating habits and weight status. As noted by Heller et al. [42], other relevant research areas include the use of longitudinal designs that "track" populations to look at weight and physical status over a lifetime, as well as those can identify factors contributing to obesity, examine medication effects and dietary out-comes, and assess the relationship of eating habits and stress.

The third area involves physical activity. Here ideas about promoting wellness are often more diffuse since little research provides a basis for hypothesis framing. However, one area of concern revolves around how to motivate people with intel-lectual disability to exercise. Heller et al. [42] have suggested that eliminating bar-riers to exercise and introducing both passive and active exercise modalities should be an important feature in promoting exercise. With this in mind, some areas for potential research include examining the effects of exercise differences among vari-ous etiologies of intellectual disability, identifying barriers to exercise and the effects of stress from "involuntary" exercise, and assessing how to best promote coordination and balance (and thus decreasing the rate of falls) through exercise. As Heller et al. [42] have noted, other research endeavors might consider examining the effects of aerobic exercise on cardiovascular functioning, assessing the efficacy of non-traditional exercise methods (for example, Tai Chi), and conducting an in-depth analysis of nutrition and exercise in terms of assessing which contributes more to physical wellness.

Lastly, on a more social level, we would suggest examining means of tying into "aging friendly communities" initiatives and their health promotion and exercise programs.[1] The Special Olympics International organization has focused on the

---

[1] 'Aging friendly communities' initiatives are when communities recognize that they are composed of a significant number of older citizens, and consequently develop and carry out plans to make their physical and social amenities and other aspects completely accessible and available to their

importance of health as an avenue to ensure that each adult can best achieve happiness, dignity, and equity in life, as well as in health by creation and broadening of its Healthy Athletes and Healthy Community programs. These efforts carried forth internationally have drawn attention to the importance of wellness, and fitness with a cross over of the need to connect to the support network, community providers of healthcare, as well as the innovative programming to ensure a sustainable and meaningful program. An example in the United States is the Special Olympics Oregon's TEAM WELLNESS program [47]. This unique, community-based health and wellness program is designed for individuals with and without intellectual disability and offers a rich range of options for engaging activities within a community context.

20.6   Some Closing Thoughts

As it has been noted, more studies are needed to document the extent and causes of health problems and the disparities in accessing health care for people with intellectual disability. Thus, the future needs to be aimed at specifically addressing this challenge. There continues to be a need for more effective education and training in the assessment, diagnosis, management and care provision of physical health in people with intellectual disability. To stimulate medical participation, reimbursement models need to be in place to help support practitioners who do treat individuals with complex healthcare needs. Internationally, the concept of a Medically Underserved Population status needs further discussion and planning to enable adults with intellectual disability in aggregate to be designated as being medically underserved. There remains a need for all professionals involved in care provision, such as community physicians, community care workers, and specialist and generic services, to be more aware of the important health issues facing adults with these lifelong disabilities. Transitioning of healthcare from pediatric to adult, and adult to geriatric healthcare services requires further education, training, research and awareness to focus more on training of the health care providers who provide these services. Postgraduate training organisations, such as universities, must incorporate the need for better education. Further scientific research is required to determine how best to inform and educate a wide range of individuals who are involved in the care of persons with intellectual disability (such as families, paid carers, general practitioners, paramedical professionals, specialists, and researchers). With the recent growth in the world wide web and better communication and initial access to information, resources are now widely available to disseminate appropriate knowledge to families, students, professionals, and organisational agencies who are involved in the care of people with intellectual disability.

Physical healthcare for people with intellectual disability remains an important area of concern and there will always be a need for better education, assessment and

---

older citizens. This may involve physical barrier removal in public and private facilities, transportation resources, and streets and sidewalks; social resource investment to develop and maintain programs and facilities for the well elderly; and provide more control in the hands of its older citizens over the physical and social fabric of their community.

management, and greater multi-disciplinary, and multi-agency service development. The future role of molecular genetics and health information technology as yet to be fully realised.

This book aims to, in part, to rectify some of the many health disparities and deficiencies in intellectual disability and point a way forward to new discoveries and practices.

References

1. Bakken TL, Martinsen H. Adults with intellectual disabilities and mental illness in psychiatric inpatient units: empirical studies of patient characteristics and psychiatric diagnoses from 1996 to 2011. Int J Dev Disabil. 2013;59:179–90. https://doi.org/10.1179/20473877 12Y.0000000006.
2. Davidson P, Prasher VP, Janicki M. Mental health, intellectual disabilities, and the aging process. Oxford: Blackwell Publishing; 2003.
3. Gomez A, Ismet K. Psychiatric disorders in adults with intellectual disabilities: A preliminary study of prevalence and associated factors. Eur Psychiatry. 2017;41(Suppl):S158–9.
4. Kyrkou M. Health issues and quality of life in women with intellectual disability. J Intellect Disabil Res. 2005;49:770–2.
5. Walsh P, Heller T. Women's health and intellectual disabilities. Oxford: Blackwell Publishing; 2002.
6. Wisdom JP, McGee MG, Horner-Johnson W, Michael YL, Adams E, Berlin M. Health disparities between women with and without disabilities: A review of the research. Soc Work Public Health. 2010;25:368–86.
7. Edgerton R. Quality of life issues: Some people know how to be old. In: Seltzer MM, Krauss MW, Janicki MP, editors. Life Course Perspectives on Adulthood and Old Age. Washington, D.C.: American Association on Mental Retardation; 1994. p. 53–66.
8. Americans With Disabilities Act of 1990. Public Law 101-336. 108th Congress, 2nd session July 26, 1990.
9. Olmstead Rights. The Olmstead supreme court decision in a nutshell. Accessed from: https://www.olmsteadrights.org/about-olmstead/.
10. Felce D. Community living for adults with intellectual disabilities: Unravelling the cost effectiveness discourse. J Policy Pract Intellect Disabil. 2017;14:187–97. https://doi.org/10.1111/jppi.12180.
11. Health Resources Services Administration (HRSA). (2016). Medically underserved areas and populations (MUA/Ps). Accessed from: https://bhw.hrsa.gov/shortage-designation/muap.
12. US Department of Health and Human Services (DHHS). Closing the gap: A national blueprint for improving the health of individuals with mental retardation. Report of the Surgeon General's Conference on Health Disparities and Mental Retardation. Washington, D.C.: U.S. Department of Health and Human Services, Office of the Surgeon General; 2002.
13. US Department of Health and Human Services. The Surgeon General's call to action to improve the health and wellness of persons with disabilities. Washington, D.C.: U.S. Department of Health and Human Services, Office of the Surgeon General; 2005.
14. National Council on Disability. The current state of health care for people with disabilities. Washington, DC: National Council on Disability; 2009. Accessed from https://www.ncd.gov/rawmedia_repository/0d7c848f_3d97_43b3_bea5_36e1d97f973d.pdf
15. Slashcheva L, Rader R, Sulkes SB. Would people with intellectual disabilities benefit for being designated "underserved"? AMA J Ethics. 2016;18:422–9.
16. National Institute on Minority Health and Health Disparities (NIMHHD). Loan repayment program. Accessed from: https://www.nimhd.nih.gov/programs/extramural/loan-repayment.html.

17. Susan G. Komen for the Cure. (2018). Research and community health grants. Accessed from: https://ww5.komen.org/ResearchGrants/ResearchandGrants.html.
18. Ackerman BM. People with intellectual disabilities must be designated a medical underserved population. Spec Care Dentist. 2013;33:207–8.
19. American Medical Association. (2010). Designation of the intellectually disabled as a medically underserved population (resolution 805-I-10). Accessed from https://www.ama-assn.org/sites/default/files/media-browser/public/about-ama/councils/Council%20Reports/council-on-medical-service/i11-cms-value-based-decision-making.pdf.
20. American Dental Association. (2004). State and community models for improving access to dental care for the underserved—a white paper. Accessed from: http://www.ada.org/~/media/ADA/Advocacy/Files/topics_access_whitepaper.ashx.
21. Kornblau BL. The case for designating people with intellectual and developmental disabilities as a medically underserved population. In: Autistic Self Advocacy Network Policy Brief, April 2014. Florida: A&M University; 2014. p. 1–19.
22. Ally S, Boyd K, Abells D, Amaria K, Hamdani Y, Loh A, Niel U, Sacks S, Shea S, Sullivan WF, Hennen B. Improving transition to adulthood for adolescents with intellectual and developmental disabilities. Can Fam Physician. 2018;64(Suppl 2):S37–43.
23. National Alliance to Advance Adolescent Health. (2018). Got transition. Accessed from: http://www.gottransition.org/.
24. Child Neurology Foundation. (2018). Transition of care. Accessed from: http://www.childneurologyfoundation.org/transitions/.
25. Children's Hospital of Philadelphia. (2017). Transitioning to adult care: supporting youth with special healthcare needs. Accessed from: https://policylab.chop.edu/evidence-action-brief/transitioning-adult-care-supporting-youth-special-health-care-needs.
26. Betz CL, Nehring WM. Transition needs of parents of adolescents and emerging adults with special health care needs and disabilities. J Fam Nurs. 2015;21:362–412.
27. Oswald DP, Gilles DL, Cannady MS, Wenzel DB, Willis JH, Bodurtha JN. Youth with special health care needs: Transition to adult health care services. Matern Child Health J. 2013;17:1744–53.
28. Carfi A, Berbabei R, Onesimo R, Zampino G, Onder G. Managing the care of adults with Down's syndrome. BMJ. 2014;349:g5596. https://doi.org/10.1136/bmj.g5596.
29. Ervin, D., Hahn, J. & Asato, M. Transitioning to adult neurologic care: Where do we go from here? Exceptional Parent, 2017;47(8):38–9.
30. Smith GF, Berg JM. Down's anomaly. In: Smith GF, Berg JM, editors. Dermatoglyphs. New York: Churchill Livingstone; 1976. p. 76–99.
31. Rafii MS, Wishnek H, Brewer JB, Donohue MC, Ness S, Mobley WC, Aisen PS, Rissman RA. The Down syndrome biomarker initiative (DSBI) pilot: proof of concept for deep phenotyping of Alzheimer's disease biomarkers in down syndrome. Front Behav Neurosci. 2015;9:239. https://doi.org/10.3389/fnbeh.2015.00239. Epub 2015 Sep 14
32. Evenhuis, H., & Nagtzaam, L.M.D. (1998). IASSID International Consensus Statement: Early identification of hearing and visual impairment in children and adults with an intellectual disability. IASSID Special Interest Research Group on Health Issues. Accessed from: https://www.iassidd.org/uploads/legacy/pdf/consensir.alg.doc.
33. Janicki MP, Heller T, Seltzer G, Hogg J. Practice guidelines for the clinical assessment and care management of Alzheimer's disease and other dementias among adults with intellectual disability. J Intellect Disabil Res. 1996;40:374–82.
34. Jokinen J, Janicki MP, Keller SM, McCallion P, Force LT, the National Task Group on Intellectual Disabilities and Dementia Practices. Guidelines for structuring community care and supports for people with intellectual disabilities affected by dementia. J Policy Pract Intellect Disabil. 2013;10(1):1–28.
35. U.S. Department of Agriculture and U.S. Department of Health and Human Services. Nutrition and Your Health: Dietary Guidelines for Americans. 5th ed. Washington D.C.: Home and Garden Bulletin No. 232; 2000.

36. Moran JA, Rafii MS, Keller SM, Singh BK, Janicki MP. The National Task Group on Intellectual Disabilities and Dementia Practices consensus recommendations for the evaluation and management of dementia in adults with intellectual disabilities. Mayo Clin Proc. 2013;88:831–40.
37. Evenhuis H, Henderson CM, Beange H, Lennox N, Chicoine B. Healthy ageing – adults with intellectual disabilities: physical health issues. J Appl Res Intellect Disabil. 2001;14:175–94.
38. Hogg J, Lucchino R, Wang KY, Janicki M. Healthy ageing - adults with intellectual disabilities: ageing and social policy. J Appl Res Intellect Disabil. 2001;14:229–55.
39. Thorpe L, Davidson P, Janicki MP. Healthy Ageing - adults with intellectual disabilities: behavioural issues. J Appl Res Intellect Disabil. 2001;14:218–28.
40. Walsh PN, Heller T, Schupf N, van Schronjenstein Lantman-de Valk H. Healthy ageing – Adults with intellectual disabilities: women's health and related issues. J Appl Res Intellect Disabil. 2001;14:195–217.
41. World Health Organization. Healthy ageing – adults with intellectual disabilities: summative report. J Appl Res Intellect Disabil. 2001;14:256–75.
42. Heller T, Janicki MP, Gill C, Factor A. Health disparities and a paradigm for health promotion: Report of the invitational symposium on health, aging, and developmental disabilities. Chicago: University of Illinois at Chicago, Department of Human Development and Disability; 2002.
43. Janicki MP, Henderson CM, Rubin L. Neurodevelopmental conditions and aging: Report on the Atlanta Study Group Charrette on Neurodevelopmental Conditions and Aging. Disabil Health J. 2008;1:116–24.
44. Watchman, K., & Janicki, M.P., and the members of the International Summit of Intellectual Disability and Dementia. The intersection of intellectual disability and Dementia: Report of the International Summit on Intellectual Disability and Dementia. Gerontologist. 2017. DOI: https://doi.org/10.1093/geront/gnx160.
45. Lee N-C, Chien Y-H, Hwu W-L. A review of biomarkers for Alzheimer's disease in Down syndrome. Neurol Ther. 2017;6(Suppl 1):69–81.
46. Manti S, Cutrupi MC, Cuppari C, Ferro E, Dipasquale V, Di Rosa G, Chimenz R, La Rosa M, Valenti A, Salpietro V. Inflammatory biomarkers and intellectual disability in patients with Down syndrome. J Intellect Disabil Res. 2018;62:382–90.
47. Special Olympics Oregon. (2018). Welcome to Oregon team wellness. Accessed from: http://www.soor.org/Sub-Page.aspx?Name=History&PID=28.

Index

A

Acceptable macronutrients distribution range (AMDR), 257, 259, 261
Activities of daily living (ADLs), 39, 42
Adult regression syndrome, *see* Down syndrome
Advanced care planning, 64
Adverse drug reactions (ADRs), 42
Advocacy skills kit (ASK), 355
Aging, 5
  cancer, 320–321
  cardiovascular disease, 316–317
  dementia, 315–316
  diabetes, 317
  Down syndrome, 319
  epidemiology
    administrative datasets, 10
    changing abilities with age, 13
    chronic conditions, 14–15
    dementia, 19–20
    epidemiological research, 20–21
    frailty, 18
    health indicators, 15–16
    health maintenance and improvement, 19
    health related outcomes, 10
    incidence, 12, 13
    international data sets, 9
    learning disabilities, 11
    levels of disability, 12
    physical health, 17
    psychosocial/mental health issues, 17–18
    public health surveys, 16
    terminology, 12
  epilepsy, 315
  facets, 305–306
  gastrointestinal and eating problems, 317–318
  genetic disorders, 312
  health inequalities and health disparity, 308
  health service delivery, 324–326
  hypertension, 316
  illness-related lifestyle health risks
    European POMONA data, 310
    interventions and recommendations, 312–313
  life expectancy, 309
  life-course-development, 309–310
  multimorbidity, 321–322, 324
  obesity, 311, 312
  overweight, 311
  polypharmacy, 322–324
  population, 307
  skeletal disorders, 319
  tobacco use, 311
  vision and hearing, 313–314
Alpha-linolenic acid (ALA), 262
Alzheimer's disease (AD), 40, 123, 124
American Academy of Developmental Medicine and Dentistry (AADMD), 400
American Association on Intellectual and Developmental Disabilities (AAIDD), 11
American Heart Association (AHA), 228
American Medical Association (AMA), 229
Amyloid precursor protein (APP), 40
Ankle and foot orthosis (AFO), 97
Anticonvulsants, 32, 97, 99, 206, 213
Antidepressants, 339
Antiepileptic drugs, 133, 190, 338
Anti-inflammatory medication, 96
Antioxidant system, 270